Immune Response and the Eye

Chemical Immunology

Vol. 73

Series Editors   *Luciano Adorini*, Milan
Ken-ichi Arai, Tokyo
Claudia Berek, Berlin
J. Donald Capra, Oklahoma City, Okla.
Anne-Marie Schmitt-Verhulst, Marseille
Byron H. Waksman, New York, N.Y.

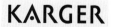

KARGER   Basel · Freiburg · Paris · London · New York ·
New Delhi · Bangkok · Singapore · Tokyo · Sydney

....

Immune Response and the Eye

Volume Editor   *J. Wayne Streilein*, Boston, Mass.

20 figures, 7 in color, and 14 tables, 1999

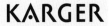 KARGER   Basel · Freiburg · Paris · London · New York ·
New Delhi · Bangkok · Singapore · Tokyo · Sydney

Chemical Immunology

Formerly published as 'Progress in Allergy'
Founded 1939 by Paul Kallos

••••••••••••••••••••••••

J. Wayne Streilein, M.D.

President and Director of Research, The Schepens Eye Research Institute,
Professor and Vice-Chair for Research, Department of Ophthalmology,
Harvard Medical School, Boston, Mass., USA

Bibliographic Indices. This publication is listed in bibliographic services, including Current Contents® and Index Medicus.

Contents

Contents

....
Preface

The eye shares with other organs the need for immune protection against exogenous and endogenous pathogens. Immune protection usually comes with a price in which inflammation produces bystander injury to cells within tissues. For some tissues – skin is a good example – immunogenic inflammation is reasonably well tolerated. While severe inflammation in the skin can lead to scarring, this does not often lead to loss of the skin's basic integrity and the viability of the host is not threatened. For the eye, immunogenic inflammation poses a much more serious problem. The delicate visual axis must be maintained in its precise anatomic state in order for light images to fall accurately and precisely on the retina. Relatively minor distortions in this axis causes major disruption of the image that reaches the retina. Reduced vision – even blindness – can result. Immune responses that encompass inflammation – even small amounts – within the eye result in visual impairment, and when of sufficient magnitude threaten host viability. The Introduction by Ohashi defines this circumstance, especially from a clinical viewpoint.

To save life as well as sight, the eye and the immune system have had to strike a physiologic compromise such that immune protection is afforded, but vision is spared. The experimental expression of the success of this compromise is immunologic privilege, anterior chamber associated immune deviation (ACAID), and the intraocular immunosuppressive microenvironment. As in all compromises, something is relinquished so that something can be gained. The chapter by Streilein relates immune privilege as an extreme example of the phenomenon of regional immunology.

The primary purpose of this volume on Immune Responses and the Eye is to describe, explain and speculate on what is currently known and understood about the consequences of the eye:immune system compromise – from the eye's standpoint. The past two decades of research have witnessed remarkable advances in our knowledge of the physiology of ocular immune privilege. The chapters by Liu, Keane-Myers, Tai & Ono, by Niederkorn, and by Taylor address this remarkable body of knowledge. A considerable amount of new information has also been gained concerning the mechanisms responsible for ocular inflammation secondary to viral, autoimmune and other immunopathogenic processes. The chapters by Magone & Whitcup, by Hendricks, and by Forrester & McMenamin summarize this information. Finally, recently gained understanding of immune responses in normal and inflamed eyes is used in the chapters by Chen & Ksander, by Streilein, and by Kaplan, Tezel, Berger & Del Priore to explain the immunologic processes involved in the growth of ocular tumors, and in the success and failure of transplants of cornea and retina.

At best, this volume can serve as a status report. So much more remains to be learned about ocular immune responses than is now at hand, and the field is growing exponentially. It is worthwhile to stop and take a 'pulse' of this young field, the but real fun is still ahead.

J. Wayne Streilein

Streilein JW (ed): Immune Response and the Eye.
Chem Immunol. Basel, Karger, 1999, vol 73, pp 1–10

....

Introduction:
All for Saving the Visual Axis

Yuichi Ohashi

Department of Ophthalmology, Ehime University School of Medicine, Shigenobu,
Ehime, Japan

The eye is an extremely elegant and delicate organ designed to transmit light images of the world onto the retina, and to transduce and then transmit these images faithfully to the brain for recognition and interpretation. The eye consists of the eyeball, the conjunctival mucosa, adnexal structures which contain the tear-forming apparatus, including the lacrimal gland, the nasolacrimal duct, and the palpebral and orbital tissues that surround and provide cover for the ocular surface. Light images are transmitted to the retina through the optical axis, which is comprised of the cornea, anterior chamber, lens, and vitreous body. For the fidelity of the images that fall on the retina, it is of paramount importance that this axis be transparent. To achieve this goal, the optical axis is devoid of blood vessels. Moreover, these ocular tissues are also deficient in lymphoreticular cells of the immune system. This simple construction – elimination of blood vessels and lymphoreticular cells from the components of the optical axis – not only renders the axis transparent, but has the secondary effect of effectively disengaging the optical axis from the cellular mediators of the immune system and of inflammation. The consequences of this disengagement account largely for why immune responses and inflammation in the eye are different from other sites in the body. The term 'immune privilege', originally used to describe prolonged acceptance of foreign grafts in the anterior chamber of the eye, now embraces the deviant and atypical immunity that occurs in the eye. Immunity of this type is the topic of this volume.

The Unusual Nature of Ocular Immunity and Inflammation

The unusual and distinctive nature of immune responses in the eye is not solely dependent upon the absence of blood vessels among the components of the optical axis. The existence of a restrictive blood:tissue barrier in other compartments of the eye that do possess vascular beds interferes with the expression of immunity in the eye. Except for the uveoscleral pathway, there is no lymphatic drainage pathway from the internal compartments of the eye, and this situation limits the ability of antigenic material to escape and reach draining lymph nodes. In addition to these unique anatomical features, other factors have also been implicated in the eye's ability to regulate local immune responses. First, the vascularized tissues of the eye possess bone marrow-derived cells with the potential to capture and present antigens to immune cells [1–3, Chapter 9 of this volume]. But under normal circumstances these cells are curiously impaired in their ability to activate T cells. Second, the presence of a variety of immunosuppressive substances in the aqueous humor, such as transforming growth factor-β (TGF-β, α-melanocyte-stimulating hormone (α-MSH), vasoactive intestinal peptide (VIP), and macrophage migration inhibitory factor (MIF), act singly or in concert to modulate ocular immune responses [4–9, Chapter 5 of this volume]. Third, ocular parenchymal tissues constitutively express cell surface molecules, such as CD95 ligand [10, 11], CD59, and CD46 [12], which directly inhibit effector T cells and complement components, thereby saving the visual axis from lethal tissue damage.

The unusual anatomic, cellular and molecular features of the eye just described also have an impact on systemic immune responses to eye-derived antigens. Anterior chamber-associated immune deviation (ACAID) is the term applied to the distinctive systemic immune response to intracameral introduction of foreign antigens [13–16]. ACAID is characterized by impaired antigen-specific delayed-type hypersensitivity and reduced production of complement fixing antibodies, but unaffected or even enhanced production of noncomplement-fixing antibodies and primed cytotoxic T cells. Because this stereotypic immune response is deficient in the effector modalities enumerated, ACAID is thought to permit certain invading pathogens to persist in the eye for considerable periods of time without elimination. According to Streilein, the significance of ACAID has been explained as an eye-protective mechanism that acts systemically to maintain the transparency of the optical axis [17, 18].

Immune Mechanisms Where the Blood: Ocular Barrier Meets the General Circulation

The blood:ocular barrier, which limits access of blood-borne molecules and cells into the internal compartments of the eye, is maintained, on the one hand, by tight junctions among retinal pigment epithelium, secretory ciliary epithelium, and ocular surface epithelium, and, on the other hand, by tight junctions among endothelial cells of the retinal and iridial microvasculatures. Thus, the anterior chamber, the vitreous cavity, and the retina and subretinal space are sequestered from the systemic circulation, residing in a zone that is relatively immunologically silent. Beyond this barrier, on the surface of the eye, the mucosal lymphoid system, termed CALT [19] conjunctiva-associated lymphoid tissue – combats foreign invaders with the aid of IgA antibodies, and a striking array of nonspecific and selective antimicrobial substances. As with other mucosal surfaces, the conjunctival stroma contains IgE-laden mast cells, and this system can lead to a variety of conjunctival allergic disorders.

The intersection of the conjunctiva with the cornea (the limbus) is one of the most immunologically active sites in the eye. The peripheral cornea is constantly bathed with plasma components that escape via the limbal vessels [20], and the limbal epithelium is replete with Langerhans' cells [21, 22], professional antigen presenting cells. Through the relatively leaky barrier of the conjunctival epithelium, Tennon's capsule serves as an efficient barrier which traps invading foreign materials and antigens. A broad network of lymphatic channels forms throughout the conjunctiva, and these channels connect with the lymph nodes of the cervical and periauricular regions. The immune and inflammatory reactivity of the limbus is reflected in a variety of disorders that can be found at this area, including marginal corneal infiltrates/ ulcers, corneal phylectenules, and episcleritis.

The blood:ocular barrier at the posterior pole of the eye resembles the limbus functionally in that it interacts with another immunologically dynamic tissue – the choriocapillaris (choroid). Since choroidal vessels are freely fenestrated, blood-borne cells and molecules of the immune system can be delivered directly to the 'door' of the blood:retinal barrier. The stroma separating the choroid from the retinal pigment epithelium is well endowed with MHC class II-positive dendritic cells and macrophages with the potential to capture and present antigens to the immune system [3]. Moreover, the choroid is supplied with lymphatic channels, which means that antigenic information can readily escape from this site. As an expression of the choroid's blood and lymphatic connections, immune and inflammatory conditions occur frequently at this region, and can have a debilitating effect on vision.

Little is known about the immunological nature of the orbital tissues which cover the posterior surface of the eyeball. Clinically, a variety of lymphoproliferative disorders can occur in this area. *Pseudotumor orbitae* and malignant lymphoma are almost exclusively of B-lymphocyte origin [23], implying the presence in this region of unknown immune mechanisms that govern humoral immunity.

Corneal Endotheliitis and Its Related Disorders

Corneal endotheliitis is a disease caused by viruses of the herpes family, specifically herpes simplex (HSV) and varicella zoster (VZV). In this disease, corneal endothelial cells are destroyed by infection, eventually leading to permanent corneal endothelial decompensation. The hallmark of this disease is a progressive, corneal stromal edema starting at the periphery, with the formation of a line or cluster of keratic precipitates located at the leading edge of the edema. The anterior chamber reaction is surprisingly minimal in spite of active virus propagation in the endothelium [24, 25]. We have postulated that early in this disorder a small amount of virus (HSV or VZV) is shed into the anterior chamber, and this in turn induces virus-specific ACAID. The disease becomes manifest when large amounts of virus are reactivated at the trabecular meshwork. Despite the presence of specific antibodies, the disease gradually progresses from the periphery to the center of the cornea by way of cell-to-cell viral spread. The absence of virus-specific delayed hypersensitivity enables the virus in its pathologic migration to the center of the cornea. In support of this hypothesis, a similar corneal endothelial lesion has been successfully established in rabbits with virus-specific ACAID in whom live HSV was injected intracamerally [26].

Fuchs' heterochromic iridocyclitis and the Posner-Schlossman syndrome are probably the same clinical entity, since both diseases are characterized by a unilateral, recurrent form of corneal inflammation with mild reaction in the anterior chamber. The depressed delayed hypersensitivity skin responses of patients with Posner-Schlossman syndrome to cutaneous challenge with VZV antigen further supports the hypothesis that ACAID is operative in the pathogenesis of these corneal inflammatory disorders [27].

Tears as 'Trojan Horses' Bearing Ocular Pathogens

The lacrimal gland is a multifunctional organ that continuously secretes tears, and simultaneously provides the ocular surface with a variety of antimicrobial substances. The gland consists of secretory acinar cells, a ductal system, and clusters of lymphoreticular cells scattered in the interstitial spaces. The tear fluids are produced by acinar cells as an ultrafiltrate of plasma, and during this process IgA antibodies (predominantly) which are secreted locally by plasma cells are transported into the tears. Despite this local immune capability, the lacrimal gland appears to be a target of a variety of infectious pathogens. For example, survey by polymerase chain reaction (PCR) of tears from patients with ocular surface disorders has disclosed that numerous herpes viruses are typically present – Epstein-Barr virus, HSV, VZV, cytomegalovirus, HHV-6, and HHV-7. The lacrimal gland, along with its complement of lymphoreticular cells, may be a potent source of these agents. In fact, EBV genomes have been demonstrated in ductal epithelial cells, and its relevance to Sjögren's syndrome has been strongly suggested [28, 29]. In addition, recurrent epithelial disorders of unknown origin, such as Thygeson's SPK, which is characterized by oval epithelial opacities scattered throughout the cornea, may be of viral origin. The clinical manifestations of this disorder closely resemble the lesion seen in adenoviral punctate superficial keratitis. Thus, there is strong circumstantial evidence that corneal inflammatory diseases which lead to clouding of the optical axis may be caused by inadvertent inoculation of the corneal surface epithelium by pathogenic agents carried via the tears.

By the same token, HVB, HCV and HIV are not uncommon inhabitants of the tears in patients infected systemically with these agents [30–32]. PCR examination of tears from patients in the active phase of their disease revealed that the genomes of these viruses are present, indicating that the lacrimal gland may serve as a conduit for the local delivery of these hematogenously spreading viruses. In this sense, a recent report on the simultaneous occurrence of Mooren's ulcer in patients with active HCV infection [33] offers the possibility that a certain group of ocular surface disorders may be secondary to primary infections at distant sites of the body. Further experimental work in this area will undoubtedly shed new light on our understanding of the pathogenesis of ocular surface disorders now thought to be idiopathic.

Allergic Conjunctival Disorders

The incidence of allergic conjunctival diseases has been steadily increasing all over the world. Although IgE-mediated, type I hypersensitivity is presumed to lie at the heart of these disorders, type IV hypersensitivity (represented typically by delayed hypersensitivity) may be partly responsible for proliferative changes seen in the palpebral and perilimbal conjunctiva. Unlike vernal keratoconjunctivitis (which is self-limited by 20 years of age), atopic keratoconjunctivitis (AKC) tends to run a prolonged clinical course throughout life. AKC can cause a profound disruption of the entire ocular surface, including limbal stem cell deficiency, foreshortening of the forniceal conjunctiva, and persistent epithelial defects [34]. Patients with AKC are also prone to develop cataracts and retinal detachments. Abnormal cytokine production by conjunctival epithelial cells has been postulated as one of the pathogenic mechanisms. The increased incidence of allergic conjunctival disorders may correlate paradoxically with the general improvement in living conditions around the world.

Th1 responses, dominated by delayed hypersensitivity T cells, are mandatory for protecting humans from life-threatening infectious diseases observed in less well-developed countries. As the incidence of these infections falls in developed countries, Th2-type responses – which lead directly to IgE production and allergic manifestations – are becoming more dominant. If true, then it can be expected that AKC may develop in the next century into one of the major blinding disorders, especially within the well-developed countries. It is worth noting that the recent success of a multicentered study of the efficacy of topical FK-506 ointment to treat atopic dermatitis encourages the development of similar therapies for AKC [35, 36].

The Battle Against Cicatrizing Ocular Surface Disorders

Although novel therapeutic procedures, developed in the past two decades, have made it possible to control many blinding corneal diseases, the cicatrizing ocular surface disorders have remained an unresolved challenge to the corneal surgeon. The primary ocular surface disorders, such as ocular cicatricial pemphigoid, and Stevens-Johnson syndrome, and the secondary disorders, such as chemical and thermal burns, post-trachoma cicatrization, and radiation keratopathy represent the major challenges. These disorders are characterized by an absence of limbal stem cells, and, as a consequence, conjunctival epithelium invades onto the corneal surface, bringing with it a varied degree of subconjunctival fibrosis.

In order to reconstruct the epithelium of the ocular surface in these diseases, corneal epithelial cells must be supplied either by limbal transplantation, or by keratoepithelioplasty [37]. The source of tissue for these procedures is human donor eyes, and therefore the transplants are allografts. Not surprisingly, epithelial rejection has provided a major barrier to success. Although the postoperative outcome has been improved remarkably with the recent introduction of amniotic membrane transplantation and the topical or systemic use of cyclosporin A [38, 39], a more specific and selective therapeutic regimen is sorely needed.

Preemptive induction of ACAID has been proposed as a treatment option in this situation. Yao et al. [40] have shown in rats that intracameral injection of allogeneic lymphocytes not only induces alloantigen-specific ACAID, but also significantly suppresses epithelial rejection following keratoepithelioplasty in an animal model. Moreover, ACAID has been generated in vivo by incubating alloantigen-bearing mononuclear cells in vitro with TGF-β [41]. Since it has recently been shown that regulatory T cells can be created in vitro by stimulating naive T cells with TGF-β-exposed mononuclear cells, it may be possible to return these 'in vitro-educated' lymphocytes to a recipient of an allogeneic keratoepithelioplasty. An alternative possibility could be the introduction though genetic engineering of the CD95 ligand gene into tissues to be used for keratoepithelioplasty, thereby conferring on the graft resistance to transplantation rejection. I believe that in the not too distant future we will resolve the challenge of intractable cicatrizing ocular surface disorders with exciting protocols of this type.

Molecular Mimicry and Autoimmune Diseases of the Eye

Mooren's ulcer is a devastating corneal disorder that is characterized by progressive, circumferential and peripheral ulceration with an undermined edge. The exact cause of this disease is unknown. However, the disease is thought to occur via an autoimmune mechanism. An interesting report from Africa indicates that Mooren's ulcer patients have a high incidence of helminth infection [42], and that the eye disease ceases as systemic treatment effectively eliminates the helminth infection. This raises the possibility that there might be a cross-reactive antigen – a molecular mimicry between a putative helminth antigen, and a presumed corneal autoantigen. Infrequently, Mooren's ulcer patients have a history of previous corneal injury, bacterial keratitis, or intraocular surgery. It is possible that, upon injury to the cornea, the cornea-specific autoantigen is released (unmasked), and therefore becomes available to trigger a systemic immune response. A mechanism similar to this has been proposed for the pathogenesis of stromal keratitis in patients with HSV infections of the cornea [43]. Sympathetic ophthalmia and lens-induced endophthalmitis are probably additional examples of similar breakdowns of immune tolerance and ignorance for ocular autoantigens.

Antigen/Pathogen Clearance and Connective Tissue Destruction

The capsule of the eye, predominately the sclera, consists of a collagen-rich, tendon-like tissue. The capsule serves as an anatomical barrier that provides the resistance which enables intraocular pressure to rise sufficiently to keep the optical axis in perfect alignment with the retina. Inflammatory, and presumably immune, reactions take place in this tissue since it contains a very modest blood and lymph vasculature. It has occurred to some investigators that antigen and pathogen clearance from the sclera may be inefficient, and this inefficiency may promote sustained local inflammation and injury. A good example is often seen in patients with rheumatoid arthritis in whom pre-formed immune complexes preferentially deposit at distinct connective tissue sites [44]. Interestingly, the periphery of the cornea and the anterior portion of the sclera represent two such deposit sites. In the worst cases, necrotizing scleritis or corneal perforation occurs after the connective tissue is degraded by prolonged inflammation. The process of degradation may be rapid, and typically resists any mode of therapy. The field needs a novel weapon to either protect the ocular capsule from deposition of harmful antigen-antibody complexes, or to promote their resorption before inflammation leads to connective tissue breakdown.

Concluding Remarks

The chapters comprising this volume address many important blinding diseases of the eye for which an immune response – either innate or adaptive – has been implicated as a key participant. I have described in this Introduction additional blinding disorders for which no effective remedy now exists. The careful reader may be able to probe into these chapters, looking for an idea or insight that may lead to an improvement in the current situation. While this volume amply describes the remarkable advances in ocular immunology that have marked research conducted over the past 30 years, there remains an impressive set of idiopathic eye diseases in which inflammation and immunity probably contribute to the pathogenesis. We would indeed be fortunate if the first three decades of the new millennium witness progress in research of ocular immunity that is comparable to that of the last three decades.

References

1   Williamson JSP, Bradley D, Streilein JW: Immunoregulatory properties of bone marrow derived cells in the iris and ciliary body. Immunology 1989;67:96–102.
2   Wilbanks GA, Mammolenti M, Streilein JW: Studies on the induction of anterior chamber-associated immune deviation (ACAID). II. Eye derived cells participate in general blood borne signals that induce ACAID. J Immunol 1991;146:3018–3024.
3   McMenamin PG, Forrester J: Dendritic cells in the central nervous system and eye and their associated supporting tissues; in Lotze MT, Thomson AW (eds): Dendritic Cells: Biology and Clinical Applications. San Diego, Academic Press, 1999, pp 205–254.
4   Streilein JW, Wilbanks GA, Tylor A, Cousins S: Eye-derived cytokines and the immunosuppressive intraocular microenvironment: A review. Curr Eye Res 1992;11(suppl):41–47.
5   Cousins SW, McCabe MM, Danielpour D, Streilein JW: Identification of transforming growth factor-beta as an immunosuppressive factor in aqueous humor. Invest Ophthal Vis Sci 1991;32: 2201–2211.
6   Taylor A, Streilein JW, Cousins S: Identification of alpha-melanocyte-stimulating hormone as a potential immunosuppressive factor in aqueous humor. Curr Eye Res 1992;11:1199–1206.

7   Taylor A, Streilein JW, Cousins S: Immunoreactive vasoactive intestinal peptide contributes to the immunosuppressive activity of normal aqueous humor. J Immunol 1994;153:1080–1086.
8   Taylor AW, Yee DG, Streilein JW: Suppression of nitric oxide generated by inflammatory macrophages by calcitonin gene-related peptide (CGRP) in aqueous humor. Invest Ophthal Vis Sci 1998; 39:1372–1378.
9   Apte RS, Niederkorn JY: MIF, a novel inhibitor of NK cell activity in the anterior chamber of the eye. J Allergy Clin Immunol 1997;99:S467.
10   Griffith TS, Yu X, Herndon JM, Green DR, Ferguson TA: CD95-induced apoptosis of lymphocytes in an immune privileged site induces immunological tolerance. Immunity 1996;5:7–16.
11   Ferguson TA, Griffith TS: A vision of cell death: Insights into immune privilege. Immunol Rev 1997;156:167–184.
12   Bora NS, Gobleman CL, Atkinson JP, Pepose JS, Kaplan HJ: Differential expression of the complement regulatory proteins in the human eye. Invest Ophthalmol Vis Sci 1993;34:3579–3584.
13   Streilein JW: Immune regulation and the eye: A dangerous compromise. FASEB J 1997;1:199–208.
14   Streilein JW, Niederkorn JY, Shadduck JA: Systemic immune unresponsiveness induced in adult mice by anterior chamber presentation of minor histocompatibility antigens. J Exp Med 1980;152: 1121–1125.
15   Niederkorn JY: Immune privilege and immune regulation in the eye. ACAID review. Adv Immunol 1990;48:191–226.
16   Streilein JW: Ocular immune privilege and the Faust dilemma. Invest Ophthal Vis Sci 1996;37: 1940–1950.
17   Kaplan HJ, Stevens TR: A reconsideration of immunologic privilege within the anterior chamber of the eye. Transplantation 1975;19:302–307.
18   Streilein JW: Anterior chamber-associated immune deviation: The privilege of immunity in the eye. Surv Ophthalmol 1990;35:67–73.
19   Chandler JW, Axelrod AJ: Conjunctiva-associated lymphoid tissue; a probable component of the mucosa-associated lymphoid tissue; in O'Connor GR (ed): Immunologic Diseases of the Mucous Membranes: Pathology, Diagnosis and Treatment. New York, Masson, 1980, pp 63–70.
20   Marreu F, Boisjoly HM, Wagner E: Long-term culture and characterization of human limbal microvascular endothelial cells. Exp Eye Res 1990;51:645–650.
21   Gillette TE, Chandler JW, Greiner JV: Langerhans' cells of the ocular surface. Ophthalmology 1982;89:700–711.
22   Jager MJ: Langerhans' cells and ocular immunology. Reg Immunol 1992;4:186–195.
23   Mederios LJ, Harris NL: Lymphoid infiltrates of the orbit and conjunctiva: A morphologic and immunologic study of 99 cases. Am J Surg Pathol 1989;13:459–471.
24   Khodadoust AA, Attarzadeh A: Presumed autoimmune corneal endotheliopathy. Am J Ophthalmol 1982;93:718–722.
25   Ohashi Y, Yamamoto S, Nishida K, Okamoto S, Kinoshita S, Hayashi K, Manabe R: Demonstration of herpes simplex virus DNA in idiopathic corneal endotheliopathy. Am J Ophthalmol 1991;112: 419–423.
26   Zheng XD, Yamaguchi M, Okamoto S, Ohahi Y: Herpetic corneal endotheliitis in rabbits. Invest Ophthalmol Vis Sci 1997;38:S873.
27   Tanaka Y, Harino S, Danjo S, Hara J, Yamanishi K, Takahashi M: Skin test with varicella-zoster virus antigen for ophthalmic herpes zoster. Am J Ophthalmol 1984;98:7–10.
28   Pflugfelder SC, Crouse C, Pereira I, Atherton SS: Amplication of Epstein-Barr virus genomic sequences in blood cells, lacrimal glands, and tears from primary Sjögren syndrome patients. Ophthalmology 1993;97:976–984.
29   Pflugfelder SC, Crouse C, Monroy D: Epstein-Barr virus and the lacrimal gland pathology of Sjögren syndrome. Am J Pathol 1993;143:49–64.
30   Ablashi DV, Sturzenegger S, Hunter EA: Presence of HTLV-III in tears and cells from the eyes of AIDS patients. J Exp Pathol 1987;3:693–703.
31   Su CS, Bowden S, Fong LP, Taylor HR: Detection of hepatitis B virus DNA in tears by polymerase chain reaction. Arch Ophthalmol 1994;112:621–625.

32   Feucht HH, Polywka S, Zollner B, Laufs R: Greater amount of HCV-RNA in tears compared to blood. Microbiol Immunol 1994;38:157–158.
33   Wilson SE, Lee WM, Murakami C, Weng J, Moninger GA: Mooren-type hepatitis C virus-associated corneal ulceration. Ophthalmology 1994;101:736–745.
34   Liesegang TJ: Atopic keratoconjunctivitis; in Pepose JS, Holland GN, Wilhelmus KR (eds): Ocular Infection and Immunity. St Louis, Mosby, 1996, pp 376–390.
35   Ong CS: Tacrolimus ointment for atopic dermatitis. N Engl J Med 1998;10:1788–1789.
36   Nakagawa H, Etoh T, Ishibashi Y, Higaki Y, Kawashima M, Torii H, Harada S: Tacrolimus ointment for atopic dermatitis. Lancet 1994;24:883.
37   Kinoshita S, Manabe R: Chemical burns; in Brightbill FS (ed): Corneal Surgery. St Louis, Mosby, 1986, pp 370–379.
38   Shimazaki J, Yang HY, Tsubota K: Aminiotic membrane transplantation for ocular surface reconstruction in patients with chemical and thermal burns. Ophthalmology 1997;104:2068–2076.
39   Tsubota K, Satake Y, Ohyama M, Toda I, Takano Y, Ono M, Shinozaki N, Shimazaki J: Surgical reconstruction of the ocular surface in advanced ocular cicatoricial pemphigoid and Stevens-Johnson syndrome. Am J Ophthalmol 1996;122:38–52.
40   Yao YF, Inoue Y, Hara Y, Kiritoshi A, Tano Y, Ohashi Y: Suppression of graft rejection in rat keratoepithelioplasty by anterior chamber inoculation of donor lymphocytes. Jpn J Ophthalmol 1994;38:345–352.
41   Okamoto S, Hara Y, Streilein JW: Induction of anterior chamber-associated immune deviation with lymphoreticular allogeneic cells. Transplantation 1995;59:377–381.
42   Van der Gaag R, Abdillahi H, Stilma JS, Vetter JC: Circulating antibodies against corneal epithelium and hookworm in patients with Mooren's ulcer from Sierra Leone. Br J Ophthalmol 1983;67: 623–628.
43   Zhao ZS, Granucci F, Yeh L, Schaffer PA, Cantor H: Molecular mimicry by herpes simplex virus-type 1: Autoimmune disease after viral infection. Science 1998;279:1344–1347.
44   Hylkema HA, Rathman WM, Kijlstra A: Deposition of immune complexes in the mouse eye. Exp Eye Res 1983;37:257–265.

Dr. Yuichi Ohashi, Department of Ophthalmology, Ehime University School of Medicine, Onsen-gun, Shigenobu, Ehime 791-0295 (Japan)
Tel. +81 89 960 5361, Fax +81 89 960 5364, E-Mail ohashi@m.ehime-u.ac.jp

Streilein JW (ed): Immune Response and the Eye.
Chem Immunol. Basel, Karger, 1999, vol 73, pp 11–38

....

Regional Immunity and Ocular Immune Privilege

J. Wayne Streilein

Schepens Eye Research Institute, Harvard Medical School, Boston, Mass., USA

Introduction

Beyond the most primitive of oligocellular creatures, all animals possess the capacity to defend themselves against invading pathogens. In vertebrates, defense against pathogens is accomplished by two independent, but complementary, response systems: innate immunity and adaptive immunity. Innate immunity is thought to be phylogenetically older and is comprised of a set of cells and molecules which, in a stereotypic manner detect, respond to, and, often, eliminate pathogens. By contrast, adaptive immunity is comprised of cells (lymphocytes) that throughout life generate unique receptor molecules that recognize with extraordinary specificity molecules expressed by invading pathogens. In advanced vertebrates, the innate and adaptive immune systems interact coordinately in responding and destroying invading pathogens.

Principles of Immune Responses

The discovery of immunity in our time occurred in the 1880s, based on pioneering work of Pasteur, von Behring, Kitazawa, Ehrlich, Koch and Metchnikoff [1]. Almost immediately a controversy emerged over the question of specificity for antigen. One group of scientists, especially Pasteur and Ehrlich, argued in favor of an immunity that had exquisite specificity for the initiating pathogen. The logic of vaccination turned on this view. Another group, championed by Metchnikoff, favored the view that leukocytes possessed the capacity to phagocytize and thereby eliminate pathogens, irrespective of antigenic specificity. These two lines of investigation have resulted in our current view of immunity as a collaboration between the innate immune system (Metchnikoff's view) and the adaptive immune system (the other view). We now appreciate that neither system exists independent of the other, and that the cells and molecules of innate immunity interact with their counterparts in the adaptive immune system to achieve immediate and long-term protection against pathogens.

Innate Immunity

Animals completely devoid of an adaptive immune system still retain the capacity to resist many infectious agents [1–3]. This capacity rests largely among a set of leukocytes and plasma proteins that are able to detect and destroy pathogens. The leukocytes include monocytes/macrophages, dendritic cells, granulocytes (neutrophils, basophils, eosinophils), and lymphocytes (natural killer cells) that lack the receptors for antigen that are typical of the adaptive immune response. The plasma proteins include members of the complement cascade, members of the clotting cascade, some of the acute phase reaction proteins (e.g. C-reactive protein, mannose-binding protein), and a variety of proteases and substrates (e.g.kallikrein system, plasminogen activators). Acting alone, together, and/or in concert with the cells and molecules of the adaptive immune system, components of the innate immune system can and do provide immediate, intermediate, and even long-term protection against infectious diseases. Moreover, cells and molecules of the innate immune system contribute to immunopathogenic disease when the response is excessive or inappropriate.

Cells and molecules of the innate immune system possess receptors that enable them to detect pathogens. Janeway and Medzhitov [2, 3] have championed the view that all pathogens express stereotypic surface structures called pathogen-associated molecular patterns (PAMPs). These structures represent the major targets of innate immune system recognition. PAMPs include bacterial lipopolysaccharides (LPS) on gram-negative microbes, lipotechoic acid on gram-positive microbes, as well as mannan and glycans. This list is incomplete and new structures are being added on a continuing basis. An interesting and provocative recent discovery is that molecules expressed on the surface of mammalian cells undergoing apoptosis resemble PAMPs [4]. If true, this may account, on the one hand, for the ability of macrophages to phagocytose apoptotic cells rapidly, and, on the other hand, for the participation of macrophages in the process of tissue differentiation as apoptotic cell death contributes to tissue molding.

The cell surface molecules that recognize PAMPs have been termed 'pattern recognition receptors' (PRRs). To date, very few of these structures have been identified, cloned and sequenced. Ulevitch and Tobias [5] have speculated that the Fcγ receptor for immunoglobulin G acts as a recognition structure that arms innate effector cells. Stahl and Ezekowicz [6] have deduced that the mannose-binding protein, an acute phase reactant secreted by the liver, and present constitutively in serum and amniotic fluid, resembles C1q. It has a collagen-like region, and a carbohydrate bind region, and can function as an opsonin. Other PRRs include CD36, scavenger receptors, and CD14.

Recognition of pathogens by PRRs triggers immediate responses among the cells expressing these receptors. Neutrophils are activated, leading them to phagocytose, to generate reactive oxygen intermediates, and to release their lytic granules. Macrophages are similarly activated, and in addition the so-called immediate early gene program is set in motion, chiefly through NFκB. This process enables the cells to acquire effector functions that lead to phagocytosis and death of pathogens.

It has recently become clear that the innate immune response plays a critical role in initiating the adaptive immune response. We have learned in the last decade that professional antigen-presenting cells (APC), chiefly dendritic cells and macrophages, bear the responsibility of capturing antigens and preparing them for presentation to T (and B) lymphocytes [7, 8]. And we have learned that successful presentation of antigen by APC requires that the cells themselves be activated – not only to process antigenic peptides, but to display costimulatory signals that are required for T-cell activation. There is now increasingly good evidence to indicate that innate immunity serves to 'activate' APC in peripheral tissues, and it is this activation signal that enables the cells to differentiate into effective activators of T cells. Molecules such as LPS and lipotechoic acid are good examples of agents able to 'activate' dendritic cells and macrophages.

The innate immune response is characterized by its proinflammatory nature, and by its capacity for immediate reactivity. Since the system lacks the specificity of the adaptive immune system, host tissues and organs may suffer indiscriminately the deleterious consequences of innate effector mechanisms. One need only contemplate the wide-ranging and potentially lethal consequences of injection of LPS into susceptible animals and humans to appreciate the threat that unregulated or excessive activation of innate immunity represents. Not surprisingly, elaborate regulatory mechanisms have been devised evolutionarily in an effort to insure that the innate immune response does not proceed to pathology. Both the complement and clotting cascades are regulated by inhibitors, soluble as well as cell membrane associated, which limit initial activation, amplification, and effector function. Similarly, activated macrophages are constrained by molecules such as transforming growth factor-β, and natural killer (NK) cells are inhibited by macrophage migration inhibitory factor.

Inflammation is a profound threat to vision, and it comes as no surprise that the eye has acquired a variety of local strategies to contain and control the cells and molecules of the innate immune system [9–17]. Aqueous humor itself inhibits complement activation, suppresses nitric oxide production by LPS-activated macrophages, and interferes with lysis by NK cells. The animal model of experimental endotoxin-induced uveitis has proven to be a valuable source of new knowledge concerning the interaction between the eye and innate immune mechanisms.

Adaptive Immunity

Early in vertebrate evolution, specialized leukocytes (lymphocytes) acquired the ability to create unique receptor molecules from a limited repertoire of genetic elements. These novel molecules, termed antibodies and T-cell receptors for antigen, arise in almost limitless variety and display the capacity in the aggregate of recognizing virtually all molecules of biologic interest. Two subsets of lymphocytes possess this capacity: B lymphocytes which produce antibodies, and T cells which produce T-cell receptors for antigen. In the absence of any exogenous stimulation, T and B cells spontaneously generate these recognition structures and display them as receptors on the cell surface. Each lymphocyte expresses thousands of these receptors on its surface, but on any given lymphocyte, all of the receptors are molecularly identical. Therefore, the ability of the adaptive immune system to recognize billions of different molecules rests in its ability to generate complementary sets of billions of B and T lymphocytes, each with the capacity to recognize a different molecule.

B and T lymphocytes generate this enormous diversity of cell surface receptors spontaneously during differentiation, i.e. in the absence of exogenous stimulation. Once receptor-bearing lymphocytes have matured, they are poised through these receptors to recognize biologically important molecules. However, each cell remains silent, locked in G_0 of the cell cycle, until or unless it encounters a molecule for which it has the complementary ability to bind with high affinity. By convention, molecules that have the capacity to bind lymphocyte receptors with high affinity are called *antigens*. Thus, in the native state, mature vertebrates contain large numbers of T and B lymphocytes, each of which expresses on its surface a monotonous array of a single, unique receptor for a different antigen. It is only when antigen is introduced into the system that T and B lymphocytes with receptors capable of binding that antigen with high affinity are activated. And antigen-triggered activation of these cells initiates an immune response. If the antigen is a molecule borne by a pathogen, activation leads to the pathogen's elimination. On the contrary, if the antigen is a molecule of the responding host's own tissue, then activation may lead to tissue injury and disease. The ability to distinguish between foreign (and therefore pathogenic) antigens and self (and presumably nonpathogenic) or autoantigens is an existential one made by the immune system, since the genome confers on each individual the potential to create antibodies or T-cell receptors for antigen that bind autoantigens with high affinity. Regulation of autoimmune reactivity is crucial to an individual's survival.

Since mature individuals already contain quiescent T and B lymphocytes with the capacity to recognize the entire range of biologically important molecules, introduction of a particular antigen allows for a selection process to take place in which B or T cells that express a surface receptor with sufficiently high affinity for the antigen are aroused. If the antigenic stimulus is of appropriate magnitude, the 'aroused' T and B lymphocytes become activated. One important consequence is that the cells enter into replicative cycles, leading eventually to the emergence of 'clones' of T and B lymphocytes distinguished primarily by their unique ability to recognize the initiating antigen. In stochastic terms, the simple act of proliferation of antigen-triggered T and B lymphocytes changes the adaptive immune system forever; compared to other (unactivated) T and B lymphocytes in the system, the frequency of cells triggered by this particular antigen is increased. Consequently, if the same antigen is reintroduced at a later date, the elevated frequency of antigen-specific lymphocytes enhances the likelihood of interaction with antigen and therefore the likelihood of an immune response. To a certain extent, the existence of memory in the adaptive immune system reflects the increased frequency of antigen-specific lymphocytes generated by an initial encounter with antigen.

Proliferation in response to antigen stimulation is only one dimension of the way in which B and T lymphocytes are triggered by specific antigen. Arousal of antigen-specific lymphocytes by antigen leads to the development of a response that is designed to eliminate the antigen-bearing pathogens. Thus, lymphocytes aroused by their specific antigen also differentiate into effector function. In the case of B lymphocytes, differentiation enables the activated cell to synthesize its antibody molecule in a secretory form, and as a consequence, soluble antibodies specific for the initiating antigen appear in the systemic circulation and in other body fluids. In the case of T lymphocytes, differentiation equips the cell responding to antigen to secrete a spectrum of cytokines that have an enormously wide array of effects on other cells, including cells of the innate immune system, and parenchymal cells of various solid organs and tissues. In this manner, the adaptive immune T cell commands other leukocytes and parenchymal cells in an attack that leads to elimination of the pathogen. Thus, adaptive immunity is expressed in two major ways: in the form of so-called 'humoral immunity' mediated by soluble antibodies produced by B lymphocytes, and in the form of so-called 'cellular immunity' mediated by T lymphocytes.

Memory, or anamnesia, in the immune system is revealed when an antigen is reintroduced into an individual that previously encountered the same antigen. The capacities of that individual to (a) produce large amounts of specific antibody in a rapid fashion, (b) mobilize a powerful effector force, and (c) eliminate the antigen-bearing pathogen before it has a chance to cause disease are all expressions of immunologic memory. Moreover, the fact that only the original antigen, not a molecularly unrelated antigen, can trigger this memory response reveals one of the most important features of the adaptive immune response: its specificity. Together, activation of preexisting T and B lymphocytes, memory for the original antigen that triggered them, and the specificity inherent in that memory reveal three cardinal features of the adaptive immune response: (a) it is acquired, (b) it is specific, and (c) it is remembered through time.

There are two additional features of the adaptive immune response that set it apart from all other responses to environmental stimuli. Adaptive immunity can be transferred from an individual that has been immunized by an antigen to an individual who has never previously encountered that antigen. Antibodies obtained from the plasma of an immunized individual can transfer humoral immunity to that antigen when injected into a 'naive' individual. Similarly, T lymphocytes from an immunized individual can transfer cell-mediated immunity if injected into an individual that never previously encountered the same antigen. Thus, the ability of immunity to be transferable is a fourth cardinal feature of the response.

For certain antigens – of which autoantigens are good examples – the adaptive immune responses also expresses 'tolerance'. Tolerance is defined as the specific *inability* of a mature individual to mount an immune response to a particular antigen. An individual who is tolerant of antigen A is not tolerant of other antigens, and when immunized, will respond to all other antigens except antigen A. In a sense, tolerance is the mirror image of immunity; it is acquired, specific, remembered – and sometimes, even transferable from a 'tolerant' individual to a naive one. Therefore, the ability to acquire antigen-specific unresponsiveness, i.e. tolerance, represents the fifth cardinal feature of the adaptive immune response.

The Immune Reflex Arc

Enumerating the five cardinal features of the adaptive immune response only begins to express the complicated, elaborate nature by which this type of immunity arises and is expressed. The very fact that the same antigen can induce either protective immunity or tolerance reveals that factors well beyond

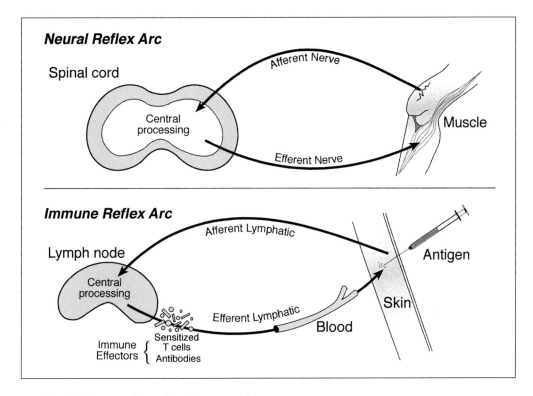

Neural Reflex Arc

Spinal cord

Afferent Nerve

Central
processing

Muscle

Efferent Nerve

Immune Reflex Arc

Afferent Lymphatic

Lymph node

Antigen

Central
processing

Efferent Lymphatic

Skin

Blood

Immune { Sensitized
Effectors { T cells
Antibodies

Fig. 1. Elements of neural and immune reflex arcs.

antigen alone govern the type of immunity that is generated. In order to understand the elemental rules of immunity, immunologists have resorted to an analogy between the immune response and the neural reflex arc (fig. 1). In a highly predictable and stereotypic manner, the physician's hammer strikes the patellar tendon of the quadriceps muscle of the leg of a seated patient, and elicits the muscle's contraction, pulling the lower leg forward. No conscious thought on the part of the patient contributes to this response, and it is therefore a 'reflex'. In a similar manner, injection of antigen leads to a highly predictable immune response, and this response occurs without 'thought' on the part of the responding individual. Neuroscientists consider the neural reflex an 'arc' that is comprised of an afferent limb (which carries the sensory stimulus to the spinal cord), a central processing mechanism (that converts the sensory signal into a motor nerve impulse), and an efferent limb (which delivers the impulse to the muscle, causing it to contract). Immunologists similarly divide the immune response into an afferent limb (in which antigenic signals are captured and transmitted to secondary lymphoid organs), a central processing mechanism (in which the antigenic signal is transduced into effector modalities – antibodies and effector T cells), and an efferent limb (in which the effectors are delivered via the blood to the site of antigen, leading to its elimination). When the immune reflex arc functions conventionally, conventional immunity emerges. However, disruption or modification of the reflex arc leads either to an unconventional immune response, or even its failure. Regional immunity and immune privilege represent immune responses that occur when the conventional immune reflex arc is altered by tissue-restricted factors. A brief description of the three components of the immune reflex arc helps to explain and understand both regional immunity and immune privilege.

Afferent Limb

The afferent limb encompasses the interval from introduction of antigen into the body, and its presentation to antigen-specific T and B lymphocytes. Naive lymphocytes can only be activated in organized secondary lymphoid organs, such as lymph nodes, spleen, Peyer's patches, tonsils, etc. Under normal circumstances, antigens first enter the body through a cutaneous or mucosal surface. The afferent limb bridges the gap between point of tissue entry of antigen to point of presentation of antigen to lymphocytes. While antigens that penetrate the skin can flow via tissue lymph to draining lymph nodes, this is by no means the only, or perhaps even the more common, mode of delivery. Instead, skin and other solid tissue organs contain bone marrow-derived cells that have the responsibility of capturing tissue-derived antigens and delivering them via the lymph to draining lymph nodes. Both macrophages, which have the property of phagocytosis of particulate material, and dendritic cells, which have the capacity to endocytose large amounts of extracellular fluid, perform these functions. Langerhans' cells in the epidermis belong to the dendritic cell lineage. Together with macrophages, dendritic cells are considered to be 'professional' APC [8]. Not only do APC capture antigen introduced into the body, but their mobility enables them to migrate out of tissues and organs via lymph channels and flow to draining lymphoid organs. Within these organs, cells of this type come to rest in parafollicular areas, regions adjacent to specialized postcapillary venules which deliver to the site large numbers of T and B lymphocytes from the blood. APC display yet another function that makes immune responses possible: APC that have migrated from a peripheral tissue upregulate on their surfaces an array of molecules that function as ligands for co-ligands expressed on T and B lymphocytes. These ligands are referred to as 'costimulatory' molecules because activation of resting lymphocytes by antigen can only be accomplished if antigen recognition occurs simultaneously with costimulation. These requirements indicate a critical feature of lymphocyte activation: proper activation of T and B lymphocytes occurs only if the responding cell receives two independent signals. The first, usually referred to as signal 1, is delivered when the receptor for antigen on the lymphocyte engages antigen displayed by an APC. The second, referred to as signal 2, is delivered when costimulatory stimuli are perceived by the responding lymphocyte. APC prepare two types of costimulatory signals – membrane-bound ligands expressed on their surface, and cytokines that they secrete. In conventional immune responses, APC that have captured an antigen and migrated to a draining lymphoid organ present that antigen to specific lymphocytes while simultaneously (a) expressing surface molecules such as CD80, CD86, ICAM-1, LFA-3, and CD40, and (b) secreting cytokines, such as IL-12 and IL-1β. The responding lymphocytes, having received both signals 1 and 2, respond by proliferating and differentiating.

Before leaving this discussion, it is necessary to point out that APC that capture antigen bear the responsibility of presenting that antigen to specific T and B lymphocytes. However, the rules of presentation during immune induction to a new antigen are different for the two different lymphocyte types. For responding B cells, APC merely present the native antigen molecule on their surface, a variety of nonspecific molecular interactions being responsible for the expression. For responding T cells, the antigen must be partially degraded within the APC, and then, as peptide fragments, loaded onto special molecules encoded by genes within the major histocompatibility complex (MHC). These special molecules, termed class I and class II, are able, respectively, to bind peptides derived from protein molecules degraded in the cytoplasm (class I) or in endocytic and phagocytic vesicles (class II). Thus, antigen presented by APC to B cells is the native antigen molecule itself, whereas antigen presented by APC to T cells is a breakdown product of the native antigen. These differences reflect the different manners in which receptors for antigen on B and T lymphocytes recognize and bind to antigenic material.

Central Processing Mechanism

The process of converting the antigenic signal into an effector immune response begins when specific T and B cells recognize antigen on the surfaces of APC in the parafollicular regions of the cortex of secondary lymphoid organs. Providing that the APC present antigen plus costimulation, lymphocytes that recognize the antigen are activated. In usual circumstances, the first cells to respond are CD4+ T cells. These cells, which recognize antigenic peptides presented in the context of class II MHC molecules, proliferate and secrete cytokines such as IL-2, IL-3, GM-CSF, IFN-γ, and IL-4. In turn these cytokines act as 'helper' factors which 'help' the responses of other cells in the immediate environment. IL-2 is a growth factor for T cells, and as responding T cells begin to express IL-2 receptors, the cells enter mitosis and replicate.

IL-3 and GM-CSF also promote T- and B-cell growth. IFN-γ and IL-4 have differing effects, depending upon the target cells that bear their receptors. For example, IFN-γ acts on the APC to enhance its production of IL-12 and expression of CD40, both of which drive the responding CD4+ T cell in a direction that favors proliferation, and production of IFN-γ and TNF-α. IL-4 promotes the proliferation and differentiation of CD4+ cells in a somewhat different direction in which the resultant cells produce IL-4, IL-5, IL-6 and IL-10, but little or no IFN-γ or TNF-α. In addition, IL-2, IFN-γ, and IL-4 promote the activation and differentiation of CD8+ T cells that eventually become cytotoxic. CD8+ T cells recognize antigen-derived peptides in the context of class I MHC molecules. Upon antigen-dependent activation, CD8+ T cells not only carry out lytic function, but they produce cytokines, especially IFN-γ, which have 'helper-type' as well as proinflammatory effects on surrounding cells. Finally, the cytokines secreted by CD4+ T cells provide 'help' to the activation of B lymphocytes. If the cytokines produced by CD4+ T cells are predominately IFN-γ and IL-2, then the responding B cells produce IgG antibodies that fix complement. Alternatively, if the helper CD4+ T cells produce primarily IL-4, IL-5, IL-6 and IL-10, then the responding B cells produce IgG antibodies that do not fix complement, and/or the B cells produce IgE or IgA antibodies.

Thus, central processing allows the antigenic signal received by the lymph node or spleen to be converted into immune effectors, including CD4+ and CD8+ T cells, and B cells secreting a range of different immunoglobulins. All of these effectors share the property of displaying surface receptors that are highly specific for the eliciting antigen. Moreover, as antigen-specific T and B cells proliferate and differentiate in the lymph node or spleen, their progeny, as well as secreted antibody molecules, are delivered via lymph into the bloodstream where they are disseminated throughout the circulation. Some of the lymphocytes that emerge from the central processing mechanism will function as effector cells, while others will function as memory cells, having converted into long-lived cells with the capacity to recirculate repeatedly throughout the blood and various tissues.

Efferent Limb

Hematogenous dissemination of immune effectors generated during central processing makes it possible for these effectors to gain access to all tissues and organs served by blood vessels. A typical site of infection or immunization is usually inflamed, and the blood vasculature at the site is usually leaky. Because of this state, and because immune effector T cells display receptors that bind to ligands on activated vascular endothelial cells, immune effectors tend to localize at sites of inflammation, injury, etc. If the relevant antigen is present at the site, then antigen recognition takes place, the effector cells that invade the site are terminally activated, and the final act of immune elimination is triggered. For effector T cells, the ability to recognize antigen at the peripheral site still requires that the antigen be presented by an APC. Professional APC within the inflamed site may serve this function, but often, under the influence of IFN-γ, parenchymal cells (such as epithelial cells, fibroblasts, and even vascular endothelial cells) upregulate class I and class II MHC expression and present antigenic epitopes to T cells. No such requirements exist for specific antibodies that penetrate into the inflamed, antigen-containing site.

While interaction with antigen is the initial step in the process that leads to immune elimination, under most circumstances the actual destruction of the antigen/pathogen is accomplished by the effectors of innate immunity. For example, effector CD4+ T cells have little capacity directly to eliminate antigen-bearing target cells. Instead, antigen presentation triggers these cells to secrete lymphokines, such as IFN-γ and TNF-α, which recruit to the site monocyte/macrophages and NK cells. Activation of these cells leads to the generation of cytotoxic products, to the phagocytosis of the offending pathogen, and to activation of the capacity to kill the target cell. In the case of antibody, interactions with antigen and then complement components leads to elimination of the target antigen via direct lysis of cells, and by recruitment of neutrophilic granulocytes that destroy the offending pathogen/antigen. Thus, in the expression of immunity, antigen-specific immune effectors usually bring about neutralization and elimination of the invading pathogen by enlisting the aid of the effectors of innate immunity, i.e. nonspecific defense mechanisms.

Immune Regulation, Tolerance, and the Immune Reflex Arc

Each of the three components of the immune reflex arc represents the concerted interactions of diverse cells and molecules. Consequently, regulation of immunity can be exerted during the afferent limb, central processing and efferent limb by different mechanisms that act on the unique dimensions of each of these three components. In general, regulation of immunity is usually thought to mean inhibition or lack of an immune response to an antigen. The general term 'tolerance' refers to that aspect of the immune response where an antigen challenge fails to lead to a detectable antigen-specific response. In order for tolerance to be expressed, antigen-specific T and/or B cells must have been silenced. Since the original discovery of tolerance experimentally in the early 1950s, numerous silencing mechanisms have been described, including clonal deletion, clonal anergy, T-cell suppression, immune deviation, and immunologic ignorance.

During lymphocyte development, fully functional T cells (and B cells) with receptors that recognize *Self* molecules with high affinity are not generated. The lack of these cells appears to be due to a process of clonal deletion that takes place within the organs in which these lymphocytes are maturing. In the case of T cells, potentially self-reactive thymocytes that encounter APC expressing self-encoded molecules are triggered to undergo apoptosis. As a consequence, the thymocytes that mature and disseminate into the periphery as mature T cells are largely devoid of self-reactivity. This is, however, an affinity issue, since T cells with relatively low affinity for self molecules can be detected in the peripheral blood of normal individuals. Thymic elimination of self-reactive T cells seems primarily to affect cells of the highest affinity. Moreover, thymic elimination can only apply to T cells that recognize antigens expressed within the gland. Many tissue-specific antigens (especially eye-restricted molecules) are not expressed intrathymically. Therefore, T cells with high-affinity receptors capable of recognizing tissue-restricted antigens can be readily found in the blood.

The existence of self-reactive T cells in the peripheral blood means that the potential exists for induction and expression of autoimmunity. This is one important reason why mechanisms of regulation exist in the periphery to contain and prevent the activation of self-reactive T cells. Unless these cells are constrained, autoimmunity and autoimmune disease are a threat. Whereas clonal deletion seems to be the primary mechanism by which self-tolerance is achieved within the thymus, other mechanisms are involved in regulation of immunity in the periphery. It is useful to consider immune regulatory mechanisms in the context of the immune reflex arc.

During induction of immunity, i.e. the afferent limb, the key activity is to capture, process and present antigen. Since these are largely the functional properties of APC, regulation of immune induction is exerted primarily via these cells. Various mechanisms can operate to prevent APC from presenting antigen to T cells. First, antigen can be sequestered or prevented from gaining access to APC. Physical barriers can accomplish this, or the APC itself (or auxiliary phagocytic and degrading cells) can be rendered incapable of capturing antigen from the microenvironment. Second, APC can be inhibited from degrading antigen into immunogenic peptides, and/or inhibited from loading these peptides onto MHC molecules in the endoplasmic reticulum, and/or inhibited from expressing peptide-loaded MHC molecules on the cell surface. Third, antigen-bearing APC may be inhibited from migrating from the somatic tissue of origin to draining lymphoid organs where naive T cells are first encountered. Fourth, the capacity of APC to upregulate costimulatory molecules may be suppressed. In general, these inhibitions of APC function result in a kind of immunologic ignorance in which naive T cells with specificity for the antigen in question are never confronted by the antigen in immunogenic form.

But, other types of APC regulation during immune induction actually lead to 'tolerance'. APC are functionally plastic, and the cytokine milieu in which they reside often dictates the type of functional properties they display. Following high-dose UVB radiation of skin, APC come under this damaging influence, and begin to secrete IL-10 rather than IL-12. As a consequence, the cells acquire accessory properties that favor the activation of Th2 rather than Th1 cells, i.e. immune deviation [18, 19]. Similarly, APC within immuno-suppressive microenvironments of immune privileged sites (such as the eye) display an unusual array of costimulatory properties, and as a consequence they fail to activate effector CD4+ T cells. Instead, they activate regulatory T cells – another form of immune deviation [20–22].

Many mechanisms have been implicated in regulation of central processing of the antigen-specific signal. The initial encounter between a naive T cell and an antigen-bearing APC is particularly vulnerable to disruption. Activation of CD4+ and CD8+ T cells requires that immunogenic peptide be presented in the context of MHC molecules, and that costimulation be elaborated by the APC. In fact, this costimulation works bidirectionally in a process that further amplifies the costimulatory signals emanating from the APC. Lack of costimulation in the presence of antigen-specific stimulation can render responding T cells anergic, i.e. unable thereafter to respond to the same antigen, even in the presence of intense costimulation [23]. Alternatively, intense costimulation in the presence of high-antigen dose can induce profound T-cell activation, followed quickly thereafter by apoptosis among the responding T cells. Both anergy and apoptosis of T cells leads to a state of tolerance in which response to the antigen in question is missing. In addition, APC with unusual costimulatory molecules, such as the APC from privileged sites [20–22], or the APC that process orally ingested antigens, can distort the functional program of responding T cells, deflecting them toward regulatory cells that, on the one hand, secrete TGF-β, and, on the other hand, resemble Th2 cells. When this occurs, the antigen-specific T cells that leave the draining lymph node act to regulate, rather than effect, cell-mediated immunity to the initiating antigen. Since these regulatory T cells disseminate widely throughout the body, they can modify the immune response in an antigen-specific way in whatever organ or tissue the original antigen is eventually encountered.

The final level of control that expresses itself as tolerance is exerted at the efferent limb. For effector T cells, regulation of the consequences of their interaction with antigen in the periphery can take one of several forms. The most dramatic, perhaps, is the capacity of antigen-bearing targets either to induce apoptosis among effector T cells, or to render the cells anergic. Effector

T cells express CD95, and if they are confronted by antigen-bearing cells in the periphery that express CD95 ligand, the former cells can be triggered to undergo programmed cell death [24]. Other molecular mechanisms can also induce T-cell apoptosis, including TNF-α production at the site of antigen encounter. In expression of T-cell-mediated immunity in the periphery, the requirement for T-cell activation still holds, namely that antigenic peptides must be presented by local APC in the context of class I or II MHC molecules. If the APC express inappropriate costimulatory molecules, the responding T cells may become anergic. Whether effector T cells are lost via apoptosis, or their function is dissipated via anergy, tolerance is expressed. Effector T cells can also be regulated by distinctive properties of the peripheral microenvironment. T cells that encounter antigen in the context of MHC molecules on APC that are simultaneously secreting IL-10 or TGF-β often fail to carry out their effector function. To the contrary, the functions of these T cells may even undergo reprogramming, and what emerges are T cells that secrete immunosuppressive cytokines. That is, under certain circumstances, a microenvironment can convert effector T cells into regulatory cells which end up further promoting unresponsiveness and tolerance.

Concept of Regional Immunity

It is axiomatic that all organs and tissues of the body, irrespective of their specific biologic function, require immune protection against exogenous and endogenous pathogens. It is also well appreciated that different pathogenic agents use distinctive virulence strategies to gain advantage over the host, and that these distinctive strategies are tissue- and organ-specific. The diversity of immune effector mechanisms, ranging from functionally distinct subsets of T cells to functional distinct immunoglobulin isotypes, addresses the wide range of virulence strategies employed by pathogenic organisms. As a consequence, certain immune effectors tend to work best at certain regions of the body. For example, IgA antibodies are particularly effective at protecting the mucosal surfaces from attack by pathogenic bacteria and viruses that attempt to invade via these surfaces. Delayed hypersensitivity T cells are particularly effective at ridding the skin of pathogenic organisms that have invaded across the cutaneous surface. Whereas IgA is virtually without effect in protecting the skin against its pathogens, T cells that mediate delayed hypersensitivity can protect mucosal surfaces against invading pathogens, but the damage caused by the inflammation that accompanies this response may be unacceptably great. The concept that different organs and tissues (regions) are protected by specialized immune effectors has given rise to the term 'regional immunity'

[25, 26]. The thesis of regional immunity is that individual organs and tissues interact with the systemic immune apparatus, selecting immune effectors that match the virulence strategies of pathogens that threaten each region, while at the same time requiring these immune effectors to interfere as little as possible with the physiologic functions of each individual region.

Components of Regional Immune Systems

Each regional immune system contains a stereotypic set of components that ensure that regional immune responses occur, are effective, and appropriate. These components include (a) a tissue-restricted microenvironment that is created by factors and molecules secreted by the region's parenchymal cells; (b) tissue-distributed bone marrow-derived cells that provide the region with indigenous, albeit replaceable, APC; (c) tissue-distributed accessory cells that provide the region with nonspecific, innate defense mechanisms, such as macrophages, mast cells, NK cells; (d) tissue-tropic T and B lymphocytes that express surface ligands (cell adhesion molecules) that bind preferentially to co-ligands on endothelial cells of a region's microvasculature, and that recirculate ceaselessly from blood to tissue to lymph to blood; (e) blood:tissue barriers that regulate access of blood-borne molecules and cells into the interstitium of a region; (f) lymph drainage networks that enable migrating APC from a region to carry antigen captured within the region to draining secondary lymphoid organs, and (g) nerves which bring to the region neuropeptides and transmitters that modify the functional properties of parenchymal cells, adventitial cells, accessory cells, APC, and recirculating T and B lymphocytes. Much remains to be learned concerning how each of these components interacts in a manner that produces immune protection in a region without compromising local physiologic function, but some understanding is beginning to emerge. For the benefit of the following discussion, table 1 lists the regional immune components that have now been defined for immune privilege in the eye: an extreme form of regional immunity.

Examples of Regional Immune Systems

The first regional immune system to be appreciated was called GALT – gut-associated lymphoid tissues [27]. Through time, investigators have appreciated that GALT serves not only the surfaces of the gastrointestinal tract, but all other mucosal surfaces as well. Unique features of the so-called mucosal-associated lymphoid tissues (MALT) [28] include (a) localized accumulations of lymphocytes and accessory cells immediately beneath epithelial surfaces, (b) specialized mechanisms for transport of antigenic material from the lumen, across the epithelium, into the lymphoid cell accumulations, (c) B cells that secrete IgA antibodies specific for these antigens, and (d) IgA-secreting B cells

Table 1. Regional immune components in ocular immune privilege

Type	Ocular component
Tissue-restricted microenvironment	Aqueous humor produced by ciliary epithelium
Local antigen presenting cells	Dendritic cells and macrophages in stroma of iris, ciliary body, trabecular meshwork and stroma of choriocapillaris; retinal microglia
Innate defense cells	Macrophages in stroma of iris, ciliary body and choroid
Tissue-tropic T and B lymphocytes	Not yet described
Blood:tissue barrier	Vascular endothelium of iris and retinal vessels; tight junctions among secretory epithelium of ciliary body and pigment epithelium of retina
Lymph drainage network	Virtually absent, except uveoscleral pathway, and lymphatics of choroid
Nerves	Sympathetics, parasympathetics in iris, ciliary body, choroid; corneal C-type fibers

and CD4+ Th2 cells that recirculate preferentially to MALT. Immunity generated through one mucosal surface is, in this manner, available for all mucosal surfaces. In this sense, the mucosal surfaces represent a 'region', and MALT represents the specialized immune system that serves and protects this region.

The second regional immune system to be described was called SALT – skin-associated lymphoid tissues [29]. In many ways, SALT is the polar opposite of MALT. Far from promoting antigen transfer across the skin, the superficial epidermis is designed to prevent invasion by microbial organisms. For pathogens that succeed, a vast network of dendritic APC (Langerhans' cells) maximizes the likelihood that antigenic material will be captured and prepared for presentation to T and B cells. Whereas the secondary lymphoid tissues serving mucosal surfaces are located adjacent to the surface epithelium, the secondary lymphoid organs (lymph nodes) serving skin are situated at a distance, and are connected via lymphatic drainage pathways. Thus, whereas antigenic material that crosses the mucosa is immediately detectable by antigen-specific T and B lymphocytes, cutaneous APC must retain a 'snapshot' of antigenic materials that penetrate the epidermis, and the APC must deliver this image faithfully to T and B cells present in the draining nodes. The primary effector mechanisms that serve the skin are skin-seeking CD4+ T cells that mediate delayed hypersensitivity, CD8+ cytotoxic T cells, and antibodies of the IgG isotypes. Delayed hypersensitivity T cells and complement-fixing IgG antibod-

Table 2. Immune privileged tissues and sites

Sites	Tissues
Eye (anterior chamber, vitreous cavity subretinal space)	Cornea, lens
	Liver
Brain	Ovary
Testis	Testis
Adrenal cortex	Cartilage
Pregnant uterus	Fetoplacental unit
Tumors	Tumors

ies eliminate pathogens by recruiting nonspecific host defenses which produce intense inflammatory responses. Tissue injury of the innocent bystander type is typical of cutaneous immune responses. Apparently, the virulence of pathogens that invade the skin is such that only the most intense immunogenic inflammation serves to nullify the threat. While these reactions often lead to local scarring, the overall capacity of skin to retain its functional integrity is rarely threatened by this type of protective immunity.

Immune Privilege – Extreme Regional Immunity

The phenomenon of immune privilege was described more than 100 years ago [30], but our understanding of its immune basis dates to the seminal work of Medawar in the 1940s [31]. Medawar, who had recently worked out the immune basis of transplantation rejection, understood that immune privilege was a special circumstance where the 'rules' of transplantation immunology were suspended. He defined immune privilege experimentally as the prolonged, often indefinite, survival of organ or tissue grafts at special sites in the body – immune privileged sites. Later, Medawar's student, R.E. Billingham, and his colleague, C.F. Barker, extended the definition to include special organs or tissues which, as grafts, enjoyed prolonged, often indefinite, survival when placed at conventional body sites [32]. Through the years, a surprisingly large number of sites and organs/tissues have come to be regarded as immune privileged (table 2).

Medawar's description of the immune basis of privilege arose long before our current understanding of regulatory mechanisms that shape the expression of immunity. Medawar studied the anterior chamber of the eye and the brain as examples of immune privileged sites. Since both sites were known to reside outside blood:tissue barriers, and since lymphatic drainage pathways had not yet been described for either the anterior chamber or the brain, Medawar came to the conclusion that immune privilege resulted from immunologic ignorance. That is, Medawar postulated that antigens from foreign tissue grafts placed in privileged sites could not escape the eye or the brain, because no lymph drainage existed. Since both eye and brain were further protected from blood-borne molecules and cells by strict barriers, he concluded that grafts in privileged sites were sequestered from the immune system. He reasoned, as a consequence, that the immune system never became aware of the existence of the grafts. For the past three decades, the validity of this concept has been repeatedly challenged, and at present virtually all investigators agree that immune privilege is a dynamic state, rather than a merely passive one, in which immunoregulatory forces combine with anatomical features to maintain the vitality of grafts in privileged sites, and of privileged organs and tissues as grafts [33–38].

The Eye as a Site of Immune Privilege

The original experiments of Dooremal, and the later experiments of Medawar, using human cancer cells, and rabbit skin grafts, respectively, amply demonstrated that the anterior chamber of the eye functions as an immune privileged site. Immune privilege is an extreme form of regional immunity, and the components of this system within the eye are presented in table 1. The knowledge summarized in table 1 has accumulated from studies that marked the modern renaissance of ocular immune privilege that was launched by Kaplan and his collaborators in the early 1970s. In an elegant series of experiments, these investigators demonstrated that allografts of skin and thyroid placed in the anterior chamber of rat eyes enjoyed prolonged survival [39]. Shortly thereafter, Niederkorn and Streilein [33] injected allogeneic tumor cells in the anterior chamber of mouse eyes and found that the cells formed progressively growing tumors. Even more recently, Jiang and Streilein [40, 41] placed allogeneic neuronal retinal tissue, as well as retinal pigment epithelial cells, into the anterior chamber and observed prolonged survival. While all of these experiments confirmed the existence of immune privilege in the anterior chamber, they also defined the limits of that privilege. For example, the ability of allogeneic tumor cells to grow progressively in the anterior chamber was influenced by the strength of the antigens expressed on the tumor cells: tumors expressing MHC-encoded alloantigens enjoyed only transiently extended survival, whereas tumors expressing only weak transplantation antigens persisted indefinitely [42]. These findings underscore the fact that immune privilege is a dynamic, rather than a passive state, and that active factors are important in creating and sustaining privilege. If one or more of these factors falter, then the privileged state may collapse.

In addition to the existence of privilege in the anterior chamber, privilege also exists in the vitreous cavity and in the subretinal space [43, 44]. Although considerably fewer in number, experiments similar to those conducted in the anterior chamber have demonstrated that (a) allogeneic tumor cells grow progressively in both the vitreous cavity and the subretinal space, and (b) that foreign neuronal retinal tissue and retinal pigment epithelial cells also experience prolonged survival in these ocular compartments.

The Eye as a Source of Immune Privileged Tissues

Certain tissues within the eye possess unique immunologic properties that enable them to be classified as 'immune privileged tissues'. The cornea is a good example [45]. The extraordinary success of corneas as orthotopic allografts cannot be ascribed solely to the fact that the site into which they are grafted – the anterior surface of the anterior chamber – is immunologically privileged. Corneal tissue itself resists immune destruction. Perhaps the most dramatic evidence to support this statement comes from a recent series of experiments conducted by Hori and Streilein [46] in which corneal tissue fragments were placed beneath the capsule of the kidney – a site known by transplantation immunologists not to be immune privileged. Whereas allogeneic conjunctival and skin grafts placed beneath the kidney capsule were rejected quickly, corneal tissue survived indefinitely at this site. But cornea may not be the only ocular immune privileged tissue. Recent experiments by Wenkel and Streilein [submitted], similar in design to those conducted by Hori and Streilein, have revealed that allogeneic retinal pigment epithelial cells survive indefinitely when placed beneath the kidney capsule, and it may even prove to be true that neuronal retinal tissue has the property of 'immune privileged' status.

The findings which indicate that, on the one hand, the eye contains immunologically privileged sites, and, on the other hand, eye-derived tissues function as immune privileged tissues, reflect a more general property of the phenomenon of immune privilege. Numerous sites in the body have now been defined as immune privileged (table 2). Similarly, numerous tissues of the body have been found to resist immune rejection, and therefore qualify as immune privileged (also in table 2). Thus, when one considers 'immune privilege' in the eye, it must be remembered that both forces may be acting. For example, when cornea grafts are placed orthotopically in the eye, both the graft and the site have the inherent properties of immune privilege. Undoubtedly, this conspiracy accounts for the extraordinary success of keratoplasties in human beings.

Factors Known to Be Important in Immune Privilege

The original hypothesis, advanced by Medawar, to explain immune privilege emphasized anatomic features as key elements: the existence of a blood:tissue barrier, and the absence of afferent lymphatic drainage pathways. This emphasis led him directly to postulate that immune privilege resulted from

Table 3. Factors responsible for ocular immune privilege

Passive	Active
Blood:tissue barrier	Cell surface CD95 ligand, CD59, MCP, DAF, Class Ib
Deficient lymphatics	Immunosuppressive
Tissue fluids drain IV	Microenvironment:
Reduced expression of MHC class I and II molecules	TGF-β, α-MSH, VIP CGRP, MIF, IL-1ra
Reduced APC with altered function	Free cortisol

sequestration of antigenic material within the privileged site. However, studies over the past 30 years have revealed that immune privilege is dynamically created and maintained, although microanatomical features remain important. Even today, the list of relevant factors operating in immune privilege is incomplete. Nonetheless, the list of known factors is formidable (table 3). We now recognize both active and passive features of immune privileged sites and tissues that contribute to the privileged status. The absence of bone marrow-derived cells that function within tissues as APC, combined with the reduced expression of MHC-encoded transplantation antigens, renders immune privileged tissues decidedly less immunogenic than other tissues. In a sense, this reemphasizes the capacity of immune privileged tissues to survive because of 'immunologic ignorance'. However, immune privileged tissues also express cell surface molecules that selectively inactivate immune effectors – such as CD95L (which can delete CD95 + T cells that threaten a tissue's viability), and CD59, CD46, and other membrane-bound inhibitors of complement (which render complement-fixing antibodies ineffective). In addition, tissues such as the cornea have been found to secrete immunosuppressive factors that inhibit T-cell activation. The ability of ocular parenchymal cells to secrete immunosuppressive and anti-inflammatory factors, thereby creating a microenvironment inhospitable to immunogenic inflammation, makes a major contribution to the immune privilege observed in the anterior chamber, the vitreous cavity and the subretinal space.

Understanding the Mechanisms of Immune Privilege: Influence of Immune Privilege on the Immune Reflex Arc

The following section is designed to pick up the individual threads that represent the distinctive elements of immune privilege and weave them into the context of the immune reflex arc. The goal is to illuminate how the unique features of immune privilege act on the three phases of the immune response, shaping the final response to the benefit of the immune privileged site or tissue. Injection of antigen into the anterior chamber of the eye, similar to injection of antigen elsewhere in the body, leads to a systemic immune response. This statement alone directly refutes the Medawar hypothesis that immune privilege results from sequestration of antigen away from the immune system. However, the nature of the immune response evoked by intracamerally injected antigen differs substantially from immunity evoked by antigens injected elsewhere. This unusual systemic immune response has been termed 'anterior chamber-associated immune deviation' [47–50], and is described in detail in a subsequent paper in this volume.

Immune Privilege and the Afferent Limb

Although the cornea is devoid of bone marrow-derived cells, the iris, trabecular meshwork, and ciliary body contain a significant number of such cells – some are dendritic cells, and others resemble conventional macrophages. When antigen is injected into the anterior chamber, circumstantial evidence suggests that it is captured by indigenous APC. These cells then migrate across the trabecular meshwork into the blood, eventually reaching the spleen where the antigen is presented to specific T and B lymphocytes [20–22, 51, 52]. In a superficial sense, this process resembles that which follows the injection of antigen elsewhere in the body. Two features, however, are different. First, the antigen-bearing APC escape from the eye via the blood – not afferent lymphatics. Thus, lymph nodes are excluded from participation in the earliest phases of antigen recognition. This has a significantly negative impact on the ability of the antigen to elicit conventional cell-mediated immunity. Second, eye-derived APC display functional properties distinctly different from APC from other tissue sites. Taken directly from the eye, these cells fail to activate allogeneic T cells, and when pulsed with antigen and injected intravenously into naive mice, eye-derived APC induce ACAID, rather than conventional immunity [53–55].

Recent evidence has begun to unravel why intraocular APC function so distinctly, and so differently from APC that reside elsewhere. When APC are obtained from conventional sites, and exposed to the immunoregulatory factors in the ocular microenvironment, especially TGF-β_2, they display several unique features [22, 56, 57]. Compared to conventional APC, TGF-β_2-treated APC produce less IL-12, express CD40 poorly, and secrete increased amounts of mature TGF-β. As a consequence, when TGF-β_2-treated APC are pulsed with antigen and used to stimulate naive T cells, the responding T cells proliferate and secrete copious amounts of IL-4, trace amounts of IL-2, and no IFN-γ.

If these results based on in vitro studies reflect what happens after antigen is injected into the anterior chamber in vivo, then the antigen-specific signal that leaves the eye – and eventually generates the ACAID response – already contains immunomodulatory elements that will shape the response of T and B cells that the migrating, eye-derived APC first encounter in the spleen.

Immune Privilege and Central Processing

Injection of a heterologous protein antigen (such as ovalbumin) into the anterior chamber generates ACAID. And the spleen has been found to be the critical secondary lymphoid organ in which the blood-borne ACAID-inducing signal is transduced [51]. Spleen cells obtained from mice within 1 week after antigen injection in the anterior chamber fail to proliferate, or to secrete either Th1- or Th2-type cytokines when stimulated with antigen in vitro. Instead, a population of CD4+ T cells secretes TGF-β in response to in vitro stimulation with antigen [58]. If mice that receive an injection of antigen in the anterior chamber are immunized 1 week later with the same antigen incorporated into complete Freunds' adjuvant, many more antigen-specific T cells can be found 1 week later in both the spleen and in the lymph nodes draining the adjuvant injection site. Interestingly, the T cells from these sites secrete predominately Th2-type cytokines when stimulated in vitro with antigen. If the antigen injected in the anterior chamber is a minor histocompatibility antigen expressed on tumor cells, then one can find antigen-specific T cells in the spleen and lymph nodes, and the phenotype of these cells is of a precursor T-helper cell; when these cells are stimulated with allogeneic tumor cells in vitro, they produce only small amounts of IL-2, and no IFN-γ or IL-4 [59]. Thus, central processing of eye-derived antigen signals appears to activate an unusual population of T cells, primarily in the spleen. These cells are CD4+, and secrete IL-2 and/or TGF-β in response to antigen. If the same antigen is reintroduced with adjuvant, then the responding T cells display an intense bias toward Th2-type responses.

B-cell responses to intraocular antigen appear to form only if a second antigen exposure that includes adjuvant is administered. Under those circumstances, a unique spectrum of B cells is activated, primarily in the spleen; as these cells differentiate beyond the original IgM isotype, they switch toward the IgG1 isotype, and away from IgG2a, IgG2b, and IgG3 [60]. Cells of this type are consistent with a Th2-type response.

Recent evidence indicates that expression of CD95 and its ligand – which have already been implicated in the privileged existence of corneal allografts – also influence ACAID. Ferguson and coworkers [61, 62] have reported that mice deficient in CD95 ligand expression fail to acquire ACAID following injection of herpes simplex virus into the anterior chamber. Similarly, Gergorson and coworkers [63] have claimed that CD95-deficient allogeneic spleen cells are incapable of inducing allo-specific ACAID when injected into the anterior chamber of eyes of normal mice. In our laboratory, T. Kezuka [manuscript under review] has produced evidence which indicates that the ability of antigen-pulsed, TGF-β-treated APC to induce immune deviation when injected into naive mice requires (a) that the APC express CD95 ligand, and (b) that the recipient T cells be capable of expressing CD95. What remains unclear is the precise mechanism by which CD95/CD95 ligand interactions promote ACAID. While the simplest explanation involves the power of these interactions to delete CD95+ cells, the correct answer may be more complicated.

Immune Privilege and the Efferent Limb

Expression of systemic immunity within immune privileged sites, or when directed at immune privileged tissues, is distinctly unusual. Although the original experiments of Medawar led to the conclusion that immune expression in the anterior chamber was 'normal', a large body of recent evidence indicates that Medawar's conclusion was only partly correct. On the one hand, tumor cells injected into the anterior chamber of a mouse that had previously rejected that type of tumor fail to grow, whereas tumor cells injected into a normal mouse grow progressively. However, antigen (for example, bovine serum albumin) injected into the anterior chamber of a mouse presensitized to that antigen fails to elicit an inflammatory response, whereas an injection of the same antigen into the skin elicits an intense delayed hypersensitivity response [64]. Thus, there appear to be significant, but not complete, barriers to the expression of immunity within the eye. Much has been learned over the past decade about the factors that regulate expression of intraocular immunity, and this subject is described in detail in a subsequent paper.

If aqueous humor is taken as an example of the normal intraocular microenvironment, then the indigenous immunosuppressive properties of this site are revealed. Aqueous humor profoundly inhibits T-cell activation in vitro [9]. Moreover, aqueous humor suppresses the ability of NK cells to lyse their targets, and this ocular fluid contains soluble factors that prevent complement activation. The factors in aqueous humor that are responsible for these diverse effects are themselves diverse, and, at present, incompletely understood. Suffice to say that the ocular microenvironment – at least in normal eyes – has the capacity to suppress a wide spectrum of adaptive and innate immune effector mechanisms.

It should be emphasized that aqueous humor is not a global inhibitor of all innate and adaptive immune functions. Antibodies that neutralize viruses remain functional in the presence of aqueous humor, and cytotoxic T cells that have terminally differentiated are fully able to bind and kill their target cells in the presence of aqueous humor. It is the resistance of these effectors to local control that accounts for the extent to which immune protection acts within the eye, and it is doubtless this resistance that led Medawar to believe that immune expression in privileged sites is intact.

Rationale for Immune Privilege in the Eye

Neither the original discovery of immune privilege by Dooremal, nor the rediscovery and explanation of the meaning of immune privilege by Medawar, suggested why immune privilege exists! As the army of investigators studying immune privilege in the eye has grown over the past three decades, general agreement has been reached that the raison d'être for the existence of immune privilege is related to the vulnerability of the eye to inflammation. The function of the eye is to provide for accurate light images of the outside world to be placed precisely on the retina, and to transduce that signal in a form that can be transmitted electrically to the brain for interpretation. Both the visual apparatus that enables images to pass through the cornea to the retina, and the neuronal retinal mechanism that processes these images are highly sensitive to microanatomic and biochemical distortion. Extremely slight alterations of the visual apparatus can reduce a visual image on the retina to a blur, and very slight modifications of the microenvironment of the retina can disrupt the processing that creates the transduced image and sends it through the optic nerve to the brain. Inflammation within the eye is profoundly deleterious to both dimensions of eye function, and it is generally believed that immune privilege is the eye's strategy to avoid inflammation caused by innate and adaptive immune responses.

It is pertinent that immune privilege is not complete immunological ignorance, nor is it complete suppression of all aspects of immune responsiveness to ocular antigens. Instead, the systemic immune response to ocular antigens, and the local expression of immunity in the eye are molded in a such a manner that immune protection – against pathogens, tumors, etc. – is provided, with a minimum of attendant inflammation [65].

A compromise such as this has – as do all compromises – both positive and negative consequences. On the negative side, the existence of ocular immune privilege renders the eye vulnerable to the progressive growth of tumors that would otherwise be destroyed at nonimmune privileged sites. Similarly, immune privilege is probably responsible for the ability of viruses, such as HSV, to establish persistent infections that lead, through inflammation and neovascularization, to uveal tract and corneal scarring and blindness [66]. In addition, river blindness, in which filaria-specific immune responses are heavily biased toward the Th2 type, may be the direct consequence of the eye's tendency to convert immune protective Th1 responses into inflammation-inhibiting Th2 responses [67]. It is a naive conception that Th1 responses are proinflammatory, while Th2 responses are only anti-inflammatory. The corneal scarring which is characteristic of river blindness is clearly triggered by Th2-type cells. Thus, the eye's tendency to bias T-cell responses toward Th2-type effects can actually be deleterious to vision.

On the positive side, immune privilege undoubtedly contributes to the amazing success of orthotopic corneal allografts – by far the most successful of all solid organ transplants performed in human beings today. More subtly, experimental evidence implicates immune privilege in protecting the cornea from irreversible destruction during the course of herpes infections of the anterior segment of the eye [68]. Finally, immune privilege may contribute to the low incidence of autoimmune diseases that occur in the eye [69]. The eye contains a large number of proteins that are uniquely produced by genes within the eye, and these proteins have been found to be potent immunogens. The fact that most individuals, even those who suffer ocular trauma and infection, do not develop autoimmune eye disease may be related to the success of ocular immune privilege.

Acknowledgments

Supported by USPHS grant EY05678.

References

1 Janeway CA Jr, Travers P: Immunobiology: The Immune System in Health and Disease. New York, Garland Publishing, 1997.
2 Medzhitov R, Janeway CA Jr: Innate immunity: The virtues of a nonclonal system of recognition. Cell 1997;91:295–298.
3 Medzhitov R, Janeway CA Jr: Innate immunity: Impact on the adaptive immune response. Curr Opin Immunol 1997;9:4–9.
4 Korb LC, Ahearn JM: C1q binds directly and specifically to surface blebs of poptotic human keratinocytes. J Immunol 1997;158:4525–4528.
5 Ulevitch RJ, Tobias PS: Recognition of gram-negative bacteria and endotoxin by the innate immune system. Curr Opin Immunol 1999;11:19–22.
6 Stahl P, Ezekowitz RAB: The mannose receptor is a pattern recognition receptor involved in host defense. Curr Opin Immunol 1998;10:50–55.
7 Steinman RM: The dendritic cell system and its role in immunogenicity. Annu Rev Immunol 1991; 9:271–296.
8 Austyn JM, Larsen CP: Migration patterns of dendritic leukocytes. Implications for transplantation. Transplantation 1990;48:1–9.
9 Kaiser CJ, Ksander BR, Streilein JW: Inhibition of lymphocyte proliferation by aqueous humor. Reg Immunol 1989;2:42–49.

10   Granstein R, Stszewski R, Knisely T, Zeira E, Nazareno R, Latina M, Albert D: Aqueous humor
      contains transforming growth factor-β and a small (< 3,500 daltons) inhibitor of thymocyte prolifera-
      tion. J Immunol 1990;144:3021–3027.
11   Cousins SW, McCabe MM, Danielpour D, Streilein JW: Identification of transforming growth
      factor-beta as an immunosuppressive factor in aqueous humor. Invest Ophthal Vis Sci 1991;32:
      2201–2211.
12   Taylor AW, Streilein JW, Cousins SW: Identification of alpha-melanocyte-stimulating hormone as
      a potential immunosuppressive factor in aqueous humor. Curr Eye Res 1992;11:1199–1206.
13   Taylor AW, Streilein JW, Cousins SW: Vasoactive intestinal peptide contributes to the immuno-
      suppressive activity of normal aqueous humor. J Immunol 1994;153:1080–1086.
14   Apte RS, Niederkorn JY: Isolation and characterization of a unique natural killer cell inhibitory
      factor present in the anterior chamber of the eye. J Immunol 1996;156:2667–2673.
15   Apte RS, Niederkorn JY: MIF, a novel inhibitor of NK cell activity in the anterior chamber of the
      eye. J Allergy Clin Immunol 1997;99:S467.
16   Taylor AW, Yee DG, Streilein JW: Suppression of nitric oxide generated by inflammatory macro-
      phages by calcitonin gene-related peptide in aqueous humor. Invest Ophthal Vis Sci 1998;39:
      1372–1378.
17   Goslings WRO, Prodeus AP, Streilein JW, Carroll MC, Jager MJ, Taylor AW: A small molecular
      weight factor in aqueous humor acts on C1q to prevent antibody dependent complement activation.
      Invest Ophthalmol Vis Sci 1998;39:989–995.
18   Araneo BA, Dowel T, Moon HB, Dayes RA: Regulation of murine lymphokine production in vivo.
      Ultraviolet radiation exposure depresses IL-2 and enhances IL-4 productions by T cells through
      an IL-1 dependent mechanism. J Immunol 1989;143:1737–1745.
19   Mosmann TR, Coffman RL: Th1 and Th2 cells: Different patterns of lymphokine secretion lead
      to different functional properties. Annu Rev Immunol 1989;7:145–173.
20   Wilbanks GA, Streilein JW: Studies on the induction of anterior chamber associated immune
      deviation (ACAID). I. Evidence that an antigen-specific, ACAID-inducing, cell-associated signal
      exists in the peripheral blood. J Immunol 1991;146:2610–2617.
21   Wilbanks GA, Mammolenti MM, Streilein JW: Studies on the induction of anterior chamber
      associated immune deviation (ACAID). II. Eye-derived cells participate in generating blood-borne
      signals that induce ACAID. J Immunol 1991;146:3018–3024.
22   Wilbanks GA, Mammolenti MM, Streilein JW: Studies on the induction of anterior chamber
      associated immune deviation (ACAID). III. Induction of ACAID depends upon intraocular trans-
      forming growth factor-β. Eur J Immunol 1992;22:165–173.
23   Jenkins MK, Pardoll DM, Mizguchi J, Chused T, Schwartz R: Molecular events in the induction
      of a non-responsive state in interleukin-2 producing helper lymphocyte clones. Proc Natl Acad Sci
      USA 1987;84:5409–5412.
24   Nagata S, Golstein P: The Fas death factor. Science 1995;267:1449–1456.
25   Streilein JW: Regional immunology; in Dulbecco R (ed): Encyclopedia of Human Biology, ed 2.
      San Diego, Academic Press, 1997, vol 4, pp 767–776.
26   Streilein JW: Regional immunology of the eye; in Pepose JW, Holland GN, Wilhemus KR (eds):
      Ocular Infection and Immunity. Philadelphia, Mosby-Year Book, 1996, pp 19–33.
27   Parrott DM: The gut as a lymphoid organ. Clin Gastroenterol 1976;5:211.
28   Brandtzag P: Overview of the mucosal immune system. Curr Top Microbiol Immunol 1989;146:13–28.
29   Streilein JW: Skin-associated lymphoid tissues (SALT): The next generation; in Bos J (ed): The
      Skin Immune System (SIS). Boca Raton, CRC Press, 1993, pp 226–248.
30   Van Dooremall JC: Die Entwicklung der in fremden Grund versetzten lebenden Gewebe. Albrecht
      Van Graefes Arch Ophthalmol 1873;19:358–373.
31   Medawar P: Immunity to homologous grafted skin. III. The fate of skin homografts transplanted
      to the brain, to subcutaneous tissue and to the anterior chamber of the eye. Br J Exp Pathol 1948;
      29:58–69.
32   Barker CF, Billingham RE: Immunologically privileged sites. Adv Immunol 1977;25:1–54.
33   Niederkorn J, Streilein JW, Shadduck JA: Deviant immune responses to allogeneic tumors injected
      intracamerally and subcutaneously in mice. Invest Ophthalmol Vis Sci 1980;20:355–363.

34 Streilein JW: Immune regulation and the eye: A dangerous compromise. FASEB J 1987;1:199–208.
35 Niederkorn JY: Immune privilege and immune regulation in the eye. Adv Immunol 1990;48:191–226.
36 Ksander BR, Streilein JW: Regulation of the immune response within privileged sites; in Granstein R (ed): Mechansims of Regulation of Immunity Chemical Immunology. Basel, Karger, 1993, pp 117–145.
37 Tompsett E, Abi-Hanna D, Wakefield D: Immunological privilege in the eye: A review. Curr Eye Res 1990;9:1141–1150.
38 Streilein JW: Unraveling immune privilege. Science 1995;270:1158–1159.
39 Kaplan HJ, Stevens TR, Streilein JW: Transplantation immunology of the anterior chamber of the eye. J Immunol 1975;115:800–804.
40 Jiang LQ, Streilein JW: Immunologic privilege evoked by histoincompatible intracameral retinal transplants. Reg Immunol 1991;3:121–130.
41 Jiang LW, Jorquera M, Streilein JW: Immunologic consequences of intraocular implantation of retinal pigment epithelial allografts. Exp Eye Res 1994;58:719–728.
42 Niederkorn JY, Streilein JW: Immunogenetic basis for immunologic privilege in the anterior chamber of the eye. Immunogenetics 1981;13:227–236.
43 Jiang LQ, Streilein JW: Immune privilege extended to allogeneic tumor cells in the vitreous cavity. Invest Ophthal Vis Sci 1990;32:224–228.
44 Wenkel H, Streilein JW: Analysis of immune deviation elicited by antigens injected into the subretinal space. Invest Ophthal Vis Sci 1998;39:1823–1834.
45 Streilein JW: Immune privilege and the cornea; in Pleyes U, Hartmann C, Sterry W (eds): Proceedings of Symposium on Bullous Oculo-Muco-Cutaneous Disorders. Buren, Aeolus Press, 1997; pp 43–52.
46 Hori J, Streilein JW: Corneal tissues inherently possess immune privilege due in part to constitutive expression of Fas ligand. Invest Ophthal Vis Sci 1998;39:S455.
47 Kaplan HJ, Streilein JW: Immune response to immunization via the anterior chamber of the eye. 1. F_1 lymphocyte-induced immune deviation. J Immunol 1977;118:809–814.
48 Kaplan HJ, Streilein JW: Immune response to immunization via the anterior chamber of the eye. II. An analysis of F_1 lymphocyte induced immune deviation. J Immunol 1978;120:689–693.
49 Streilein JW, Niederkorn JY, Shadduck JA: Systemic immune unresponsiveness induced in adult mice by anterior chamber presentation of minor histocompatibility antigens. J Exp Med 1980;152:1121–1125.
50 Streilein JW, Ksander BR, Taylor AW: Commentary: Immune privilege, deviation and regulation in the eye. J Immunol 1997;158:3557–3560.
51 Kaplan HJ, Streilein JW: Do immunologically privileged sites require a functioning spleen? Nature 1974;251:553–554.
52 Hara Y, Caspi RR, Wiggert B, Dorf M, Streilein JW: Analysis of an in vitro generated signal that induced systemic immune deviation similar to that elicited by antigen injected into the anterior chamber of the eye. J Immunol 1992;149:1531–1538.
53 Williamson JSP, Bradley D, Streilein JW: Immunoregulatory properties of bone marrow derived cells in the iris and ciliary body. Immunology 1989;67:96–102.
54 Steptoe R, Holt PG, McMcnamin PG: Functional studies of major histocompatibility class II-positive dendritic cells and resident tissue macrophages isolated from the rat iris. Immunology 1995;85:630–637.
55 McMenamin PG, Forrester JV: Dendritic cells in the central nervous system and eye and their associated supporting tissues; in Lotze MY, Thomson AW (eds): Dendritic Cells: Biology and Clinical Applications. San Diego, Academic Press, 1999, pp 205–254.
56 Takeuchi M, Kosiewicz MM, Alard P, Streilein JW: On the mechanisms by which TGF-β_2 alters antigen presenting abilities of macrophages on T cell activation. Eur J Immunol 1997;27:1648–1656.
57 Takeuchi M, Alard P, Streilein JW: TGF-β promotes immune deviation by altering accessory signals of antigen presenting cells. J Immunol 1998;160:1589–1597.
58 Kosiewicz MM, Alard P, Streilein JW: Alterations in cytokine production following intraocular injection of soluble protein antigen: Impairment in IFN-γ and induction of TGF-β and IL-4 production. J Immunol 1998;161:5382–5390.

59 Bando Y, Ksander BR, Streilein JW: Characterization of specific T helper cell activity in mice bearing alloantigenic tumors in the anterior chamber of the eye. Eur J Immunol 1991;21:1923–1932.

60 Wilbanks GA, Streilein JW: Distinctive humoral responses following anterior chamber and intravenous administration of soluble antigen. Evidence for active suppression of IgG_{2a}-secreting B-cells. Immunology 1990;71:566–572.

61 Griffith TS, Brunner T, Fletcher SM, Green DR, Ferguson TA: Fas ligand-induced apoptosis as a mechanism of immune privilege. Science 1995;270:1189–1192.

62 Griffith TS, Yu X, Harndon JM, Green DR, Ferguson TA: CD95-induced apoptosis of lymphocytes in an immune privileged site induces immunological tolerance. Immunity 1996;5:7–16.

63 Kawashima H, Yamagami S, Tsuru T, Gregerson DS: Anterior chamber inoculation of splenocytes without Fas/Fas ligand interaction primes for a delayed-type hypersensitivity response rather than inducing anterior chamber-associated immune deviation. Eur J Immunol 1997;27:2490–2494.

64 Cousins SW, Trattler WB, Streilein JW: Immune privilege and suppression of immunogenic inflammation in the anterior chamber of the eye. Curr Eye Res 1991;10:287–297.

65 Streilein JW: Ocular immune privilege and the Faustian dilemma. Invest Ophthal Vis Sci 1996;37:1940–1950.

66 Streilein JW, Dana MR, Ksander BR: Immunity causing blindness: Five different paths to herpes stromal keratitis. Immunol Today 1997;18:443–449.

67 Pearlman E, Lass HJ, Bardenstein DS, Kopf M, Hazlett FE Jr, Diaconu E, Kazura JW: Interleukin-4 and T-helper type 2 cells are required for development of experimental onchocercal keratitis (river blindness). J Exp Med 1995;182:931–940.

68 McLeish W, Rubsamen P, Atherton SS, Streilein JW: Immunobiology of Langerhan's cells on the ocular surface. II. Role of central corneal Langerhans' cells in stromal keratitis following experimental HSV-1 infection in mice. Reg Immunol 1989;2:236–243.

69 Gery I, Streilein JW: Autoimmunity in the eye and its regulation. Curr Opin Immunol 1994;6:938–945.

J. Wayne Streilein, MD, Schepens Eye Research Institute, Harvard Medical School,
20 Staniford Street, Boston, MA 02114-2500 (USA)
Tel. +1 617 912 7422, Fax +1 617 912 0115, E-Mail waynes@vision.eri.harvard.edu

Streilein JW (ed): Immune Response and the Eye.
Chem Immunol. Basel, Karger, 1999, vol 73, pp 39–58

....

Molecular and Cellular Aspects of Allergic Conjunctivitis

Grace Liu, Andrea Keane-Myers, Dai Miyazaki, Albert Tai, Santa J. Ono

Laboratory of Molecular Immunology, Schepens Eye Research Institute &
Committee on Immunology, Harvard Medical School, Boston, Mass., USA

Introduction

One of the most common immunologically mediated diseases of the eye is allergic conjunctivitis (AC). Over 14% of the population of the USA suffers from some form of this disease [1] typified by red, itchy, watery eyes and which can have results ranging in severity from discomfort to potential blindness. Seasonal allergic conjunctivitis, the mild and nonthreatening form of the disease, is a recurrent disorder caused by allergic sensitity to a variety of airborne allergens, such as pollen, mold, mites, and animal dander. The acute phase of the disease is characterized by itching, erythema, and edema of the conjunctiva. Seasonal allergic conjunctivitis is usually associated with allergic rhinitis (hay fever) and is typically seasonal. Perennial allergens, such as mold and animal dander, however, can cause signs and symptoms to occur perenially as well.

In contrast to seasonal allergic conjunctivitis, atopic keratoconjunctivitis (AKC) and vernal keratoconjunctivitis (VKC) display more severe and chronic symptoms and can involve the cornea (fig. 1). The ocular counterpart of atopic dermatitis, AKC produces tearing, itching, and photophobia associated with eczema. The conjunctiva is usually erythematous due to capillary congestion and a diffuse papillary hypertrophy may be visible on the lower palpebral conjunctival surface [2] (fig. 2). Corneal and conjunctival scarring may be observed when the disease is prolonged, and may be accompanied by cataracts or keratoconus.

VKC is a disease that develops primarily in young males during childhood but rarely lasts beyond 30 years, tending to resolve spontaneously after several years. It occurs more often in warm climates and is generally worse during

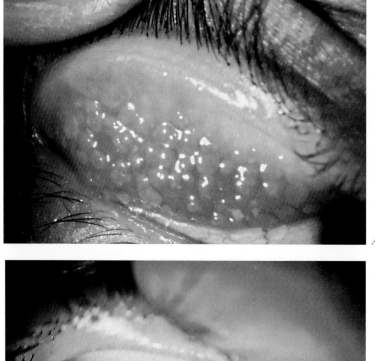

A

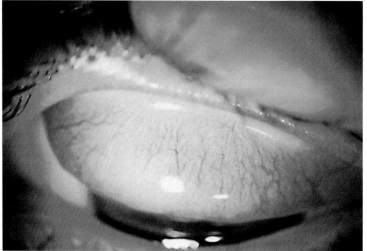

B

Fig. 1. A Upper tarsal conjunctiva in a VKC patient showing marked cobblestone formation. *B* Upper tarsal conjunctiva of a normal patient.

spring and summer. Patients experience severe tearing, itching, and photophobia and have a stringy mucous discharge from the eyes. Cobblestone-like giant papillae develop on the upper palpebral conjunctiva due to hypertrophy of the connective tissue [2]. In both AKC and VKC, Trantas' dot may be observed in the marginal cornea. In severe cases, corneal ulcers may develop in the central cornea, causing scarring and visual loss.

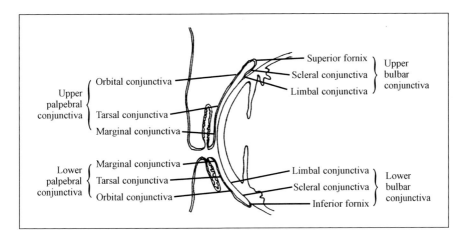

Fig. 2. Anatomy of the conjunctiva.

Table 1. Elevation of tissue-specific and general atopy within the Schepens ocular allergy study

Probands, n	117
First-degree relatives, n	559
Atopic family members, %	64
Family members with ocular allergy, %	47
Family members with other allergies, %	20
Nonatopic family members, %	36
Atopy within general US population, %	25
General US population with ocular allergy, %	14.8

These allergic eye diseases can and have been used as models to study the genetics of allergic diseases and their treatments. As can be seen in table 1, we have determined that in addition to general atopy genes, there are genes which 'target' the allergic response to the conjunctiva. This can be seen in the profound elevation of the incidence of AC in family members of probands we are studying. Elevated serum immunuglobulin E (IgE) levels, a hallmark of all allergic diseases [3], exhibit strong familial patterns of inheritance [4], a fact that has spurred intense efforts to identify potential atopy genes. The approach in our laboratory has been to characterize regulatory pathways that influence the immune response to allergens with the rationale that these are likely to involve atopy genes. Our research has focused on two multigene families associated with the allergic response: the class II major histocompatibility complex (MHC) genes and the interleukin (IL)-4 cluster of cytokine genes [5, 6]. Since serum IgE levels are associated with particular alleles of the IL-4 locus [7, 8], we study the activation of the human IL-4 gene and the related transcription factors as mechanisms which may contribute to the overexpression of the IL-4 gene in atopic individuals. These efforts to identify atopy genes will also identify possible targets for the design of new anti-inflammatory drugs and treatments [9].

Animal Models

Many researchers have attempted to develop an animal model to further study the pathophysiology of AC and to test the effectiveness of new antiallergic drugs. Models of actively induced AC have used allergens such as keyhole limpet hemocyanin (KHL) [10], ovalbumin (OVA) [11], or DNP conjugated to a hapten [12]. Additional animal models used either the physical act of eye-rubbing [13], or dithiothreitol (DTT) [11], a mucolytic agent, to disrupt the conjunctival barrier prior to antigen challenge.

In a model of topically induced ocular anaphylaxis in rats, investigators immunized rats with intraperitoneal injections of egg albumin and alum and topically challenged with egg albumin after pretreating the eyes with DTT. It was found that treatment without DTT led to no disease formation, and repeated challenges did not increase edema or mast cell degranulation from those challenged by one egg albumin application [11]. However, another rat model using DNP hapten was able to induce an allergic response without pretreatment with DTT. Daily repeated topical applications of antigen in this model, intended to mimic the situation faced by the human conjunctiva during the pollen season, revealed that response was higher with one challenge than with multiple challenges, and thus could be attenuated [12].

Some adjuvants, which are usually used for effective induction of immune responses, tend to induce cellular immunity, while others enhance humoral responses [14–16]. Results indicated that adjuvants were necessary to induce disease as well as cellular and humoral immunity. Alum and complete Freund's adjuvant, which promote higher T-helper type 1 (Th1) cell infiltration, induced stronger disease and cellular immunity than incomplete Freund's adjuvant, which tends to promote higher T-helper type 2 (Th2) cell induction [17].

Compound 48/80, a nonimmunologic mast cell degranulator, has been used as an alternative treatment in antigen-antibody-dependent systems for eliciting anaphylaxis. It has been found that a threshold dose is necessary to induce degranulation. However, once maximal degranulation is achieved, higher levels of compound 48/80 will not increase the level or change the type of degranulation [18]. Similar to the DNP hapten model, a study of multiple versus single applications of compound 48/80 showed that clinical response was the most marked after one application of compound 48/80, and repeated daily applications reduced that response [19]. An interval of 7 days between challenges was found to be sufficient to cause a clinical response similar to that observed on the first dose. It was unclear whether this was due to the continued presence of 48/80 in the mast cell, or if the mast cells themselves were affected [20].

One experimental model of ocular allergy developed in the guinea pig used topical exposure of ragweed to nasal and conjunctival mucosae, followed by subsequent challenge with ragweed on the conjunctiva [21]. Ocular anaphylaxis has been reported in guinea pigs after passive transfer of serum containing two types of homocytotropic antibodies, IgG1 and IgE [22]. Allansmith and coworkers [23] established the necessity for these IgE and IgG antibodies in the allergic response by developing a guinea pig model in which immediate hypersensitivity reactions were passively induced in response to systemic sensitization with normal rabbit serum containing IgE and IgG homocytotropic antibodies.

The development of a mouse model of AC has been especially useful due to the extensive array of reagents available for study and manipulation of their immune parameters. In one model, female SWR/J mice were immunized each day for 5 days and then on the 8th day challenged topically on the nasal and conjunctival mucosae using ragweed pollen powder without adjuvant [24]. Ragweed pollen is the most common airborne allergen responsible for causing AC, but requires that the investigator wear gloves, a dust mask, and goggles for protection [24]. A more recent model reduces contact between the researcher and the highly allergenic ragweed. Female SWR/J mice were sensitized by injection of ragweed pollen and aluminum hydroxide (alum) into the footpad, and challenged by a single topical application of 1.5 mg whole ragweed suspended in 10 μl PBS to the eye 10 days after sensitization. Disease in this model was characterized by itching, chemosis, and other clinical symptoms, as well as cellular infiltration of neutrophils, macrophages, and eosinophils following mast cell degranulation. Lymphocytes taken from popliteal lymph nodes of immunized animals showed marked [^{3}H]thymidine incorporation in the presence of ragweed extract. Cytokine analysis of lymphocyte cultures derived from the popliteal lymph nodes exhibited an allergic-specific increase in the Th2-associated cytokines IL-4 and IL-5. It also reported, however, subtle amounts of IL-2 in supernatants of cultures stimulated nonspecifically with the super-antigen ConA, a result attributed to possible self-consumption of IL-2 by the proliferating cells [25].

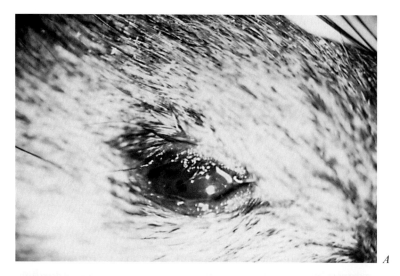

A

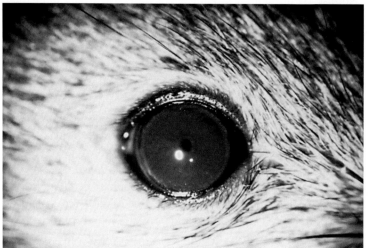

B

Fig. 3. A Murine model of AC. Mice of strain 129/SvEv were immunized with alum and Fel d1, the major antigen in cat hair. Marked tear secretion and swelling of eyelids is apparent 20 min after challenge with Fel d1. *B* FBS-immunized control mice after challenge with Fed d1.

Another murine model that we have developed in our laboratory utilizes cat dander containing known quantities of Fel d1 to sensitize A/J mice systemically in the presence of alum (fig. 3). Challenge was performed through topical application of 6.5 µg cat dander in 5 µl PBS on the conjunctival mucosae 1 and 3 weeks after sensitization. Fel d1, a 35-kDa protein, is the major allergen produced by cats and is the most common allergen worldwide. It has an unusual stability conferred by its heterodimer antiparallel configuration, which allows it to remain present and active long after cat removal and cleaning. Treated mice showed photosensitivity, itching, conjunctival swelling and redness. Histology of conjunctival cross-sections revealed mast cell degranulation 1 h postchallenge, followed by significant infiltration of eosinophils that peaked 24 h after antigen challenge. T lymphocytes from spleens and cervical draining lymph nodes displayed allergen-specific proliferation and a Th2-type cytokine profile, characterized by levels of IL-4, IL-5, IL-10, and interferon-γ (IFN-γ). Serum levels of the Th2-dependent antibodies IgE and Fel d1-specific IgG1 were increased at both 1 and 24 h after antigen challenge [26].

Clinical Studies

Early clinical models of acute AC involved histamine [27], compound 48/80 [28], or arachidonic acid [29] administered topically to the eye, and were employed to study allergic ocular disease, but did not have the clinical validity of antigen-induced mast cell degranulation. Abelson's group modified the conjunctival provocation test of Moller et al. [30] for the evaluation of local allergic response in a study design that minimized the potential variables of the allergen challenge model [31]. It was based on ocular allergen challenge of skin-test-positive subjects. This method of allergen challenge and drug testing was reported to be effective, safe and reproducible [32].

The potential for ocular allergic patients to have a site-specific antigen sensitization was investigated using various diagnostic tests of allergen sensitivity in patients with AC. Leonardi et al. [35] found that the conjunctiva could be uniquely sensitized in allergic patients. Because of the poor correlation between systemic and local ocular sensitivity, local tests, such as conjunctival scraping, allergen challenge, and measurement of tear-specific IgE, may be useful in the diagnosis of AC in patients with equivocal signs and symptoms. Because eosinophils ordinarily are not found in the conjunctiva of nonallergic individuals, the presence of a single eosinophil or eosinophil granule in a conjunctival scraping is compelling evidence of allergic conjunctivitis [21].

Mechanism of the Allergic Reaction

Response to allergens in AC is an immediate, or type I, hypersensitivity reaction. Following dissolution and movement of airborne allergens such as pollen and animal dander through the tear film to the conjunctiva, the allergens are processed by antigen presenting cells (APC) and presented to T-helper cells in conjunction with class II MHC. Th2 in turn produce mediators such as IL-4 and IL-13, which favor IgE synthesis by B cells [34–36]. Another Th2-associated cytokine, IL-5, promotes B-cell growth and differentiation, as well as eosinophil infiltration. IgE binds to specialized receptors on conjunctival mast cells and activates them; this results in intracellular calcium mobilization and mast cell degranulation and release of preformed mediators such as histamine and kinins, while cell membrane phospholipids synthesize arachidonic acid metabolites such as prostaglandins and leukotrienes. This complex inflammatory cascade continues and results in vasodilation, increased conjunctival vascular permeability, inflammatory cell infiltration, itching, chemosis and edema [37] (fig. 4).

The differential expression of cell adhesion molecules (CAMs) under various inflammatory conditions is thought to be responsible for the preferential adhesion and infiltration of different populations of cells, such as lymphocyte homing [38] or the selective deployment of memory T cells and effector leukocytes in inflammation [39]. A study to evaluate the conjunctival expression of leukocyte CAMs in the different clinical subtypes of allergic eye disease found that expression of intercellular adhesion molecule-1 (ICAM-1), E-selectin, and vascular cell adhesion molecule (VCAM-1) were increased to varying degrees in different allergic eye diseases. Positive correlations were found between the levels of ICAM-1 and E-selectin expression and the degree of granulocyte and lymphocyte infiltration, although VCAM-1 expression correlated most closely with eosinophil numbers [40]. Increased levels of CAMs and their regulating factors, such as mast cells mediators [41], are potentially responsible for the infiltration of cells bearing their ligands and may play a role in perpetuating the allergic inflammation.

Timecourse of Response

During the development of allergy, two phases, the early phase reaction (EPR) and the late phase reaction (LPR) are observable. EPR is marked by erythema and edema that develop minutes after exposure to antigen [42] and is due to upregulation of vascular permeability caused by the degranulation of mast cells and the release of histamines [11, 26, 43], and other preformed or rapidly synthesized molecules. The EPR has been studied extensively in allergic responses in the skin [44, 45], lung [46, 47] and nasal mucosae [48].

The LPR is induced by cytokine-related cellular infiltration [19, 49]. It develops 3–12 h after the initial response and can last up to 24 h. The LPR is characteristic of a number of atopic diseases and heterogeneous patterns of

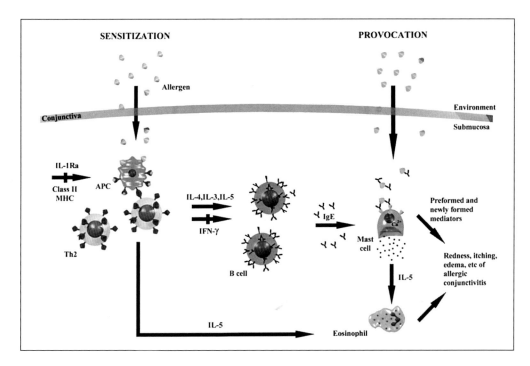

Fig. 4. Allergens penetrate the conjunctiva mucosal surface, and are taken up by local APC for processing and presentation to T-helper cells. The IL-1 receptor antagonist, a potential treatment against AC being investigated by our laboratory, downregulates APC function, and thus may prevent T-helper cell activation and the subsequent allergic response. Th2 cells release mediators such as IL-4, which promoted B-cell proliferation and differentiation to produce allergen-specific IgE. In provocation, allergen cross-links surface-bound IgE of sensitized mast cells, causing mobilization of intracellular calcium and degranulation of the mast cells to release preformed and newly formed mediators such as histamine, kinins, prostaglandin D_2, and TAME-esterase activity. IL-5 produced by Th2 cells and mast cells promotes eosinophil growth and differentiation. Eosinophil infiltration and the inflammatory mediators released by the degranulated mast cells produce the clinical effects of AC.

clinical LPRs have been described for systemic anaphylaxis, cutaneous, nasal, and asthmatic reactions [50]. It is marked by an infiltration of inflammatory cells including eosinophils, neutrophils and lymphocytes [21, 51, 52] most likely due to an upregulation of chemokines such as RANTES and eotaxin, both of which are highly selective for eosinophils. Table 2 summarizes the major features of the early and late phase responses.

Using a cellular LPR described in a rat model of topically induced ocular anaphylaxis, investigators found that, similar to the analogous reaction in human skin, a strong early response to antigen is required for the development

Table 2. Early vs. late phase allergic responses

Early phase response
Immediate hypersensitivity
Antigen-specific IgE cross-linked on mast cells
Degranulation and release of mediators
  (histamine, prostaglandins, and leukotrienes)

Late phase response
8–12 h after antigen challenge
Leukocyte infiltration (eosinophils and basophils)
Release of proinflammatory mediators

---

of a late phase ocular response to the rat [53]. Further evidence of an ocular LPR was provided in the clinical observation of periorbital swelling 6–7 h after the EPR [23], and in the observation of increased levels of degranulated mast cells, neutrophils, eosinophils, basophils, lymphocytes and macrophages in the conjunctival substantia propria of guinea pigs undergoing ocular anaphylaxis [50]. This high percentage of degranulated mast cells and mixed infiltrate present from 3 to 24 h after the initial reaction are likely to sustain the observed clinical LPR. Both of these studies also found that whereas guinea pigs manifested clinical LPR with biphasic, multiphasic, and prolonged patterns, anaphylactic stimulation of rat ocular tissues produced an LPR at the histologic level but did not show clinical changes [23, 50].

T-Cell Involvement

CD4+ T-helper cells have been found to influence outcome in a variety of diseases, including the allergic response. These cells can be divided into two subpopulations, Th1 and Th2, depending on the cytokine profile expressed by the cells. Th1 cells produce IL-2 and IFN-γ, and are responsible for both humoral and cell-mediated immune responses including macrophage activation and delayed-type hypersensitivity [54, 55]. Conversely, Th2 cells produce IL-4, IL-5, IL-6, IL-10, and IL-13, and are essential for B-cell class switching to the IgG1 and IgE isotypes, and for eosinophil recruitment and proliferation [56]. It is these later responses of the Th2 cells that are especially important in the development of the allergic phenotype. Table 3 describes the important cytokines related to allergic eye disease.

Carreras et al. [57] reported that conjunctival infiltration of activated T cells, which are specific to antigen, plays an important role in the pathogenesis

---

Table 3. Functions of major T-cell cytokines [adapted from 85]

Cytokine	Source	Effects on:			
		B cells	T cells	Macrophages	Hematopoetic cells
(IL-1)	Ubiquitous	Activation	Activation	Activation	Activates natural killer cells
(IL-2)	Th0, Th1, some cytotoxic lymphocytes	Stimulates growth and J-chain synthesis	Growth	–	Stimulates natural killer cell growth
(IL-4)	Th2	Activation, growth, increases MHC class II induction	Growth, survival	Inhibits macrophage activation	Increases mast cell growth
(IL-5)	Th2	Differentiation, IgA synthesis	–	–	Increases eosinophil growth and differentiation
(IL-6)	Ubiquitous; mostly macrophages, fibroblasts	Growth, differentiation	Growth	–	General growth factor
(IL-10)	Th2	Increases MHC class II	Inhibits Th1, growth factor activity	Inhibits cytokine release	Costimulates mast cell growth (with IL-4 and IL-3)
(IL-13)	Th2	Proliferation, differentiation, increases MHC class II	–	–	–
(IFN-γ)	Th1, cytotoxic T lymphocytes	Differentiation, IgG2a synthesis	Kills	Activates, increases MHC class I and class II	Activates natural killer cells

of AC. In a study of the induction of experimental blepharoconjunctivitis (EAC) in rats, investigators transferred T cells from immunized rats into naive syngeneic recipients and found that EAC is transferable by immune cells. Therefore, cellular immunity is actively involved in the effector phase of development of this disease. In contrast, cellular infiltration could not be induced by adoptive transfer of immune serum, similar to the finding by Sorkness et al. [cf. 17], that adoptive transfer of a monoclonal IgE antibody could not induce LPR in an allergic asthma model.

An investigation of the prevalence of T-cells and expression of T-cell surface antigens in different allergic eye conditions found increased numbers of CD4 +, CD45R0 +, and HLA-DR + T cells in the conjunctiva of AC patients and a corresponding upregulation of markers present on APC [58]. This agrees with an earlier study, in which T-cell clones obtained from conjunctival infiltrates of patients with VC displayed the CD4 + CD8 – phenotype [59].

T-Cell-Derived Mediators and Cytokines

The pathophysiology of chronic allergic eye disease cannot be explained by type I hypersensitivity alone, and T-cell-mediated inflammation has been strongly implicated as a possible additional mechanism. Romagnani and co-workers [54] showed that T-cell clones derived from the conjunctiva of patients with allergic eye disease demonstrated increased production of IL-4 and decreased production of IFN-γ compared with normal subjects, whereas the production of IL-2 was unchanged. These T cells were better able to provide help for B cell-IgE synthesis than peripheral blood T cells from the same patients [59]. Similar data of cytokine production indicating a Th2-like response was obtained in studies using other models of AC [36, 60]. Higher levels of IL-4 and IgE have been detected in AC patients [34, 35].

Further studies examining the cytokine profile of T cells found that allergic tissue of AC patients express increased levels of mRNA for the Th2-associated cytokines IL-3, IL-4 and IL-5 when compared with normal tissue [61]. The biologic actions of the Th2-related cytokines – the promotion of IgE production and the increased survival, activation, and recruitment of eosinophils and mast cells – reinforces that they are likely to play a role in allergic inflammation. Results also showed a Th2-like T-cell cytokine array in subjects with VKC and giant papillary conjunctivitis (GPC), but a shift in cytokine profile toward a Th1-like pattern in AKC, potentially because of differences in chronicity of the disorders. Whether the variations in T-cell function can be directly related to clinical characteristics, such as the greater conjunctival cicatrization or the insidious nature of the corneal disease in AKC compared with other chronic allergic eye diseases, remains to be seen [61].

Levels of serum eosinophil cationic protein (ECP) were increased in patients with allergic disease [62]. ECP is a cytotoxic preformed mediator stored in eosinophil granules and released under various conditions to interact with blood coagulation and fibrinolytic factors activating tissue fibroblasts. The level of ECP serum is affected only by the type of sensitization, such that persistent natural exposure to a sensitizing allergen is responsible for a measurable increase in serum ECP levels in patients with allergy. A test for ECP is a possible complement for current IgE tests for allergy [62].

In VC patients, plasma levels of nerve growth factor (NGF) were reported to be elevated and correlated to the number of conjunctival mast cells. NGF displayed an inverse correlation to the number of circulating eosinophils and to increased serum levels of eosinophil cationic protein [63]. NGF is a member of the neurotrophin family and is essential for survival, differentiation, and function of peripheral sympathetic and sensory neurons and basal forebrain cholinergic neurons in the central nervous system. NGF also promotes mast cell proliferation and release of soluble biological mediators, enhances survival, phagocytosis, and superoxide production of neutrophils, causes mediator release from basophils, suppresses leukotriene C4 formation from eosinophils, stimulates T- and B-lymphocyte proliferation, and stimulates B-cell differentiation into immunoglobulin-secreting plasma cells. A similar increase in NGF serum levels was detected in a later study which established that with more than one allergic disease (asthma and/or rhinoconjunctivitis and/or urticaria-angioedema) had higher NGF serum values than those with a single disease [64].

Chemokines are considered to contribute to the development of immunopathogenesis of AC. RANTES ('regulated on activation, normal T-cell expressed and secreted'), which attracts eosinophils, CD45R0, and memory T lymphocytes, are produced by cultured human conjunctival epithelial cells in response to inflammatory stimuli such as tumor necrosis factor-α (TNF-α), the production of which is increased by IFN-γ [65]. In the murine model of AC that we have developed, upregulation of eotaxin, MIP-1α, and IP-10 have been observed [unpubl. observ.].

Mast Cells and Mast Cell Mediators

The number of mast cells in the ocular and adnexal tissues of one human eye has been estimated at 50 million [66]. Mast cells in the normal human conjunctival epithelium, cornea, iris, and optic nerve are scarce [67] and have a connective tissue phenotype containing the mast cell protease tryptase [68, 69]. The substantia propria contains larger numbers of mast cells [67] which are primarily mucosal mast cells containing tryptase, chymase, cathepsin G, and human mast cell carboxypeptidase [68, 69]. Patients with AC display a mildly increased number of mast cells in the substantia propria [67], and demonstrate a more significant increase in the number of epithelial conjunctival mast cells [70, 71].

In the inflammatory cascade, mast cells are activated by cross-linking of antigen to the surface-bound IgE and respond by degranulating to release histamines and other proinflammatory mediators (fig. 5). Mast cell activation in AC is evidenced by an increase in tryptase levels in unstimulated tear fluid [72]. Clinical response to conjunctival provocation with allergen is associated with increases in the levels of the inflammatory mediators (e.g. histamines, kinins, prostaglandin D$_2$, albumin and TAME-esterase activity) in tears [73]. The cytokines IL-4, IL-5, IL-6 and TNF-α have been localized to mast cells in normal and allergic conjunctiva, suggesting that conjunctival mast cells can

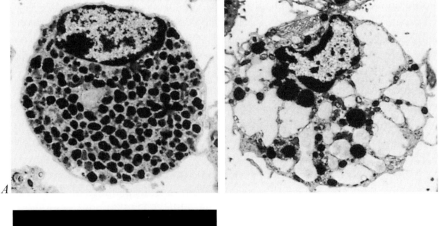

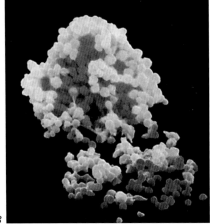

Fig. 5. A Electron micrograph of a mast cell before (left) and after cross-linking of allergen to surface-bound IgE. The mast cell responds by releasing its contents, including histamines, prostaglandins, leukotrienes and other inflammatory mediators. *B* A colored scanning electron micrograph of a degranulating mast cell. Granules are shown in grey.

store a range of multifunctional cytokines for release during active disease [74].

Histamine is a short-lived, vasoactive amine which causes an immediate increase in local blood flow and permeability, as well as mast cell chymase, tryptase, and serine esterase. Histamine also stimulates phosphoinositide (PI) turnover in human conjunctival epithelial (HCE) cells, driving inositol phosphate generation and rapidly mobilizing intracellular calcium [37]. These effects were antagonized potently by H1-antagonists but weakly by H2- and H3-antagonists. Inflammatory cytokine secretion from HCE cells after stimulation by histamine may be linked with intracellular signaling mechanisms and topically active H1-antagonists or antiallergic agents (e.g. levocabastine, emedastine, olopatadine) may be helpful for treating ocular allergic and inflammatory diseases [37].

Treatment of Allergic Conjunctivitis

The most successful treatment is to avoid contact with the specific allergens. To reduce ocular signs and symptoms, topical administration of mast cell stabilizers or nonsteroidal anti-inflammatory drugs (NSAID) [75] is usually employed. In severe cases, topical corticosteroids may be necessary. Despite their adverse side effects, oral administration of corticosteroids is helpful.

Cyclosporine A, a powerful immunosuppressant which inhibits the production of IL-2 by CD4+ T cells and the production and release of other cytokines, was also reported to inhibit mast-cell-mediated conjunctivitis in a mouse model [76]. The topical administration of cyclosporine A, which does not cause undesirable delivery into the eyeball because of its poor penetration, is successfully used as adjunct therapy in refractory cases [77]. Its systemic administration may be used as an alternative therapy [78].

IL-1 receptor antagonist (IL-1ra), a naturally occurring IL-1 isoform with no agonist activity, was suggested to have a profound downregulatory effect on the acute phase cytokine cascade [79]. Endogenous IL-1ra is produced in numerous experimental animal models of disease, as well as in human autoimmune and chronic inflammatory diseases. It is an important natural anti-inflammatory protein in arthritis, colitis, and granulomatous pulmonary disease [80]. Preclinical research by the laboratory of Dana [81] has shown the profound capacity of IL-1ra to suppress corneal transplant rejection, corneal and ocular surface inflammation [82], expression of adhesion molecules and recruitment of inflammatory cells [83], and APC function [83]. Treatment with IL-1ra is expected to downmodulate IL-1 activity and downregulate APC function, thereby preventing T-helper cell activation and the subsequent allergic response.

In recently completed studies using our mouse model, we found that treatment with IL-1ra significantly reduced the clinical symptoms observed in IL-1ra-treated and allergen-challenged animals. In addition, RNAse protection assays revealed a significant reduction in allergen-induced chemokine production in both the cervical draining lymph nodes and in the matrix surrounding the conjunctiva. In particular, there was a significant reduction in the chemokines RANTES, MIP-1α, and eotaxin, causing significant reduction in eosinophil infiltration and other allergen-induced infiltration [84]. These studies suggest that IL-1ra administration may feature in future immunotherapy to combat AC.

Concluding Remarks

The human cost of eye allergies can be assessed directly in terms of mediation needs, sleep loss, and impaired work and learning ability. The frequency of allergic forms of conjunctivitis and the hazards associated with topical steriods have led to the need for alternatives in new anti-allergic and anti-inflammatory compounds that can be safely used in the eye. Further research into the biological patterns of allergic early and late phase responses and their pharmocologic modulation may facilitate the identification of new therapeutic agents.

In addition, efforts to identify the factors and their genes involved in conjunctival allergy may help in selecting between multiple potential atopy genes identified thus far. This will in turn advance our understanding of the molecular basis of the allergic response and the strong familial component of atopic diseases. The application of this new information to the clinical setting would benefit not only those individuals suffering from AC, but also the approximately 30% of all individuals who develop allergic reactions to inocuous materials.

References

1   King T: Chemical and biological properties of some atopic allergens. Adv Immunol 1976;23:77–105.
2   Friedlaender MH: Immunologic aspects of diseases of the eye. JAMA 1992;268:2869–2873.
3   Marsh D, Bias W, Ishizaka K: Genetic control of basal serum IgE level and its effect on specific reagenic sensitivity. Proc Natl Acad Sci USA 1974;71:3588–3592.
4   Gerrard J, Rao D, Morton N: A genetic study of immunoglobulin E. Am J Hum Genet 1978;20:46–58.
5   Ono SJ: Transcriptional regulation of the genes of the human major histocompatibility complex; in Chicz, R, Urban R (eds): The Major Histocompatibility Complex. Austin, Landes, 1995.
6   Marsh D, Neely J, Breazeale D, Ghosh B, Friedhoff L, Errlich-Kautzky E, Schou C, Krishnaswamy G, Beaty T: Linkage analysis of IL-4 and other chromosome 5q31.1 markers and total serum immunoglobulin E concentrations. Science 1994;264:1152–1156.
7   Meyers D, Postma D, Panhuysen C, Amelung P, Levitt R, Bleecker E: Evidence for a locus regulating total serum IgE levels mapping of chromosome 5. Genomics 1994;26:464–470.
8   Casolaro V, Georas S, Ono SJ: Regulation of interleukin-4 synthesis. Int J Immunopathol Pharm 1997;10:1–5.
9   Ono SJ: Molecular genetics of IgE-mediated inflammation. J Allergy (in press).
10 Hahn L, Cornell-Bell A, Martin-Ellis C, Allansmith M: Conjunctival basophil hypersensitivity lesions in guinea pigs. Invest Ophthalmol Vis Sci 1986;27:1255–1260.
11 Trocme S, Trocme M, Bloch K, Allansmith M: Topically induced ocular anaphylaxis in rats immunized with egg albumin. Ophthalmic Res 1986;18:68–74.
12 Barney N, Kleinman R, Trocme S, Bloch K, Allansmith M: Attenuation of rat conjunctival response by repeated hapten applications. Curr Eye Res 1988;7:843–848.
13 Greiner J, Peace D, Baird R, Allansmith M: Effects of eye rubbing on the conjunctiva as a model of ocular inflammation. Am J Ophthalmol 1985;100:45–50.

14   Germann T, Szeliga J, Hess H, Storkel S, Podlaski F, Gately M, Schmitt E, Rude E: Administration of interleukin-12 in combination with type II collagen induces severe arthritis in DBA/1 mice. Proc Natl Acad Sci USA 1995;92:4823–4827.

15   Trinchieri G: Interleukin-12: A proinflammatory cytokine with immunoregulatory functions that bridge innate resistance and antigen-specific adaptive immunity. Annu Rev Immunol 1995;13:251–276.

16   Mauri C, Williams RO, Walmsley M, Feldmann M: Relationship between Th1/Th2 cytokine patterns and the arthritogenic response in collagen-induced arthritis. Eur J Immunol 1996;26:1511–1518.

17   Fukushima H, Yoshida H, Iwamoto O, Yoshida O, Ueno H: The role of cellular immunity both in the induction and effector phases of experimental allergic blepharoconjunctivis in rats. Exp Eye Res 1997;65:631–637.

18   Allansmith M, Baird R, Barney N, Ross R, Bloch K: Determination of the interval during which one application of compound 48/80 to the rat conjunctiva influences the response to a second application. Ophthalmic Res 1990;22:137–143.

19   Abelson M, Allansmith M, Friedlander M: Effects of topically applied ocular decongestants and antihistamines. Am J Ophthalmol 1980;90:254–257.

20   Udell I, Abelson M: Animal and human ocular surface response to a topical nonimmune mast cell degranulating agent (compound 48/80). Am J Ophthalmol 1981;91:226–230.

21   Merayo-Lloves J, Calonge M, Foster CS: Experimental model of allergic conjunctivitis to ragweed in guinea pig. Curr Eye Res 1995;14:487–494.

22   Dwyer R StC, Turk J, Darougar S: Immediate hypersensitivity in the guinea pig conjunctiva. I. Characterization of the IgE and IgG1 antibodies involved. Int Arch Allergy Appl Immunol 1974;46:910–924.

23   Saiga T, Briggs R, Allansmith M: Clinical and cytologic aspects of ocular late-phase reaction in the guinea pig. Ophthalmic Res 1992;24:45–50.

24   Merayo-Lloves J, Zhao TZ, Dutt J, Foster CS: A new murine model of allergic conjunctivitis and effectiveness of nedocromil sodium. J Allergy Clin Immunol 1996;97:1129–1140.

25   Magone MT, Chan CC, Rizzo L, Kozhich A, Whitcup S: A novel murine model of allergic conjunctivitis. Clin Immunol Immunopathol 1998;87:75–84.

26   Keane-Meyers A, Cheung-Chau KW, Bond J, Ono SJ: Th2 cytokines influence both the early and late phase reactions in an experimental model of allergic conjunctivitis (submitted).

27   Allansmith M, Baird R, Ross R: Morphologic evidence that compound 48/80-challenged rat eyelid mast cells differ in their states of maximal degranulation. Ophthalmic Res 1989;21:206–215.

28   Allansmith M, Baird R, Barney N, Ross R, Bloch K: Response of rat conjunctival mast cells to multiple versus single applications of compond 48/80. Ophthalmic Res 1989;21:392–400.

29   Abelson M, Butrus S, Kliman G, Larson D, Corey EJ, Smith L: Topical arachidonic acid: A model for screening anti-inflammatory agents. J Ocul Pharmacol 1987;3:63–75.

30   Moller C, Bjorksten B, Nilsson G, Dreborg S: The precision of the conjunctival provocation test. Allergy 1984;39:37–41.

31   Abelson M, Smith L: The conjunctival provocation test: A new method for the evaluation of therapeutic agents (abstract). Invest Ophthalmol Vis Sci 1988;29(suppl):45.

32   Abelson M, Chambers W, Smith L: Conjunctival allergen challenge – A clinical approach to studying allergic conjunctivitis. Arch Ophthalmol 1990;108:84–88.

33   Leonardi A, Battista M, Gismondi I, Fregona A, Secchi A: Antigen sensitivity evaluated by tear-specific and serum-specific IgE, skin tests, and conjunctival and nasal provocation tests in patients with ocular allergic disease. Eye 1993;7:461–464.

34   Finkelman F, Katona I, Urban J, Holmes J, Ohara J, Tung J, Sample J, Paul W: Interleukin-4 is required to generate and sustain in vivo IgE responses. J Immunol 1988;141:2335–2341.

35   Fujishima H, Shinozako N, Takeuchi T, Saito I, Tsubota K: Interleukin-4 and IgE in seasonal allergic conjunctivitis. Ophthalmologica 1996;210:325–238.

36   Fujishima H, Saito I, Takeuchi T, Shinozaki N, Tsubota K: Measurement of interleukin-4 and histamine in superficial cells of conjunctiva in patients with allergic conjunctivitis. Curr Eye Res 1996;15:209–213.

37   Sharif N, Xu SX, Magnino P, Pang IH: Human conjunctival epithelial cells express histamine-1 receptors coupled to phosphoinositide turnover and intracellular calcium mobilization: Role in ocular allergic and inflammatory diseases. Exp Eye Res 1996;66:169–178.

38   Picker L, Kishimoto T, Smith C, Warnock-Butcher E: ELAM-1 is an adhesion molecule for skin-homing T cells. Nature 1991;349:796–799.

39   Shimizu Y, Shaw S, Graber N, Gopal TV, Horgan KJ, Van Seventer GA, Newman W: Activation-independent binding of human memory T cells to adhesion molecule ELAM-1. Nature 1991;349: 799–802.

40   Bacon A, McGill J, Anderson D, Baddeley S, Lightman S, Holgate S: Adhesion molecules and relationship to leukocyte levels in allergic eye disease. Invest Ophthalmol Vis Sci 1998;39:322–330.

41   Meng H, Tonnensen M, Marchese M, Clark R, Bahou W, Gruber B: Mast cells are potent regulators of endothelial cell adhesion molecule ICAM-1 and VCAM-1 expression. J Cell Physiol 1995;165: 40–53.

42   Allansmith M, Lee J, McClellan B, Dohlman C: Evaluation of a sustained release hydrocortisone ocular insert in humans. Trans Am Acad Ophthalmol Otolaryngol 1975;79:128–136.

43   Leonardi A, Bloch K, Briggs R, Allansmith M: Histology of ocular late-phase reaction in guinea pigs passively sensitized with IgG1 antibodies. Ophthalmic Res 1990;22:209–219.

44   Rapuano C, Webster G: Conjunctivitis and blepharitis; in Mannis M, Macsai M, Huntley A (eds): Eye and Skin Disease. Philadelphia, Lippincott-Raven, 1996, pp 637–647.

45   Matsuda H, Watanabe N, Geba G, Sperl J, Tsudzuki M, Hiroi J, Matsumoto M, Ushio H, Saito S, Askenase P, Ra C: Development of atopic dermatitis-like skin lesion with IgE hyperproduction in NC/Nga mice. Int Immunol 1997;9:461–466.

46   Keane-Meyers A, Gause W, Linsley P, Chen SJ, Willis-Karp M: B7-CD28/CTLA-4 costimulatory pathways are required for the development of T helper cell 2-mediated allergenic airway responses to inhaled antigens. J Immunol 1997;158:2042–2049.

47   Gavett S, O'Hearn D, Li X, Huang SK, Finkleman F, Willis-Karp M: Interleukin-12 inhibits antigen-induced airway hyperresponsiveness, inflammation, and Th2 cytokine expression in mice. J Exp Med 1995;182:1527–1536.

48   Naclerio R, Soloman W: Rhinitis and inhalent antigens. JAMA 1997;278:1842–1848.

49   Zweiman B: The late-phase reaction: Role of IgE, its receptor and cytokines. Curr Opin Immunol 1993;5:950–955.

50   Leonardi A, Secchi A, Briggs R, Allansmith M: Conjunctival mast cells and the allergic late phase reaction. Ophthalmic Res 1992;24:234–242.

51   deSchazo R, Levinson A, Dvorak H: The late phase skin reaction: Paradigm or epiphenomena? Ann Allergy 1983;51:166–172.

52   Behrens B, Clark R, Feldstein D, Presley D, Glezen L, Graves J, Larsen G: Comparison of the histopathology of immediate and late asthmatic and cutaneous responses in a rabbit model. Chest 1985;87:153S–155S.

53   Trocme S, Bonini S, Barney N, Bloch K, Allansmith M: Late-phase reaction in topically induced ocular anaphylaxis in the rat. Curr Eye Res 1988;7:437–443.

54   Prete G, Maggi E, Parronchi P, Chretien I, Tiri A, Macchia D, Ricci M, Banchereau J, Vries J, Romagnani S: IL-4 is an essential factor for the IgE synthesis induced in vitro by human T cell clones and their supernatants. J Immunol 1988;145:3796–3806.

55   Street N, Mossmann T: Functional diversity of T lymphoctes due to secretion of different cytokine patterns. FASEB J 1991;5:171–177.

56   Finkelman F, Katona I, Mossman T, Coffman R: IFN-γ regulates the isotypes of Ig secreted during in vivo humoral responses. J Immunol 1988;140:1022.

57   Carreras I, Carreras B, McGrath L, Rice A, Easty D: Activated T cells in an animal model of allergic conjunctivitis. Br J Ophthalmol 1993;77:509–514.

58   Metz D, Bacon A, Holgate S, Lightman S: Phenotypic characterization of T cells infiltrating the conjunctiva of chronic allergic eye disease. J Allergy Clin Immunol 1996;98:686–696.

59   Maggi E, Biswas P, Del Prete G, Parronchi P, Macchia D, Simonelli C, Emmi L, De Carli M, Tiri A, Ricci M, Romagnani S: Accumulation of Th-2 like helper T cells in the conjunctiva of patients with vernal conjunctivitis. J Immunol 1991;146:1169–1174.

60   Fujishima H, Saito I, Takeuchi T, Shinozaki N, Tsubota K: Characterization of cytokine mRNA transcripts in conjunctival cells in patients with allergic conjunctivitis. Invest Ophthalmol Vis Sci 1997;39:1350–1357.

61   Metz D, Hingorani M, Calder V, Buckley R, Lightman S: T-cell cytokines in chronic allergic eye disease. J Allergy Clin Immunol 1997;100:817–824.

62   Tomassini M, Lagrini L, Petrillo G, Adriani E, Bonini S, Balsano F, Bonini S: Serum levels of eosinophil cationic protein in allergic diseases and natural allergen exposure. J Allergy Clin Immunol 1996;97:1350–1355.

63   Lambiase A, Bonini S, Bonini S, Micera A, Magrini L, Bracci-Laudiero L, Aloe L: Increased plasma levels of nerve growth factor in vernal keratoconjunctivitis and relationship to conjunctival mast cells. Invest Ophthalmol Vis Sci 1995;36:2127–2132.

64   Bonini S, Lambiase A, Bonini S, Angelucci F, Magrini L, Manni L, Aloe L: Circulating nerve growth factor levels are increased in humans with allergic diseases and asthma. Proc Natl Acad Sci USA 1996;93:10955–10960.

65   Fukagawa K, Saito H, Tsubota K, Shimmura S, Tachimoto H, Akasawa A, Oguchi Y: RANTES production in a conjunctival epithelial cell line. Cornea 1997;16:564–570.

66   Allansmith MR: Immunology of the external ocular tissues. J Am Optom Assoc 1990;61: S16–S22.

67   Irani AM, Butrus SI, Tabbara KF, Schwartz LB: Human conjunctival mast cells: Distribution of MCT and MCTC in vernal conjunctivitis and giant papillary conjunctivitis. J Allergy Clin Immunol 1990;86:34–40.

68   Irani MA, Bradford TR, Kepley CL, Schechter NM, Schwartz LB: Detection of MCT and MC$_{TC}$ types of human mast cells by immunohistochemistry using new monoclonal anti-tryptase and anti-chymase antibodies. J Histochem Cytochem 1989;37:1509–1515.

69   Irani MA: Tissue and developmental variation of protease expression in human mast cells; in Caughey GH (ed): Mast Cell Proteases in Immunology and Biology. New York, Dekker, 1995, p 12.

70   Baddeley SM, Bacon AS, McGill JI, Lightman SL, Holgate ST, Roche WR: Mast cell distribution and neutral protease expression in acute and chronic allergic conjunctivitis. Clin Exp Allergy 1995; 25:41–50.

71   Morgan SJ, Williams JH, Walls AF, Church MK, Holgate ST, McGill JI: Mast cell numbers and staining characterisitcs in the normal and allergic human conjunctiva. J Allergy Clin Immunol 1991;87:111–116.

72   Butrus SI, Ochsner KI, Abelson MB, Schwartz LB: The level of tryptase in human tears: An indicator of activation of conjunctival mast cells. Ophthalmology 1990;97:1678–1683.

73   Proud D, Sweet J, Stein P, Settipane RA, Kagey-Sobotka A, Frielaender MH, Lichtenstein LM: Inflammatory mediator release on conjunctival provocation of allergic subjects with allergen. J Allergy Clin Immunol 1990;85:896–905.

74   Macleod J, Anderson D, Baddeley S, Holgate S, McGill J, Roche W: Immunolocalization of cytokines to mast cells in normal and allergic conjunctiva. Clin Exp Allergy 1997;27:1328–1334.

75   Tauber J, Raizman MB, Ostrov CS, Laibovitz RA, Abelson MB, Betts JG, Koester JM, Gill D, Schaich L: A multicenter comparison of the ocular efficacy and safety of diclofenac 0.1% solution with that of ketorolac 0.5% solution in patients with acute seasonal allergic conjunctivitis. J Ocul Pharmacol Ther 1998;14:137–145

76   Whitcup SM, Chan CC, Luyo DA, Bo P, Li Q: Topical cyclosporine inhibits mast cell-mediated conjunctivitis. Invest Ophthalmol Vis Sci 1996;37:2686–2693.

77   Bleik JH, Tabbara KF: Topical cyclosporine in vernal keratoconjunctivitis. Ophthalmology 1991; 98:1679–1684.

78   Hoang-Xuan T, Prisant O, Hannouche D, Robin H: Systemic cyclosporine A in severe atopic keratoconjunctivitis. Ophthalmology 1997;104:1300–1305.

79   Ohlsson K, Bjork P, Bergenfeldt M, Hageman R, Thompson RC: Interleukin-1 receptor antagonist reduces mortality from endotoxin shock. Nature 1990;348:550–552.

80   Arend W, Maylak M, Guthridge C, Gabay C: Interleukin-1 receptor antagonist: Role in biology. Annu Rev Immunol 1998;16:27–55.

81 Dana MR, Yamada J, Streilein JW: Topical interleukin-1 receptor antagonist promotes corneal transplant survival. Transplantation 1997;63:1501–1507.

82 Dana MR, Zhu SN, Yamada J: Topical modulation of interleukin-1 activity in corneal neovascularization. Cornea 1998;17:403–409.

83 Dana MR, Dai R, Zhu S, Yamada J, Streilein JW: Interleukin-1 receptor antagonist suppresses Langerhans cell activity and promotes ocular immune privilege. Invest Ophthalmol Vis Sci 1998; 39:70–77.

84 Keane-Myers AM, Liu G, Miyazaki D, Dekaris I, Ono SJ, Dana MR: Treatment with IL-1 receptor antagonist prevents allergic eye disease (manuscript submitted).

85 Janeway CA Jr, Travers P: Immunobiology: The Immune System in Health and Disease, ed 3. New York, Current Biology Ltd, 1997, pp 7–27.

Grace Liu, Laboratory of Molecular Immunology, Schepens Eye Research Institute and
Committee on Immunology, Harvard Medical School,
20 Staniford Street, Boston, MA 02114 (USA)
Tel. +1 617 912 2522, Fax +1 617 912 0127, E-Mail gliu@vision.eri.harvard.edu

Santa J. Ono, Laboratory of Molecular Immunology, Schepens Eye Research Institute,
Harvard Medical School, 20 Staniford Street, Boston, MA 02114 (USA)
Tel. +1 617 912 7521, Fax +1 617 912 0127, E-Mail sjono@vision.eri.harvard.edu

Streilein JW (ed): Immune Response and the Eye.
Chem Immunol. Basel, Karger, 1999, vol 73, pp 59–71

....

Anterior Chamber-Associated Immune Deviation

Jerry Y. Niederkorn

Department of Ophthalmology, University of Texas Southwestern Medical Center,
Dallas, Tex., USA

It has been recognized for over 100 years that the anterior chamber (AC) of the eye is endowed with remarkable qualities which permit the long-term survival of tissue and tumor grafts [1]. The capacity of foreign tumor and tissue grafts to survive in the AC, but not at other sites, led to the notion that a unique privilege was extended to alien tissues placed into this compartment of the eye. In the 1940s, Greene and Lund [2] took advantage of this property and used the AC as a site for propagating various human and animal tumors and as an assay for evaluating the metastatic potential of tumor biopsy specimens. The conspicuous absence of patent lymphatic vessels draining the AC of the eye led to the conclusion that tissue and tumor grafts were sequestered from the peripheral lymphoid apparatus and thereby escaped immunological recognition

It was not until the late 1970s that this perception was changed when Kaplan and Streilein [3, 4] discovered that antigenic cells placed into the AC were not only perceived by the systemic immune apparatus, but in fact, elicited a dynamic downregulation of alloimmune responses. Although AC injection of alloantigenic lymphoid cells aroused the humoral arm of the immune response resulting in the generation of hemagglutinating antibodies against donor histocompatibility antigens, the cell-mediated component was impaired as demonstrated by the significant delay in the rejection of orthotopic donor-specific skin allografts in the AC-primed hosts [3, 4]. The simultaneous activation of humoral immunity and downregulation of cellular immune function was termed 'lymphocyte-induced immune deviation' [3, 4]. Subsequent studies by Niederkorn and Streilein [5, 6] indicated that the immune deviation induced by AC priming was not a function of lymphoid cells per se, but was a characteristic of the AC. Accordingly, they coined the term 'anterior chamber-associated immune deviation' (ACAID) to emphasize the dynamic nature of this phenomenon and the fact that it required the participation of the AC [7]. Since the original observations by Kaplan and Streilein [3, 4], hundreds of publications have confirmed the presence of ACAID using a wide range of antigens including: viral proteins [8], soluble proteins [9, 10], histocompatibility antigens [5, 6, 11, 12], hapten-derivatized cells [13], and tumor antigens [14].

Characteristics of ACAID

Several laboratories have demonstrated that AC presentation of antigens elicits an array of immune responses which is characterized by the synthesis of noncomplement fixing antibodies (IgG1 isotype in the mouse), generation of cytotoxic T lymphocyte (CTL) precursors, and a conspicuous absence of normal delayed-type hypersensitivity (DTH) responses [15–18]. The impaired DTH coincides with the survival of highly immunogenic tumor allografts placed into the AC. Studies showed that DBA/2-derived P815 mastocytoma cells, which typically undergo brisk immunological rejection following subcutaneous transplantation in allogeneic BALB/c recipients, escaped immunological destruction in the AC and grew progressively [5, 6]. The fact that P815 tumor allografts were consistently rejected at extraocular sites suggested that the growth of the highly immunogenic intraocular P815 tumors was due to an active downregulation of cell-mediated immunity (CMI). Two sets of experiments indicated that two arms of CMI were affected. Within the intraocular tumor, infiltrating CD8+ CTL precursors failed to terminally differentiate and acquire cytolytic function [19, 20]. CMI was also actively downregulated systemically. This was confirmed in experiments which showed that BALB/c mice primed in the AC with P815 DBA/2 mastocytoma cells were unable to reject orthotopic DBA/2 allografts, yet were able to reject skin allografts from third-party donors [5, 6]. The inability of BALB/c mice to reject DBA/2 skin grafts indicated that the host's systemic CMI was actively inhibited. Subsequent studies from several laboratories, using a variety of antigens, demonstrated that AC priming induced the generation of regulatory T cells which suppressed DTH [15–18]. Analysis of the regulatory T cells of ACAID indicated that two functionally distinct populations were induced by AC priming. One population of T cells was CD4+ and acted at the afferent arm of the immune response, while a separate population of regulatory T cells expressed the CD8 determinant and acted at the efferent arm of the immune response [21]. The mechanism by which the regulatory T cells suppress the expression of DTH is still poorly understood. However, recent evidence indicates that the ACAID regulatory

---

Niederkorn 60

T cells secrete transforming growth factor-β_2 (TGF-β_2) which not only has anti-inflammatory properties, but can also prevent the activation of CD4+ T cells that mediate DTH [22]. Thus, AC priming appears to stimulate the generation of two separate populations of regulatory T cells which prevent the induction and expression of DTH respectively

Is ACAID a Th2 Immune Response?

The downregulation of DTH and the concomitant stimulation of IgG1 antibody synthesis are characteristic features of a Th2-dominated immune response and have prompted investigators to examine the cytokine profiles during ACAID. Li et al. [23] found that CD4+ spleen cells from animals primed in the AC with alloantigenic cells produced significantly higher levels of the Th2 cytokine, IL-10, and reduced levels of the Th1 cytokines, IL-2 and interferon-γ (IFN-γ) compared to control animals or animals immunized subcutaneously. Interestingly, CD4+ spleen cells from mice primed in the AC with alloantigens did not produce detectable IL-4 protein or mRNA. This Th2-like cell population, which elaborates IL-10 but no detectable IL-4, is reminiscent of Th2 clones which have been generated in vitro [24]. Using an ovalbumin (OVA) model of ACAID, D'Orazio and Niederkorn [25] found that ACAID was readily induced in IL-4 knockout (KO) mice, but could not be induced in IL-10 KO mice, thereby providing further evidence of a role for IL-10 in the development of ACAID.

Other investigators have used an in vitro model of ACAID to evaluate the cytokine profile of T cells exposed to ocular antigen presenting cells (APC) [26, 27]. The in vitro model of ACAID is based on the premise that cytokines, namely TGF-β_2, present in the aqueous humor alter resident APC such that they deliver antigens to T cells in a manner that leads to suppression of Th1 responses (i.e. ACAID). Using this model, Takeuchi and coworkers [26, 27] found that in vitro-generated ACAID APC induced the generation of T cells which elaborated increased amounts of IL-4, but no detectable IL-10. The supernatants from the Th2-like cells inhibited the production of IFN-γ by normal T cells; however, IL-4 was not responsible for the inhibitory effect as treatment of the supernatants with anti-IL-4 antibody did not restore IFN-γ production. Our laboratory has used the same in vitro model of ACAID and found that APC from IL-10 KO mice failed to support the generation of ACAID when transferred to normal recipients [25]. However, APC collected from normal mice and pulsed with antigen in the presence of TGF-β_2 induced ACAID when transferred to IL-10 KO mice. The latter findings suggest that IL-10 is needed for the generation of regulatory T cells, yet the regulatory T cells do not need to produce IL-10 in order to suppress DTH. Although there appears to be discrepancies in the roles of IL-4 and IL-10 in the generation of ACAID, inhibition of IFN-γ secretion is a consistent feature in three different models of ACAID reported from three independent laboratories [25–28]

Role of Antigen in the Induction of ACAID

To date, all of the soluble antigens injected into the AC have been shown to induce ACAID. These include, bovine serum albumin (BSA) [9], OVA [25], SV40 large T antigen [29], inner photoreceptor binding peptide [30], and retinal S-antigen [10]. By contrast, some cell-associated antigens induce ACAID while others do not [31–35]. AC inoculation of either DBA/2 mastocytoma cells or plastic-nonadherent, MHC class II-negative DBA/2 lymphoid cells induces ACAID in BALB/c mice [34]. By contrast, AC inoculation of highly immunogenic regressor tumor cell lines not only fails to induce ACAID, but also results in the spontaneous, T-cell-dependent rejection of the intraocular tumor cells [31, 33–35]. As mentioned above, plastic-nonadherent, MHC class II-negative allogeneic DBA/2 lymphocytes induce ACAID in BALB/c hosts [34]. By contrast, AC injection of plastic-adherent, MHC class II-positive dendritic cell inocula fails to induce ACAID in similar BALB/c hosts [34]. Particulate bacterial antigens such as *Mycobacterium* or *Listeria* fail to induce ACAID and in fact elicit robust DTH responses following AC inoculation [36, 37]. While it is unclear why some cell-associated antigens are capable of inducing ACAID and others are not, it appears that the nature of noncellular antigens determines whether or not ACAID is induced. Soluble antigens, such as BSA and OVA, induce ACAID when injected into the AC [9, 25]. However, AC inoculation of either OVA conjugated to latex beads or BSA conjugated to mouse erythrocytes fails to induce ACAID [29, 37]. Likewise, soluble SV40 large T antigen induces ACAID; however, AC inoculation of cell-associated SV40 large T antigen, in the form of SV40 T antigen-positive syngeneic tumor cells, induces strong DTH immunity [35]. Thus, the physical conformation of proteinaceous antigens introduced into the AC has a profound effect on the systemic immune response.

The mechanism which determines whether an antigen promotes ACAID or induces normal Th1 responses remains largely unknown. However, in vitro studies have shown that under the influence of the ocular cytokine, TGF-β2, soluble antigen (i.e. OVA) stimulates APC to produce IL-10 [25]. By contrast, OVA conjugated to latex beads stimulates similar APC to elaborate the Th1-inducing cytokine, IL-12 [29]. Cell-associated antigens which induce ACAID in vivo stimulate TGF-β-treated APC to produce IL-10 in vitro. Likewise, cell-associated antigens which fail to induce ACAID elicit robust IL-12 (but not IL-10) production by APC in vitro.

The fact that all of the soluble antigens tested to date induce ACAID suggests that antigens introduced into the AC are processed by APC via the endosomal pathway and are presented to T cells by MHC class II molecules. However, ACAID cannot be induced in mice deficient in β_2-microglobulin and thus, unable to assemble functional class I MHC molecules [38]. The latter observation is consistent with the hypothesis that ACAID antigens are loaded onto class I molecules of ocular APC and presented to CD8+ T cells that ultimately differentiate into downregulatory cells. However, recent results from our laboratory suggest that the lesion in the β_2-microglobulin-deficient mice that prevents the induction of ACAID is not the absence of the functional classical MHC class I molecule, but a deficiency in the expression of the nonclassical, class I-like Qa-1 molecule on antigen presenting B cells [D'Orazio and Niederkorn, submitted].

Role of the Camerosplenic Axis in ACAID

The absence of patent lymphatic vessels that directly drain the interior of the eye suggests that antigens introduced into the AC are obligated to depart via the blood vascular route. It has been suggested that delivering antigens into the AC is tantamount to an intravenous (IV) injection and that the downregulation of DTH is nothing more than a form of immune deviation that is known to be induced when soluble proteins and alloantigenic cells are injected IV [39]. However, ACAID and IV-induced immune deviation differ in two fundamentally important ways. First, one population of regulatory cells produced during ACAID, unlike those induced by IV injection of antigen, act at the efferent arm of the immune response and prevent the expression of DTH in sensitized hosts [40]. Second, ACAID can be induced in previously immunized hosts while IV injection of antigens fails to desensitize preimmune hosts [40]

Several laboratories have demonstrated that the eye plays a crucial role in the induction of ACAID as premature removal of the eye following AC injection prevents the development of ACAID. AC injection of herpes simplex virus (HSV) induces suppression of virus-specific DTH in mice [8, 28]. However, enucleation of HSV-injected eyes up to 3 days after AC injection prevents the induction of ACAID [28]. A simple explanation to account for the obligatory role of the intact eye is that it serves as a depot for the slow and continuous release of small quantities of antigen which induce the development of Th2 cells and a concomitant downregulation of DTH. Precedence for this hypothesis comes from studies by Guery et al. [41] who showed that the prolonged release of small quantities of soluble antigens from subcutaneous osmotic pumps in mice promotes the generation of a Th2-dominated systemic immune response and suppression of DTH. However, several findings suggest that ACAID is not merely a consequence of prolonged, slow release of antigen into the bloodstream. Unlike the low-dose antigen model of Guery et al. ACAID cannot be induced in β_2-microglobulin-deficient mice [38]. Also, ACAID is readily induced in C57BL6 mice while the low-dose antigen model cannot be produced in this mouse strain [41]. Moreover, removal of an eye 24 h after AC injection of HSV not only prevents the induction of ACAID, but also results in the development of positive DTH responsiveness, even without further extraocular immunization [28]. By contrast, removal of an HSV-injected eye 4 days after AC injection of HSV fails to prevent ACAID. These findings suggest that HSV antigens can escape from the eye within 24 h of AC injection and stimulate Th1 cells; however, by 96 h an ACAID-inducing signal supersedes and culminates in the downregulation of Th1 responses [28].

It is widely accepted that an intact spleen is necessary for the induction of ACAID. Removal of the spleen within 7 days of AC injection of antigen prevents the development of ACAID and leads to the generation of positive DTH [15–18]. To date, the cellular mechanisms within the spleen that contribute to the generation of ACAID have been largely neglected. We are attracted to the hypothesis that antigen-specific signals – either itinerant ocular APC or blood-borne antigen – are focused in the spleen after leaving the eye. We further propose that within the spleen, the modified antigen is released from the ocular APC and captured by splenic B cells which in turn present the antigen to T cells. The rationale for this hypothesis is based on the fact that the spleen is richly endowed with B cells which characteristically present antigens in a manner that leads to the downregulation of Th1 responses, especially DTH [42, 43]. Moreover, we have shown that ACAID cannot be induced either in mice chronically treated with anti-μ antibody to deplete B cells [44] or in B cell KO mice [D'Orazio and Niederkorn, submitted]. In vitro studies have confirmed that TGF-β-treated APC release antigens which are captured by B cells and presented to T cells which subsequently develop into regulatory cells capable of inhibiting DTH responses in vivo [D'Orazio and Niederkorn, submitted].

Role of FasL-Induced Apoptosis in ACAID

ACAID contributes to the immune privilege of the eye by inhibiting the generation of potentially destructive DTH responses to antigens delivered into the AC. In recent years it has become apparent that the eye is capable of eliminating inflammatory cells that enter the AC. Griffith et al. [45] demonstrated that the interior of the eye is decorated with Fas ligand (FasL; CD95L) which induces apoptosis of Fas+ inflammatory cells entering the AC. In addition to purging effector cells from the eye, the presence of FasL also appears to be important for the induction of ACAID. Functional FasL must be expressed in the eyes of hosts and Fas must be present on alloantigenic or hapten-derivatized cells injected into the AC in order for ACAID to be induced [28, 46]. Moreover, hapten-derivatized cells from Fas-defective lpr/lpr mice cannot induce ACAID unless they are rendered apoptotic, either by γ-irradiation or heat shock, prior to AC injection [28]

It is unclear how apoptosis contributes to the induction of ACAID with cell-associated antigens or if it is necessary for the induction of ACAID with soluble antigens. It is possible that membrane vesicles shed from apoptotic cells are more readily phagocytosed and processed by APC within the AC and that apoptosis induces the release of IL-10 from the injected cells and thereby facilitates the generation of Th2 responses. The latter explanation is particularly attractive as we have recently shown that IL-10 production by APC is a prerequisite for the induction of ACAID and that APC from IL-10 KO mice are incapable of generating an ACAID signal [18]

Diverging Hypotheses on the Induction and Expression of ACAID

ACAID has been demonstrated by several laboratories using a variety of model systems; thus, it is not surprising that there are diverging opinions as to the mechanisms that lead to the induction of ACAID. However, there is a consensus that the eye plays an active role in the induction of ACAID and that its premature removal abrogates the development of ACAID. It is also clear that the eye does not act as an antigen depot for the sustained slow release of antigen into the bloodstream resulting in a modified form of IV-induced immune deviation. In the HSV model of ACAID, viral antigens are promptly perceived by the systemic immune apparatus within 24 h of AC injection as removal of the eye within 1 day of AC injection of HSV results in positive DTH responses [28]. However, if the eye remains in place another 48 h, ACAID supersedes and DTH is actively suppressed. Similar findings have been reported with other models of ACAID indicating that significant events occur within the eye which lead to the generation of regulatory T cells. This begs the obvious question: 'What happens within the eye and what is the nature of the antigen-specific signal that is transmitted to the spleen?'

Using soluble antigens, Streilein et al. [37] have offered compelling data which indicate that within 24–48 h of AC injection of OVA, F4/80+ mononuclear cells bearing the characteristics of monocyte/macrophages can be found in the blood. Importantly, these blood-borne leukocytes are capable of inducing ACAID when transferred to naive hosts. The same investigators were able to generate similar leukocytes in vitro by incubating peritoneal exudate cells (PEC) with either aqueous humor (AH) or the AH cytokine, TGF-β_2. The in vitro-generated APC homed preferentially to the spleen and induced antigen-specific downregulation of OVA DTH that was phenotypically identical to ACAID. Ferguson and Herndon [47] have also demonstrated that a cell-associated signal of ACAID can be detected in the blood of mice immunized via the AC with the soluble antigen BSA. By contrast, AC injection of either particulate or cell-associated antigens induces the appearance of a soluble blood-borne signal which appears to be the T-cell-receptor-α chain [48]. Thus, it appears that the nature of the antigen introduced into the AC has a remarkable influence on the form which the ACAID-inducing signal assumes before leaving the eye

Results from in vitro models of the ocular component of ACAID suggest that TGF-β_2 (which is present in the AH) induces APC to produce their own TGF-β_2 which promotes the development of regulatory T cells in the spleen [22, 49]. Using the same model, our laboratory has found that incubation with TGF-β_2 induces PEC to produce IL-10 which promotes the in vitro generation of regulatory T cells which suppress the expression of DTH upon adoptive transfer to naive hosts [25]. IL-10 appears to be a crucial element in the ocular phase of ACAID because ACAID cannot be induced in IL-10 KO mice and importantly, PEC from IL-10 KO mice cannot induce the in vitro generation of regulatory T cells in the aforementioned in vitro model of ACAID [25]. The latter findings are consistent with the hypothesis offered by Ferguson and Griffith [18, 28] which suggests that apoptosis is necessary for the induction of ACAID with cell-associated antigens. The authors have proposed that within the eye, the antigenic cells undergo apoptosis and as a result, release significant quantities of IL-10. Moreover, the apoptotic cells are also much more susceptible to phagocytosis through their increased expression of cell membrane-associated phosphatidylserine and integrins [18, 50]. This proposition is also consistent with our findings which indicate that PEC pulsed with OVA in the presence of IL-10 induce ACAID when adoptively transferred to normal mice [25]. In addition to FasL-induced apoptosis, we have found that a small peptide (<10 kDa) in the AH induces macrophages to undergo apoptosis which does not peak until 72 h after in vitro exposure [D'Orazio et al., submitted]. Thus, it is plausible that ocular APC undergo delayed apoptosis after emigrating from the eye and arriving in the spleen, and release IL-10 within the spleen and thereby induce the generation of Th2 cells.

Streilein et al. [22] have offered an alternative hypothesis to explain the ocular phase of ACAID. Using the previously described in vitro model of ACAID, these investigators found that TGF-β_2 induced PEC to produce large amounts of mature TGF-β_2, which is known to be a potent inhibitor of CD4 + T cells. Moreover, PEC exposed to TGF-β_2 preferentially presented OVA to class I-restricted OVA-specific T-cell hybridoma cells [22]. The latter finding helps to explain the observation that AC priming with antigen leads to the generation of CD8 + regulatory T cells and MHC class I-restricted CTL precursors [15–18].

In trying to reconcile these divergent hypotheses for the induction of ACAID, one wonders if perhaps both scenarios are compatible. It has been previously reported that ACAID involves two distinct regulatory T-cell populations. One population is CD4 + and prevents the induction of DTH immunity (i.e. afferent suppression). The other population of regulatory T cells is CD8 + and prevents the expression of DTH in immunized hosts (i.e., efferent suppression). The development of these two regulatory cell populations might occur as follows. Following exposure to TGF-β_2 in the AC, ocular APC emigrate from the eye and accumulate in the spleen where they activate CD8 + regulatory T cells and MHC class I-restricted CTL [15–18]. The CD8 + regulatory T cells would function as the efferent suppressor cells of ACAID. APC exposed to TGF-β_2 in the eye would also be induced to produce IL-10 which would promote the development of CD4 + Th2 cells in the spleen. The Th2 cell population would prevent the generation of CD4 + Th1 cells without affecting the CD8 + cells in the spleen. We propose that at least some of the ocular APC undergo apoptosis after leaving the eye and release IL-10 along with antigen, the latter of which is captured by B cells in the spleen. In other systems, B cells are known to present antigen in a manner which leads to downregulation of DTH [42, 43]. Moreover, we have recently shown that B cells are necessary for the induction of ACAID and the generation of Th2 cells [44, D'Orazio and Niederkorn, submitted]. These CD4 + Th2 cells could act as the 'afferent suppressor cells' of ACAID. Thus, a soluble ocular factor, TGF-β_2, induces the generation of CD8 + regulatory T cells, and an ocular cell-membrane-associated factor, FasL, induces the generation of CD4 + (Th2) regulatory cells

What Is the Significance of ACAID?

ACAID is a crucial, but certainly not the only, component of immune privilege in the eye. We and others have suggested that ACAID is an adaptation for preventing the expression of immune effector mechanisms which inflict collateral damage to ocular tissues which possess only a limited capacity for regeneration [15–18]. ACAID is an elegant example of an immunological response which minimizes the generation of immune-mediated injury, while preserving protective mechanisms against potential pathogens which enter the eye. Activation of the complement cascade and expression of DTH have the potential to cause significant damage to innocent bystander cells, but are typically suppressed within the eye as a consequence of ACAID. By contrast, CTL responses can be tolerated in the AC as these effector elements exhibit exquisite precision in their mode of action and damage only those cells infected with endogenously generated proteins (e.g. viral antigens). It is noteworthy that of the limited number of pathogens that have been tested, those that fail to induce ACAID (i.e. *Mycobacterium* and *Listeria*) are potentially life-threatening and are controlled most effectively by macrophages that are activated by Th1 cytokines. That is, both *Mycobacterium* and *Listeria* are intracellular pathogens which are not affected by CTL, but are normally eliminated by macrophages activated with IFN-γ. By contrast, HSV is vulnerable to CD8+ CTL that are induced during ACAID and thus, does not pose a threat to the host's survival. It is tempting to speculate that the boundaries of ACAID encompass those antigens which represent a threat to vision but not to life

Although ACAID is believed to be an adaptation for protecting normal ocular tissues from nonspecific inflammatory injury produced by DTH responses elicited in the eye, it benefits corneal allografts. Using a mouse model of keratoplasty, Sonoda and Streilein [51] observed that hosts bearing long-term clear corneal allografts displayed an antigen-specific downregulation of DTH responses to donor alloantigens that was reminiscent of ACAID. By contrast, hosts that developed donor-specific DTH following keratoplasty invariably rejected their corneal allografts. In some rodent donor/host combinations, corneal allografts enjoy only limited immune privilege and experience a high rate of immunological rejection. However, AC inoculation of donor alloantigens prior to keratoplasty induces ACAID and results in a marked reduction in corneal graft rejection in both rat and mouse models of keratoplasty [51–54]. Moreover, maneuvers which are known to prevent the induction of ACAID, such as splenectomy [54] or systemic treatment with anti-IL-10 antibody [Niederkorn, unpubl.], also promote corneal allograft rejection. Thus, the capacity of orthotopic corneal allografts to induce immune deviation and deflect the systemic immune response away from a Th1 pathway and toward a Th2 pathway, is an integral component of the immune privilege of corneal allografts.

Thus, the eye benefits from ACAID in at least two important ways. It is shielded from immune-mediated injury induced by nominal, noninfectious antigenic agents, and it enjoys a high acceptance rate for therapeutic corneal allografts.

Acknowledgments

Supported by NIH grants EY07641 and EY05631 and an unrestricted grant from Research to Prevent Blindness, Inc., New York

References

1   Van Dooremaal JC: Die Entwicklung der in fremden Grund versetzten lebenden Gewebe. Albrecht von Graefes Arch Ophthalmol 1873;19:358–373.
2   Greene HSN, Lund PK: The heterologous transplantation of human cancers. Cancer Res 1944;4: 352–363.
3   Kaplan HJ, Streilein JW: Immune response to immunization via the anterior chamber of the eye. I. F1-lymphocyte-induced immune deviation. J Immunol 1977;118:809–814.
4   Kaplan HJ, Streilein JW, Stevens TR: Transplantation immunology of the anterior chamber of the eye. II. Immune response to allogeneic cells. J Immunol 1975;115:805–810.
5   Niederkorn J, Streilein JW, Shadduck JA: Deviant immune responses to allogeneic tumors injected intracamerally and subcutaneously in mice. Invest Ophthalmol Vis Sci 1980;20:355–363.
6   Streilein JW, Niederkorn JY, Shadduck JA: Systemic immune unresponsiveness induced in adult mice by anterior chamber presentation of minor histocompatibility antigens. J Exp Med 1980;152: 1121–1125.
7   Streilein JW, Niederkorn JY: Induction of anterior chamber associated immune deviation requires an intact, functional spleen. J Exp Med 1981;153:1058–1067.
8   Whittum J, Niederkorn JY, McCulley J, Streilein JW: Intracameral inoculation of herpes simplex virus type I induces anterior chamber associated immune deviation. Curr Eye Res 1983;2:691–697.
9   Mizuno K, Clark AF, Streilein JW: Anterior chamber associated immune deviation induced by soluble antigens. Invest Ophthalmol Vis Sci 1989;30:1112–1119.
10 Mizuno K, Altman NF, Clark AF, Streilein JW: Histopathologic analysis of experimental auto-immune uveitis attenuated by intracameral injection of S-antigen. Curr Eye Res 1989;8:113–121.
11 Okamoto S, Hara Y, Streilein JW: Induction of anterior chamber-associated immune deviation with lymphoreticular allogeneic cells. Transplantation 1995;59:377–381.
12 Niederkorn JY, Mayhew E, He YG: Alloantigens introduced into the anterior chamber of the eye induce systemic suppression of delayed hypersensitivity to third-party alloantigens through 'linked recognition'. Transplantation 1995;60:348–354.
13 Waldrep JC, Kaplan HJ: Anterior chamber associated immune deviation induced by TNP-spleno-cytes (TNP-ACAID). I. Systemic tolerance mediated by suppressor T-cell. Invest Ophthalmol Vis Sci 1983;24:1086–1092.
14 Niederkorn JY: Suppressed cellular immunity in mice harboring intraocular melanomas. Invest Ophthalmol Vis Sci 1984;25:447–454.
15 Niederkorn JY: Immune privilege and immune regulation in the eye. Adv Immunol 1990;48:191–226.
16 Streilein JW: Immune privilege as the result of local tissue barriers and immunosuppressive micro-environments. Curr Opin Immunol 1993;5:428–432.
17 Streilein JW, Wilbanks GA, Cousins SW: Immunoregulatory mechanisms of the eye. J Neuroimmu-nol 1992;39:185–200.
18 Ferguson TA, Griffith TS: A vision of cell death: insights into immune privilege. Immunol Rev 1997;156:167–184.
19 Ksander BR, Streilein JW: Failure of infiltrating precursor cytotoxic T cells to acquire direct cytotoxic function in immunologically privileged sites. J Immunol 1990;145:2057–2063.
20 Ksander BR, Bando Y, Acevedo J, Streilein JW: Infiltration and accumulation of precursor cytotoxic T cells increases with time in progressively growing ocular tumors. Cancer Res 1991;51:3153–3158.
21 Streilein JW, Niederkorn JY: Characterization of the suppressor cell(s) responsible for anterior chamber-associated immune deviation (ACAID) induced in BALB/c mice by P815 cells. J Immunol 1984;20:603–622.

22   Streilein JW, Takeuchi M, Taylor AW: Immune privilege, T-cell tolerance, and tissue-restricted autoimmunity. Hum Immunol 1997;52:138–143.

23   Li XY, D'Orazio T, Niederkorn JY: Role of Th1 and Th2 cells in anterior chamber-associated immune deviation. Immunology 1996;89:34–40.

24   Groux H, O'Garra A, Gibler M, Rouleau M, Antonenko S, de Vries JE, Rancarolo MG: A CD4+ T-cell subset inhibits antigen-specific T-cell responses and prevents colitis. Nature 1997;389:737–7442.

25   D'Orazio TJ, Niederkorn JY: A novel role for TGF-β and IL-10 in the induction of immune privilege. J Immunol 1998;160:2089–2098.

26   Takeuchi M, Kosiewicz MM, Alard P, Streilein JW: On the mechanisms by which transforming growth factor-β$_2$ alters antigen-presenting abilities of macrophages on T cell activation. Eur J Immunol 1997;27:1648–1656.

27   Takeuchi M, Alard P, Streilein JW: TGF-β promotes immune deviation by altering accessory signals of antigen-presenting cells. J Immunol 1998;160:1589–1597.

28   Griffith TS, Yu X, Herndon JM, Green DR, Ferguson TA: CD95-induced apoptosis of lymphocytes in an immune privileged site induces immunological tolerance. Immunity 1996;5:7–16.

29   D'Orazio TJ, Niederkorn JY: The nature of antigen in the eye has a profound effect on the cytokine milieu and resultant immune response. Eur J Immunol 1998;28:1544–1553.

30   Hara Y, Caspi RR, Wigert B, Chan CC, Wilbanks GA, Streilein JW: Suppression of experimental autoimmune uveitis in mice by induction of anterior chamber-associated immune deviation with interphotoreceptor retinoid-binding protein. J Immunol 1992;148:1685–1692.

31   Niederkorn JY, Meunier PC: Spontaneous immune rejection of intraocular tumors in mice. Invest Ophthalmol Vis Sci 1985;26:877–884.

32   Benson JL, Niederkorn JY: In situ suppression of delayed-type sensitivity: Another mechanism for sustaining the immune privilege of the anterior chamber. Immunology 1991;74:153–159.

33   Knisely TL, Luckenbach MW, Fischer BJ, Niederkorn JY: Destructive and nondestructive patterns of immune rejection of syngeneic intraocular tumors. J Immunol 1987;138:4515.

34   Benson JL, Niederkorn JY: The presence of donor-derived class II positive cells abolishes immune privilege in the anterior chamber of the eye. Transplantation 1991;51:834–838.

35   Ma D, Comerford S, Bellingham D, Sambrook J, Gething MJ, Alizadeh H, Anand R, Mellon J, Niederkorn JY: Capacity of simian virus 40 T antigen to induce self-tolerance but not immunological privilege in the anterior chamber of the eye. Transplantation 1994;57:718–725.

36   Li XY, Niederkorn JY: Immune privilege in the anterior chamber of the eye is not extended to intraocular *Listeria monocytogenes*. Ocul Immunol Inflamm 1997;5:245–257.

37   Streilein JW, Okamoto S, Hara Y, Kosiewicz M, Ksander B: Blood-borne signals that induce anterior chamber-associated immune deviation after intracameral injection of antigen. Invest Ophthalmol Vis Sci 1997;38:2245–2254.

38   Hara Y, Okamoto S, Rouse B, Streilein JW: Evidence that peritoneal exudate cells cultured with eye-derived fluids are the proximate antigen-presenting cells in immune deviation of the ocular type. J Immunol 1993;151:5162–5171.

39   Asherson GL, Stone SH: Selective and specific inhibition of 24-hour skin reactions in the guinea-pig. I. Immune deviation: Description of the phenomenon and the effect of splenectomy. Immunology 1965;9:205–217.

40   Wilbanks GA, Streilein JW: Characterization of suppressor cells in anterior chamber-associated immune deviation (ACAID) induced by soluble antigen. Evidence of two functionally and phenotypically distinct T-suppressor cell populations. Immunology 1990;71:383–389.

41   Guery JC, Galbiati F, Smiroldo S, Adorini L: Selective development of T helper (Th)2 cells induced by continuous administration of low dose soluble proteins to normal and β$_2$-microglobulin-deficient BALB/c mice. J Exp Med 1996;183:484–497.

42   Parker DC, Eynon EE: Antigen presentation in acquired immunological tolerance. FASEB J 1991; 5:2777–2784.

43   Eynon EE, Parker DC: Small B cells as antigen-presenting cells in the induction of tolerance to soluble protein antigens. J Exp Med 1992;175:131–138.

44   Niederkorn JY, Mayhew E: Role of splenic B cells in the immune privilege of the anterior chamber of the eye. Eur J Immunol 1995;25:2783–2787.

45   Griffith TS, Brunner T, Fletcher SM, Green DR, Ferguson TA: Fas ligand-induced apoptosis as a mechanism of immune privilege. Science 1995;270:1189–1192.

46   Kawashima H, Yamagami S, Tsuru T, Gregerson DS: Anterior chamber inoculation of splenocytes without Fas/Fas-ligand interaction primes for a delayed-type hypersensitivity response rather than inducing anterior chamber-associated immune deviation. Eur J Immunol 1997;27:2490–2494.

47   Ferguson TA, Herndon JM: The immune response and the eye: The ACAID inducing signal is dependent on the nature of the antigen. Invest Ophthalmol Vis Sci 1994;35:3085–3093.

48   Griffith TS, Herndon JM, Lima J, Kahn M, Ferguson TA: The immune response and the eye. TCR-α-chain related molecules regulate the systemic immunity to antigen presented in the eye. Int Immunol 1995;7:1617–1625.

49   Taylor AW, Alard P, Yee DG, Streilein JW: Aqueous humor induces transforming growth factor-β-producing regulatory T-cells. Curr Eye Res 1997;16:900–908.

50   Martin SJ, Reutelingsperger CP, McGahon AJ, Rader JA, van Schie RC, LaFace DM, Green DR: Early redistribution of plasma membrane phosphatidylserine is a general feature of apoptosis regardless of the initiating stimulus: Inhibition by overexpression of Bcl-2 and Abl. J Exp Med 1995;182:1545–1556.

51   Sonoda Y, Streilein JW: Impaired cell-mediated immunity in mice bearing healthy orthotopic corneal allografts. J Immunol 1993;150:1727–1734.

52   She SC, Steahly LP, Moticka EJ: Intracameral injection of allogeneic lymphocytes enhances corneal graft survival. Invest Ophthalmol Vis Sci 1990;31:1950–1956.

53   Yao YF, Inoue Y, Miyazaki D, Inoue Y, Miyazaki D, Hara Y, Shimomura Y, Tano Y, Ohashi Y: Correlation of anterior chamber-associated immune deviation with suppression of corneal epithelial rejection in mice. Invest Ophthalmol Vis Sci 1997;38:292–300.

54   Niederkorn JY, Mellon J: Anterior chamber-associated immune deviation promotes corneal allograft survival. Invest Ophthalmol Vis Sci 1996;37:2700–2707.

Jerry Y. Niederkorn, PhD, Department of Ophthalmology,
University of Texas Southwestern Medical Center, Dallas, TX 75235-9057 (USA)
Tel. +1 214 648 3829, Fax +1 214 648 9061, E-Mail jniede@mednet.swmed.edu

Streilein JW (ed): Immune Response and the Eye.
Chem Immunol. Basel, Karger, 1999, vol 73, pp 72–89

....

Ocular Immunosuppressive Microenvironment

Andrew W. Taylor

Schepens Eye Research Institute, Harvard Medical School, Boston, Mass., USA

Introduction

Activation, Function, and Regulation of Effector T Cells

Delayed-type hypersensitivity (DTH) (table 1) is initiated by primed antigen-specific T cells that recognize their antigen presented in the cleft of type II major histocompatibility complex antigens on the surface of antigen presenting cells (APC) in the tissue the T cells have migrated [1]. The responding DTH T cells express the molecule CD4 and are called T-helper (Th) cells [2]. Besides binding to their antigen, Th cells also need a second signal for activation. This second signal is usually adherence molecules expressed on the surface of the APC that bind to their corresponding surface receptors on the Th cell such as B7.1 to CD28, respectively [3–6]. This second signal is less of a requirement for primed/memory T-cell activation than naive T-cell activation [7]. Following activation, Th cells enter the growth cycle, proliferate, and produce lymphokines.

Based on their pattern of lymphokine production, Th cells are further divided into types of T-cell responders [8, 9]. It is primed type 1 Th (Th1) cells that mediate DTH following their activation by producing interferon-γ (IFN-γ) [2]. The type of lymphokine pattern produced by Th cells is influenced by antigen, type of APC, and the presence of specific lymphokines and factors when the T cells are primed. For example, stimulated primed T cells from draining lymph nodes following immunization with *Mycobacterium tuberculosis* predominantly produce IFN-γ and mediate DTH characterizing Th1 cell activity [10]. However, stimulation of primed T cells for draining lymph nodes following immunization with keyhole limpet hemocyanin characterize Th2 cell activity [11] by predominantly producing IL-4 and mediate allergic responses and antibody production by B cells. Recently, it has been found that oral

Table 1. Main stages of DTH induction

APC presentation of antigen
Activation of Th1 cell proliferation and IFN-γ production
IFN-γ activation of macrophages
Macrophage production of inflammatory factors

---

immunization induces activation of a third type of T cell that predominantly produces TGF-β and functions by suppressing activation of both Th1 and Th2 cells [12]. Autoantigen-specific Th3 cells have the ability to suppress autoimmune disease mediated by autoantigen-reactive Th1 cells, suggesting that Th3 cells are mediators of immunoregulation in the periphery.

Regulation of lymphokine production and therefore the subsequent cell-mediated immune response is not limited to the time of immunization. Three known mechanisms have been recognized which terminate T-cell-mediated immune responses after immunization and sensitization [13]. These mechanisms include induction of anergy, apoptosis, and cytokine-mediated suppression. In anergy the T cells are activated through their T-cell receptor (TcR), but either fail to receive a second signal from APC or receive an inhibitory signal initiated through another receptor such as CTLA-4 binding B7 on the APC. An anergic T cell is functionally unresponsive, but not eliminated.

Engagement of Fas antigen on the T cell to its ligand (FasL) on another cell can initiate the apoptotic cascade of cell death. Apoptosis eliminates the activated T cells. Since the ocular microenvironment constitutively expresses FasL, it has been suggested that FasL is the molecular entity that imparts onto the ocular tissue and other tissues immune privilege and tolerance [14–16]. However, this is far from being certain, since the activation of FasL/Fas-mediated apoptosis requires appropriate signals through the TcR and that aqueous humor through TGF-β_2 inhibits the signals of Fas/FasL-mediated apoptosis within lymphocytes and neutrophils [17–20, and Miyamoto and Ksander, unpubl. data]. This means that the manner by which antigen presentation occurs and the presence of specific cytokines, i.e. TGF-β_2, within the ocular microenvironment can influence the outcome of a FasL-mediated signal in T cells. Therefore, because of the nature of the normal ocular microenvironment there could be inhibition of FasL signaling with cytokine-mediated recovery of certain activated T-cell subpopulations. In contrast, it is possible that FasL expression within the eye by parenchymal cells could have a role in the pathology of ocular inflammation [20, 21].

Cytokine-mediated suppression occurs when T cells are activated in the presence of a cytokine that suppresses specific effector T-cell functions such as proliferation and/or lymphokine production. The source of the cytokines can come from other activated effector T cells. It is known that Th1 cells suppress Th2 cell activation through IFN-γ and Th2 cells suppress Th1 cells through IL-4 [22]. In addition, regulatory T cells (Th3) through TGF-β production suppresses both Th1 and Th2 cell activation [12, 23]. Since cytokine production is not limited to only lymphocytes, it is very well possible that nonlymphoid cells at the site of T-cell activation, as you will see later in this chapter, can influence the effector immune response through cytokine production. Cytokine-mediated suppression allows for a fine tuning of the immune response. The mechanisms of anergy, apoptosis, and cytokine-mediated suppression are all important in maintaining immunological homeostatis and self-tolerance [13].

The IFN-γ produced by the Th1 cells activates macrophages and other cells in the surrounding tissue [24–26]. IFN-γ-activated macrophages begin to produce biochemical substances and other inflammatory cytokines that results in induction of a cytokine storm and the observed inflammatory response. The inflammation associated with a DTH response often involves capillary breakdown, fibrosis, and cell death [27–31]. There is also cellular proliferation and tissue remodeling especially upon resolution of inflammation through the mechanisms of wound repair [32].

Inflammation in tissues such as the skin is usually handled with complete recovery of normal structure and cellular functions; whereas, in the eye where cells rarely proliferate, such inflammatory responses lead to loss of cells and structure resulting in irreversible destruction of light gathering and neural signaling activities of the eye. To prevent the induction of immunogenic inflammation, the eye has evolutionarily adapted the mechanisms of immune privilege that establishes an immunosuppressive microenvironment within the eye [33].

Immunosuppressive Ocular Microenvironment

Ocular immune privilege was first defined experimentally by Medawar [34] and his colleagues in the 1940s. They defined immune privilege as a tissue site that supports prolong survival of histoincompatible tissue grafts. This definition describes the immunological response within the eye, brain, testes, and maternal-fetal interface [35]. They explained the mechanism of immune privilege to be antigen sequestration caused by the presence of a blood-ocular barrier and the lack of direct lymphatic drainage. However, it is now known that the immune system is clearly aware and responsive to the presence of antigen within the eye, but the immunological response is far from conventional [36, 37]. Other chapters in this volume describe in detail induction of immune deviation in response to immunization through the anterior chamber. This

Table 2. Effects of aqueous humor on DTH induction

Alters manner of antigen presentation by APC
Suppresses activation of Th1 cell proliferation and IFN-γ production
Suppresses IFN-γ activation of macrophages

---

chapter will focus on the mechanisms by which the ocular microenvironment suppresses expression of efferent immune responses preventing induction of DTH.

The finding that the immune system responds even though uniquely to antigens placed into the anterior chamber opened up the possibility that the ocular microenvironment regionally manipulates the immune response to antigens. Kaiser et al. [38] found that aqueous humor, the fluid filling the anterior chamber of the eye, suppresses antigen-stimulated T-cell functions in vitro. This suppression was not cytotoxic to the T cells nor was it species-specific. They concluded that there are soluble immunosuppressive factors in aqueous humor that regulate immunological responses within the ocular microenvironment. A short time later, Niederkorn et al. [39] found that there was some sort of efferent blockade of DTH within the anterior chamber of the eye. Even though a strong DTH response could be mounted against syngeneic tumor cells placed in the skin, a conventional immune site, of an immunized mouse there is no DTH response in the eye if the tumor cells were placed in the ocular anterior chamber. This raised the possibility that the local ocular microenvironment either prevents the migration of DTH T cells into the anterior chamber or produces immunosuppressive factors actively suppressing effector T-cell activities. Cousins et al. [40] demonstrated that it is the latter mechanism. They failed to elicit a DTH response in the eye when primed T cells, that would mediate DTH when adoptively transferred with antigen and APC into the skin, were placed into the ocular anterior chamber with antigen and APC. Moreover, primed T cells first incubated with aqueous humor before being mixed with antigen and APC and adoptively transferred into the skin, also fail to mount a DTH response [40]. Therefore, the ocular microenviron-ment actively suppresses effector T-cell activities through immunosuppressive factors it produces.

Over the past decade we have found that aqueous humor can affect all stages of DTH induction (table 2). The manner of antigen presentation by APC is affected by aqueous humor and its factors [41–43]. The effect of aqueous humor on APC has been demonstrated in the induction of ACAID which is discussed in detail by Niederkorn [this volume, pp. 59–71]. Since potential APC are found between the layers of pigmented and nonpigmented epithelial cells and next to

---

neurons of the iris and ciliary body [44, 45], they are in intimate contact with the cellular sources of the immunosuppressive factors found in aqueous humor. Therefore, the APC are always in an environment of immunosuppressive factors that can influence their antigen presenting abilities.

In the presence of aqueous humor, in vitro proliferation of antigen-stimulated primed T cells is inhibited [38, 46]. However, if the in vitro assay is adapted to a serum-free culture condition, antigen-stimulated proliferation is not suppressed, but the antigen-stimulated primed T cells are suppressed in IFN-γ production [47]. This parallels the finding that primed T cells pretreated with aqueous humor cannot mediate DTH in an adoptive transfer into skin [47]. The serum-free conditions mimic as close as possible the conditions within the normal eye behind an intact blood-ocular barrier. Without serum in the in vitro conditions, blood-borne proteins and factors are not introduced into the culture conditions that may interact or combine with aqueous humor proteins and factors. In addition, degradation and neutralization of bioactive peptides in aqueous humor by serum proteases is avoided [48]. Therefore, the use of serum-free culture conditions allows for examining the full range of aqueous humor affects on effector T cells and on other cells mediating inflammation such as macrophages. Aqueous humor suppresses the ability of macrophages to generate nitric oxide when activated by IFN-γ [49]. Therefore, aqueous humor not only suppresses the production of T-cell mediators of inflammation, but also neutralizes their responding target cells. Identification of immunosuppressive factors in aqueous humor has led to understanding their role in the mechanisms of aqueous humor suppression of DTH and to their role in ocular immune privilege.

Aqueous Humor Factors That Suppress DTH

Many potential immunosuppressive factors have been detected in normal aqueous humor; however, only a few have been studied for their role in suppressing induction of DTH (table 3). The criteria for identifying a relevant immunosuppressive factor has been based on their physical presence in normal aqueous humor, their aqueous humor concentration has an in vitro immunosuppressive activity similar to whole aqueous humor, and finally neutralization of the factor also neutralizes some aspect of aqueous humor immunosuppressive activity. Based on this criteria, only TGF-β₂, α-melanocyte-stimulating hormone (α-MSH), immunoreactive vasoactive intestinal peptide (VIP), and calcitonin gene-related peptide (CGRP) have so far been identified as ocular immunosuppressors of DTH [49–53]. Other immunosuppressive factors such as somatostatin, corticosteroids, and hydrocortisone have either not been found

Table 3. 'Incomplete' list of aqueous humor factors suppressing DTH-associated APC, Th1, and macrophage activities

	APC activity	Th1 activity IFN-γ production	Macrophage inflammatory activity
TGF-β$_2$	A	S	S
α-MSH	A	S	S
VIP	?	S	?
CGRP	A	N	S

A = Alters (APC do not stimulate Th1 cell activities); S = suppresses; N = no affect; ? = unknown.

in aqueous humor or their activity in aqueous humor suppression of DTH has not been characterized [54, 55].

Transforming Growth Factor-β

The first immunosuppressive factor identified in aqueous humor was TGF-β$_2$ [50, 51, 56]. It was isolated through HPLC size fractionation where a fraction centered on 25 kDa molecular weight suppressed IL-2 production by antigen-stimulated T cells [50]. The molecular weight of the 25-kDa fraction suggested TGF-β. TGF-β is an evolutionary conserved cytokine of three isoforms in mammals. Also, TGF-β exists as either a 200-kDa latent complex or as its 25-kDa active dimmer released from its latency-associated proteins [57–60]. Only the active form of TGF-β can bind to its receptors. In normal aqueous humor the concentration of TGF-β has been reported to be between 1 and 10 ng/ml [50, 51, 56] where most ($<10\%$) of the TGF-β is latent [47]. Even though mRNA for all three TGF-β isoforms are found in cells of the eye, only TGF-β$_2$ protein is found in normal aqueous humor [50, 61, 62]. The isoform TGF-β$_2$ has also been found to be a central immunosuppressive factor in other immune privileged sites [41]. Its evolutionary conservation explains why the same TGF-β$_2$ immunosuppressive activity is observed in all samples of mammalian (human, mice, pig, rabbit) aqueous humor [46, 50].

The suppression of T-cell proliferation by aqueous humor could only be partially (80–90%) neutralized by incubating the aqueous humor with neutralizing anti-TGF-β$_2$ antibody before treating the antigen-stimulated T cells [50]. However, under serum-free in vitro conditions, aqueous humor does not suppress antigen-stimulated T-cell proliferation but does suppress IFN-γ production of which neutralization of α-MSH and VIP (see below) and not TGF-β recovers IFN-γ production [47]. This last finding suggests that the TGF-β_2 normally found in aqueous humor is latent and needs to be activated. The absence of serum proteases and cofactors [63, 64] in the serum-free conditions may slow the activation rate of TGF-β_2 to a level where it either has no affect or may mediate some other effector T-cell activity that has yet to be described. Therefore, activated aqueous humor TGF-β_2 suppresses activation of antigen-stimulated T-cell activity and based on reports that TGF-β_2 can suppress development of Th1 cells through suppression of IL-2 production [65], TGF-β_2 is a suppressor of Th1 cell activity. In addition, the presence of TGF-β_2 in aqueous humor may protect T cells from apoptotic signals, permitting T-cell survival within the ocular microenvironment [20]. Therefore, it is possible that under the influence of the other aqueous humor factors, noninflammatory T-cell effector activity can exist within the ocular miroenvironment.

The effects of TGF-β_2 on APC stimulation of T cells has been the focus of ACAID induction [66, 67]; however, there are a few findings that may suggest TGF-β_2 influences the ability for APC within the eye to activate Th1 cells. APC treated with TGF-β_2 in vitro are unable to induce a Th1 response against a DTH-inducing antigen. The APC are impaired in their production of IL-12 and expression of CD40 accessory signals [66, 67]. The APC also produce TGF-β_2 which can affect T-cell development into Th1 cells directly [66]. Therefore, APC within the ocular microenvironment are most likely altered in their production of second signals needed for activation of inflammatory T-cell activities in comparison to APC from conventional tissue sites. It is also possible that APC (monocytes and dendritic cells) within the ocular microenvironment are important sources of aqueous humor TGF-β_2.

Inflammatory macrophages are deactivated by TGF-β_2 [68–70]. The TGF-β_2-treated macophages are unable to secrete inflammatory cytokines or generate reactive oxygen intermediates making them unable to amplify the cytokine response and induce inflammation. Therefore, by the presence of TGF-β_2 in the ocular microenvironment, macrophages would also be prevented from playing their central role in the DTH response.

The effects of TGF-β_2 on APC, T cells, and macrophages indicates that the ocular microenvironment through TGF-β_2 can suppress each stage of DTH induction. However, neutralization of TGF-β_2 did not prevent aqueous humor from suppressing IL-1-induced thymocyte proliferation [51], and nor did neutralization of TGF-β_2 under serum-free conditions prevent suppression of IFN-γ production by antigen-stimulated effector T cells [47]. These non-TGF-β_2-mediated immunosuppressive activities of aqueous humor have been traced to factors in a low molecular weight (3.5 kDa) fraction of normal aqueous humor [51, 71]. Since TGF-β_2 is predominantly latent, these other immunosuppressive factors could influence effector T-cell functionality immediately upon T-cell migration into the ocular microenvironment before there is activation of TGF-β_2.

α-Melanocyte-Stimulating Hormone

The HPLC fractionation of normal aqueous humor revealed a second fraction centered on 3.5 kDa that is not associated with TGF-β_2 [51]. This low molecular weight fraction suppressed both antigen-stimulated effector T-cell proliferation and IL-1/TNF-induced thymocyte proliferation [50, 51]. The 3.5-kDa molecular weight and suppression of IL-1-induced thymocyte proliferation suggested that α-MSH may be one of the immunosuppressive factors of aqueous humor [72]. The neuropeptide α-MSH is a 13-amino acid long (1.6 kDa) protein derived from the endoproteolytic cleavage of ACTH which in turn is a proteolytic cleavage product of pro-opiomelanocortin hormone (POMC) [73, 74]. This neuropeptide originally described for its melanin-inducing activity in frogs has a fundamental role in modulating inflammatory responses in mammals [75, 76]. Endotoxin, IL-1 and TNF-induced inflammation and fever is suppressed by systemic and central injections of α-MSH [77–79]. It suppresses the induction of LPS and IFN-γ-induced reactive oxygen intermediates, nitric oxide, and inflammatory cytokines by macrophages while enhancing its receptor expression and autocrine production in macrophages [80–82]. Also, α-MSH suppresses the migration of macrophages and neutrophils [80, 83]. The sources of α-MSH are centrally derived neurons, macrophages, keratinocytes and possibly any other cell that can synthesize POMC and ACTH [82, 84, 85]. There is on average 20 pM of α-MSH in normal mammalian aqueous humor [52].

At its ocular concentration, α-MSH suppresses IFN-γ production by antigen-stimulated primed T cells under serum-free conditions with no affect on proliferation [52]. Neutralization of α-MSH activity in the low molecular weight fraction of aqueous humor recovered some of the IFN-γ production by antigen-stimulated primed T cells [52]. The other immunosuppressive factor in the low molecular weight fraction is immunoreactive VIP, discussed below [53]. Neutralization of α-MSH in whole aqueous humor contributes to neutralizing aqueous humor suppression of IFN-γ production by the antigen-stimulated primed T cells with no change in proliferation [47]. This further supports the possibility that TGF-β_2 affects some other aspect of T-cell activation. It is also possible that α-MSH induces an activity in the proliferating effector T cells of which TGF-β_2 helps. Since α-MSH has the potential to influence both APC and T cells, α-MSH pretreatment of primed T cells before antigen activation by untreated APC are potently suppressed in IFN-γ production [43]. In addition, but requiring higher levels of α-MSH, α-MSH alters the ability of APC to present antigen in a manner that induces IFN-γ production by untreated primed T cells [43]. This suppressive activity could be due to α-MSH inducing its own synthesis by the APC [82]. The α-MSH suppression of effector Th1 cell functions is similar to but independent of IL-4 activity [43]. The IL-4-like activity of α-MSH in the presence of TGF-β_2 has implications of the type of immune response that could emerge from the ocular microenvironment [86]. This issue is discussed later in this chapter. Therefore, the ocular microenvironment constitutively contains the most potent anti-inflammatory neuropeptide, α-MSH, which also influences the activation of T cells suppressing induction of Th1-associated activities.

Vasoactive Intestinal Peptide

Since α-MSH could not account for all the immunosuppressive activity of the low molecular weight fraction of normal aqueous humor, and that VIP is a neuropeptide whose immunoreactivity is abundantly found in the nerves of the iris and ciliary body [87] with immunosuppressive activity [88–94], aqueous humor was assayed for VIP. Since the antibodies for VIP have high cross-reactivity with VIP fragments and pituitary adenylate cyclase-activating polypeptide (PACAP), only immunoreactive VIP has been found in aqueous humor. The concentration of immunoreactive VIP in rabbit aqueous humor is 12 nM [53]. Whole synthetic VIP suppresses IFN-γ production by antigen-stimulated primed T cells in vitro [53]. Unlike whole aqueous humor, VIP at its aqueous humor concentration suppressed proliferation by antigen-stimulated primed T cells; however, the VIP suppression of T-cell proliferation is only 50%. It has been suggested that VIP affects selective populations of T cells [95]. Therefore, it is possible that whole aqueous humor selects for proliferative expansion of a subpopulation of effector T cells that are nonresponsive to VIP.

Even though VIP receptors have been found on monocytes [96, 97] nothing is known about the effects of VIP on antigen presentation. Also, very little is known about VIP affects on inflammatory macrophages other than the potential to suppress respiratory bursts within macrophages [98, 99]. Therefore, in the ocular microenvironment VIP could be a contributing factor to the overall suppression of DTH induction.

Calcitonin Gene-Related Peptide

Also in immuoreactive abundance in ocular nerves is CGRP [100]. CGRP, unlike VIP, cannot suppress primed T cells [101]. Mature T cells are unresponsive to CGRP; however, CGRP can influence the activity of APC and inflammatory macrophages [102, 103]. In normal aqueous humor it was found that there is a constitutive level of CGRP at 0.5 μM [49]. This concentration is 20-fold less than the concentration of CGRP found in aqueous humor of inflamed eyes [104–106]. At its constitutive level it suppresses IFN-γ/LPS-induced nitric oxide generation by macrophages, but not at its inflammatory concentration [49]. Neutralization of CGRP activity in aqueous humor by anti-CGRP prevents aqueous humor from suppressing nitric oxide generation by the inflammatory macrophages [49]. CGRP also suppresses IFN-γ-induced peroxide generation by macrophages [107]. Therefore, under normal conditions CGRP can contribute in suppressing macrophage inflammatory activity induced by IFN-γ along with TGF-β_2, and α-MSH in the ocular microenvironment. CGRP is also known to suppresses antigen presenting abilities of macrophages and dendritic cells under T-cell-mediated hypersensitivity conditions possibly by mediating a reduction in the number of class II MHC-expressing APC [102, 103, 107, 108]. The finding of CGRP activity in aqueous humor has brought to light that the ocular microenvironment not only maintains the presence of immunosuppressive factors, but also maintains them at effective concentrations that inhibit induction of DTH [49]. The presence of a constitutive amount of CGRP further strengthens the ability for the ocular microenvironment to prevent both induction of and response to Th1 cell activities.

The ocular microenvironment has adapted several cytokines and neuropeptides to mediate suppression of DTH at each stage of the response (table 3). The immunosuppressive factors TGF-β_2, CGRP, and α-MSH prevent induction of IFN-γ synthesis by altering the manner by which APC activate effector T cells. Also, TGF-β_2, α-MSH, and VIP suppress IFN-γ production by acting directly on the Th1 cells. In addition, TGF-β_2, α-MSH, and CGRP suppress macrophages from producing inflammatory mediators in response to IFN-γ. In spite of the overwhelming presence of immunosuppressive factors, there are activated T cells proliferating in the presence of aqueous humor in vitro. Therefore, is it possible that an immune response can still occur within the normal ocular microenvironment, and if possible, what is the nature of this immune response?

Immune Responses Modified by Normal Aqueous Humor

By employing serum-free culture conditions in the in vitro T-cell assays, it was discovered that normal aqueous humor, while suppressing IFN-γ production, did not suppress proliferation by TcR-stimulated primed T cells [47]. Therefore, under culture conditions that mimic as close as possible the natural and normal ocular microenvironment, some populations of primed T cells respond to TcR stimulation in the presence of whole aqueous humor. One possibility was that since α-MSH has a IL-4-like affect on T cells that maybe the proliferating cells were prompted to express type 2 activities. Culture supernatant of the

Table 4. Effector T-cell responses in the presence of aqueous humor

---

Suppression of Th1 cell activity
Induction of regulatory T-cell activity (Th3 cells)

---

primed T cells TcR-stimulated in the presence of aqueous humor do not produce IFN-γ or IL-4 [23]. In addition, when they were restimulated in the absence of aqueous humor they did not recover IFN-γ or IL-4 production. If it were not for the finding that the T cells were proliferating it could be suggested that aqueous humor induces anergy or apoptosis in the responding T cells. Therefore, T cells activated in the presence of whole aqueous humor lack the appearance of Th1, Th2, and anergic cells. A possible aqueous humor-induced T-cell activity is TGF-β production [12, 109–111]. Effector T cells TcR-stimulated in the presence of whole aqueous humor produce copious amounts of TGF-β [23]. Therefore, the factors of aqueous humor while suppressing Th1 and possibly Th2 cell responses mediate induction of TGF-β-producing T cells.

The TGF-β-producing T cells, called Th3 cells, act as regulatory cells mediating suppression of Th1 and Th2 cell activities [12]. Aqueous humor induced Th3 cells suppress IFN-γ production by other TcR-stimulated primed T cells in the absence of aqueous humor [23]. Much of this suppressive activity is mediated by the TGF-β produced by the aqueous humor induced Th3 cells. Recently it has been found that TGF-β itself and IL-4 mediate development of TGF-β-producing T cells [86]. Since, aqueous humor contains α-MSH, which has IL-4-like affects on T cells, and TGF-β₂, it is possible that these two factors mediate aqueous humor induction of Th3 cells. The induction of Th3 cells means that an immune response is induced that further contributes to the immunosuppressive nature of the immune privileged ocular microenvironment. The ability for the factors in aqueous humor to divert a population of primed T cells with a propensity to express inflammatory activities, Th1 cells, into a functioning population of Th3 cells shows that the ocular microenvironment constitutively produces potent factors that not only suppress expression of immunogenic inflammation, but also regionally coerces the immune system to respond in a manner that protects the tissue from inflammation (table 4).

Conclusions

Aqueous humor mediates suppression of DTH through factors constitutively produced by the cells of the ocular microenvironment. Each of these factors have their own distinct affects on APC, effector T cells, and inflammatory macrophages. In the collective, whole aqueous humor changes the manner by which APC present antigen, suppresses IFN-γ production by activated effector T cells, and inhibits IFN-γ-induced macrophage responses. The final result is the prevention of the induction of Th1 cells and the inflammation they mediate within the immune privileged microenvironment.

The activity of aqueous humor is not just suppressive, but is also permissive and promoting of the induction of Th3 cells that reinforces immune privilege by delivering immunosuppressive factors and by suppressing induction of Th1 cells in the ocular microenvironment. If the Th3 cells are induced to ocular autoantigens, then like in the oral tolerance models, they would prevent induction of other ocular autoantigen-reactive Th1 cells and possibly suppress autoimmune disease [12]. This would be a mechanism of peripheral tolerance through induction of ocular antigen-responsive Th3 cells within the ocular microenvironment. Therefore, by identifying which factors mediate suppression of immunogenic inflammation and induce Th3 cells, it should be possible to treat uveitic eyes with the immunosuppressive factors to suppresses inflammation, reestablish immune privilege, and possibly induce tolerance to ocular antigens. The treatment could be accomplished through gene therapy [112–114]. By delivering vectors coding for aqueous humor immunosuppressive cytokines into the uveitic eye would result in establishing sustained levels of the cytokines without repeated cytokine injections into the eye. The sustained production of the cytokines would suppress inflammation and mediate reestablishment of immune privilege. The cytokines that would be best suited for use in a cytokine gene therapy for uveitis are TGF-β$_2$ and α-MSH since the two can suppress a wide range of immunological and inflammatory activities.

The ability for the ocular microenvironment to manipulate an immune response has implications on how immunity is regulated in general and how immune responses can be manipulated in other tissues. The ocular microenvironment is an example of a tissue site that mediates termination of inflammatory T-cell activity through cytokines. It is also a tissue site that through the same anti-inflammatory cytokines promotes development of regulatory T cells. Since the mechanisms of immunoregulation is through cytokines it should be possible to use these cytokines to manipulate the immune response in other tissues. It is possible that induction of the same ocular cytokines in transplant tissues or sites of inflammation would mediate suppression of inflammation and possible tolerance to the transplanted tissue. Since normally, other tissues express some of the same cytokines as in the eye, such as α-MSH in the skin [115, 116], our understanding of their role in ocular immune privilege may suggest their systemic role in maintaining immunological and inflammatory homeostasis. Examination of the unique relationship between the ocular micro-environment and the immune system has not only giving us insight into the mechanisms of immune privilege, but also into the means that will allow for regulating and tailoring an immune response in specific tissues and to specific antigens.

Acknowledgments

Supported by USPHS grant EY10752.

References

1   Jorgensen JL, Reay PA, Ehrich EW, Davis MM: Molecular components of T-cell recognition. Annu Rev Immunol 1992;10:835–873.
2   Cher DJ, Mosmann TR: Two types of murine helper T cell clone. II. Delayed-type hypersensitivity is mediated by Th1 clones. J Immunol 1987;138:3688–3694.
3   Chen H, Hendricks RL: B7 costimulatory requirements of T cells at an inflammatory site. J Immunol 1998;160:5045–5052.
4   June CH, Bluestone JA, Nadler LM, Thompson CB: The B7 and CD28 receptor family. Immunol Today 1994;15:321–331.
5   Liu Y, Linsley PS: Costimulation of T-cell growth. Curr Opin Immunol 1992;4:265–270.
6   Lenschow DJ, Walunas TL, Bluestone JA: CD28/B7 system of T cell costimulation. Annu Rev Immunol 1996;14:233–258.
7   Dutton RW, Bradley LM, Swain SL: T cell memory. Annu Rev Immunol 1998;16:201–223.
8   Mosmann TR, Sad S: The expanding universe of T cell subsets: Th1, Th2 and more. Immunol Today 1996;17:138–146.
9   Cherwinski HM, Schumacher JH, Brown KD, Mosmann TR: Two types of mouse helper cell clones. III. Further differences in lymphokine synthesis between Th1 and Th2 clones revealed by RNA hybridization, functionally monospecific bioassays, and monoclonal antibodies. J Exp Med 1987; 166:1229–1244.
10   Rook GA, Stanford JL: Give us this day our daily germs. Immunol Today 1998;19:113–116.
11   DeKruyff RH, Fang Y, Umetsu DT: IL-4 synthesis by in vivo primed keyhole limpet hemocyanin-specific CD4+ T cells. I. Influence of antigen concentration and antigen-presenting cell type. J Immunol 1992;149:3468–3476.
12   Weiner HL: Oral tolerance: Immune mechanisms and treatment of autoimmune diseases. Immunol Today 1997;18:335–343.
13   VanParijs L, Abbas AK: Homeostasis and self-tolerance in the immune system: Turning lymphocytes off. Science 1998;280:243–248.
14   Li H, Ren J, Dhabuwala CB, Shichi H: Immunotolerance induced by intratesticular antigen priming: Expression of TGF-β, Fas and Fas ligand. Ocul Immunol Inflamm 1997;5:75–84.
15   Griffith TS, Brunner T, Fletcher SM, Green DR, Ferguson TA: Fas ligand-induced apoptosis as a mechanism of immune privilege. Science 1995;270:1189–1192.
16   Bellgrau D, Gold D, Selawry H, Moore J, Franzusoff A, Duke RC: A role for CD95 ligand in preventing graft rejection. Nature 1995;377:630–632.
17   Glickstein L, Macphail S, Stutman O: Uncoupling IL-2 production from apoptosis and TNF production by changing the signal through the TCR. J Immunol 1996;156:2062–2067.
18   Hornung F, Zheng L, Lenardo MJ: Maintenance of clonotype specificity in CD95/Apo-1/Fas-mediated apoptosis of mature T lymphocytes. J Immunol 1997;159:3816–3822.

19 Akbar AN, Salmon M: Cellular environments and apoptosis: Tissue microenvironments control activated T-cell death. Immunol Today 1997;18:72–76.

20 Chen JJ, Sun Y, Nabel GJ: Regulation of the proinflammatory effects of Fas ligand (CD95L). Science 1998;282:1714–1717.

21 De Maria R, Testi R: Fas-FasL interactions: A common pathogenetic mechanism in organ-specific autoimunity. Immunol Today 1998;19:121–125.

22 Maggi E, Parronchi P, Manetti R, Simonelli C, Piccinni MP, Rugiu FS, De Carli M, Ricci M, Romagnani S: Reciprocal regulatory effects of INF-γ and IL-4 on the in vitro development of human Th1 and Th2 clones. J Immunol 1992;148:2142–2147.

23 Taylor AW, Alard P, Yee DG, Streilein JW: Aqueous humor induces transforming growth factor-beta-producing regulatory T-cells. Curr Eye Res 1997;16:900–908.

24 Trinchieri G, Perussia B: Immune interferon: A pleiotropic lymphokine with multiple effects. Immunol Today 1985;6:131–136.

25 Farrar MA, Schreiber RD: The molecular cell biology of interferon-γ and its receptor. Annu Rev Immunol 1993;11:571–611.

26 Yoneda Y, Yoshida R: The role of T cells in allografted tumor rejection: IFN-γ released from T cells is essential for induction of effector macrophages in the rejection site. J Immunol 1998;160:6012–6017.

27 Dvorak HF, Mihm MC Jr, Dvorak AM, Johnson RA, Manseau EJ, Morgan E, Colvin RB: Morphology of delayed-type hypersensitivity reactions in man. I. Quantitative description of the inflammatory response. Lab Invest 1974;31:111–130.

28 Dvorak AM, Mihm, MC Jr, Dvorak HF: Morphology of delayed-type hypersensitivity reactions in man. II. Ultrastructural alterations affecting the microvasculature and the tissue mast cells. Lab Invest 1976;34:179–191.

29 Buchanan KL, Murphy JW: Kinetics of cellular infiltration and cytokine production during the efferent phase of a delayed-type hypersensitivity reaction. Immunology 1997;90:189–197.

30 Wangoo A, Cook HT, Taylor GM, Shaw RJ: Enhanced expression of type 1 procollagen and transforming growth factor-beta in tuberculin induced delayed type hypersensitivity. J Clin Pathol 1995;48:339–345.

31 Kimura R, Hu H, Stein-Streilein J: Delayed-type hypersensitivity responses regulate collagen deposition in the lung. Immunology 1992;77:550–555.

32 Bennett NT, Schultz GS: Growth factors and wound healing: Biochemical properties of growth factors and their receptors. Am J Surg 1993;165:728–737.

33 Streilein JW, Takeuchi M, Taylor AW: Immune privilege, T-cell tolerance, and tissue-restricted autoimunity. Hum Immunol 1997;52:138–143.

34 Medawar P: Immunity to homologous grafted skin. III. The fate of skin homografts transplanted to the brain to subcutaneous tissue, and to the anterior chamber of the eye. Br J Exp Pathol 1948; 29:58–69.

35 Barker CF, Billingham RE: Immunologically privileged sites. Adv Immunol 1977;25:1–54.

36 Kaplan HJ, Streilein JW: Transplantation immunology of the anterior chamber of the eye. II. Immune response to allogeneic cells. J Immunol 1975;115:805–810.

37 Williamson JSP, Streilein JW: Impaired induction of delayed hypersensitivity following anterior chamber inoculation of alloantigens. Regul Immunol 1988;1:15–23.

38 Kaiser C, Ksander B, Streilein JW: Inhibition of lymphocyte proliferation by aqueous humor. Regul Immunol 1989;2:42–49.

39 Niederkorn JY, Benson JL, Mayhew E: Efferent blockade of delayed-type hypersensitivity responses in the anterior chamber of the eye. Regul Immunol 1991;3:349–354.

40 Cousins SW, Trattler WB, Streilein JW: Immune privilege and suppression of immunogenic inflammation in the anterior chamber of the eye. Curr Eye Res 1991;10:287–297.

41 Wilbanks GA, Streilein JW: Fluids from immune privileged sites endow macrophages with the capacity to induce antigen-specific immune deviation via a mechanism involving transforming growth factor-beta. Eur J Immunol 1992;22:1031–1036.

42 Wilbanks GA, Mammolenti M, Streilein JW: Studies on the induction of anterior chamber-associated immune deviation (ACAID). III. Induction of ACAID depends upon intraocular transforming growth factor-beta. Eur J Immunol 1992;22:165–173.

43   Taylor AW, Streilein JW, Cousins SW: Alpha-melanocyte-stimulating hormone suppresses antigen-stimulated T cell production of gamma-interferon. Neuroimmunomodulation 1994;1:188–194.

44   Knisely TL, Anderson TM, Sherwood ME, Flotte TJ, Albert DM, Granstein RD: Morphologic and ultrastructural examination of I-A$^+$ cells in murine iris. Invest Ophthalmol Vis Sci 1991;32:2423–2531.

45   McMenamin PG, Holthouse I, Holt PG: Class II major histocompatibility complex (Ia) antigen-bearing dendritic cells within the iris and ciliary body of the rat eye: Distribution, phenotype, and relation to retinal microglia. Immunology 1992;77:385–393.

46   Streilein JW, Cousins SW: Aqueous humor factors and their effects on the immune response in the anterior chamber. Curr Eye Res 1990;9:175–182.

47   Taylor AW: Immunoregulation of the ocular effector responses by soluble factors in aqueous humor. Regul Immunol 1994;6:52–57.

48   Wilson JF, Harry FM: Release, distribution and half-life of α-melanotrophin in the rat. Endocrinology 1980;86:61–67.

49   Taylor AW, Yee DG, Streilein JW: Suppression of nitric oxide generated by inflammatory macrophages by calcitonin gene-related peptide in aqueous humor. Invest Ophthalmol Vis Sci 1998;39:1372–1378.

50   Cousins SW, McCabe MM, Danielpour D, Streilein JW: Identification of transforming growth factor-beta as an immunosuppressive factor in aqueous humor. Invest Ophthalmol Vis Sci 1991;32:33–43.

51   Granstein R, Staszewski R, Knisely TL, Zeira E, Nazareno R, Latina M, Albert DM: Aqueous humor contains transforming growth factor-β and a small (<3,500 daltons) inhibitor of thymocyte proliferation. J Immunol 1990;144:3021–3026.

52   Taylor AW, Streilein JW, Cousins SW: Identification of alpha-melanocyte stimulating hormone as a potential immunosuppressive factor in aqueous humor. Curr Eye Res 1992;11:1199–1206.

53   Taylor AW, Streilein JW, Cousins SW: Immunoreactive vasoactive intestinal peptide contributes to the immunosuppressive activity of normal aqueous humor. J Immunol 1994;153:1080–1086.

54   Knisely TL, Hosoi J, Nazareno R, Grandstein RD: The presence of biologically significant concentrations of glucocorticoids but little or no cortisol binding globulin with aqueous humor: Relevance to immune privilege in the anterior chamber of the eye. Invest Ophthalmol Vis Sci 1994;35:3711–3723.

55   Nicolai J, Larsen B, Bersani M, Olcese J, Holst JJ, Moller M: Somatostatin and prosomatostatin in the retina of the rat: An immunohistochemical, in-situ hybridization, and chromatographic study. Vis Neurosci 1990;5:441–452.

56   Jampel HD, Roche N, Stark WJ, Roberts AB: Transforming growth factor-β in human aqueous humor. Curr Eye Res 1990;9:963–969.

57   Roberts AB, Sporn MB: Transforming growth factor β. Adv Cancer Res 1988;51:107–145.

58   Miyazono K, Olofsson A, Colosetti P, Heldin, CH: A role of the latent TGF-β$_1$-binding protein in the assembly and secretion of TGF-β$_1$. EMBO J 1991;10:1091–1101.

59   Flaumenhaft R, Kojima S, Abe M, Rifkin DB: Activation of latent transforming growth factor beta. Adv Pharmacol 1993;24:51–76.

60   Flaumenhaft R, Abe M, Sato Y, Miyazono K, Harpel J, Heldin CH, Rifkin DB: Role of the latent TGF-β binding protein in the activation of latent TGF-β by co-cultures of endothelial and smooth muscle cells. J Cell Biol 1993;120:995–1002.

61   Pasquale LR, Dorman-Pease ME, Lutty GA, Quigley HA, Jampel HD: Immunolocalization of TGF-β$_1$, TGF-β$_2$, and TGF-β$_3$ in the anterior segment of the human eye. Invest Ophthalmol Vis Sci 1993;34:23–30.

62   Knisely TL, Bleicher PA, Vibbard CA, Granstein RD: Production of latent transforming growth factor-beta and other inhibitory factors by cultured murine iris and ciliary body cells. Curr Eye Res 1991;10:761–771.

63   Nunes I, Shapiro RL, Rifkin DB: Characterization of latent TGF-beta activation by murine peritoneal macrophages. J Immunol 1995;155:1450–1459.

64   Munger JS, Harpel JG, Gleizes PE, Mazzieri R, Nunes I, Rifkin DB: Latent transforming growth factor-beta: Structural features and mechanisms of activation. Kidney Int 1997;51:1376–1382.

65   Hoehn P, Goedert S, Germann T, Koelsch S, Jin S, Palm N, Ruede E, Schmitt E: Opposing effects of TGF-β₂ on the Th1 cell development of naive CD4+ T cells isolated from different mouse strains. J Immunol 1995;155:3788–3793.

66   Takeuchi M, Kosiewicz MM, Alard P, Streilein JW: On the mechanisms by which transforming growth factor-β₂ alters antigen-presenting abilities of macrophages on T cell activation. Eur J Immunol 1997;27:1648–1656.

67   Takeuchi M, Alard P, Streilein JW: TGF-β promotes immune deviation by altering accessory signals of antigen-presenting cells. J Immunol 1998;160:1589–1597.

68   Bogdan C, Paik J, Vodovotz Y, Nathan C: Contrasting mechanisms for suppression of macrophage cytokine release by transforming growth factor-β and interleukin-10. J Biol Chem 1992;267:23301–23308.

69   Chantry D, Turner M, Abney E, Feldmann M: Modulation of cytokine production by transforming growth factor-β. J Immunol 1989;142:4295–4300.

70   Tsunawaki S, Sporn M, Ding A, Nathan C: Deactivation of macrophages by transforming growth factor-β. Nature 1988;334:260–262.

71   Taylor AW: Neuroimmunomodulation in immune privilege: Role of neuropeptides in ocular immunosuppression. Neuroimmunomodulation 1996;3:195–204.

72   Cannon JG, Tatro JB, Reichlin S, Dinarello CA: α-Melanocyte-stimulating hormone inhibits immunostimulatory and inflammatory actions of interleukin-1. J Immunol 1986;137:2232–2236.

73   Lee TH, Lerner AB, Buettner-Janusch V: The isolation and structure of α- and β-melanocyte-stimulating hormones from monkey pituitary glands. J Biol Chem 1961;236:1390–1394.

74   Nakanishi S, Inoue A, Kita T, Nakamura M, Chang ACY, Cohen SN, Numa S: Nucleotide sequence of cloned cDNA for bovine corticotropin-β-lipotropin precursor. Nature 1979;278:423–427.

75   Lipton JM, Catania A: Anti-inflammatory actions of the neuroimmunomodulator α-MSH. Immunol Today 1997;18:140–145.

76   Lipton JM: Modulation of host defense by the neuropeptide α-MSH. Yale J Biol Med 1990;63: 173–182.

77   Holdeman M, Khorram O, Samson WK, Lipton JM: Fever-specific changes in central MSH and CRF concentrations. Am J Physiol 1985;248:R125-R129.

78   Watanabe T, Hiltz ME, Catania A, Lipton JM: Inhibition of IL-1β-induced peripheral inflammation by peripheral and central administration of analogs of the neuropeptide α-MSH. Brain Res Bull 1993;32:311–314.

79   Martin LW, Catania A, Hiltz ME, Lipton JM: Neuropeptide alpha-MSH antagonizes IL-6- and TNF-induced fever. Peptides 1991;12:297–299.

80   Chiao H, Foster S, Thomas R, Lipton J, Star RA: α-Melanocyte-stimulating hormone reduces endotoxin-induced liver inflammation. J Clin Invest 1996;97:2038–2044.

81   Rajora N, Ceriani G, Catania A, Star RA, Murphy MT, Lipton JM: α-MSH production, receptors, and influence on neopterin in a human monocyte/macrophage cell line. J Leukocyte Biol 1996;59: 248–253.

82   Star RA, Rajora N, Huang J, Chavez R, Catania A, Lipton JM: Evidence of autocrine modulation of macrophage nitric oxide synthase by α-MSH. Proc Natl Acad Sci USA 1995;90:8856–8860.

83   Catania A, Rajora N, Capsoni F, Minonzio F, Star RA, Lipton JM: The neuropeptide α-MSH has specific receptors on neutrophils and reduces chemotaxis in vito. Peptides 1996;17:675–679.

84   Chakraborty AK, Funasaka Y, Slominski A, Ermak G, Hwang J, Pawelek JM, Ichihashi, M: Production and release of proopiomelanocortin (POMC)-derived peptides by human melanocytes and keratinocytes in culture: Regulation by ultraviolet B. Biochim Biophys Acta 1996;1313:130–138.

85   O'Donohue TL, Dorsa DM: The opiomelanotropinergic neuronal and endocrine systems. Peptides 1982;3:353–395.

86   Seder RA, Marth T, Sieve MC, Strober W, Letterio JJ, Roberts AB, Kelsall B: Factors involved in the differentiation of TGF-β-producing cells from naive CD4+ T cells: IL-4 and IFN-γ have opposing effects, while TGF-β positively regulates its own production. J Immunol 1998;160:5719–5728.

87   Uddman R, Alumets J, Ehinger B, Håkanson R, Lorén I, Sundler F: Vasoactive intestinal peptide nerves in ocular and orbital structures of the cat. Invest Ophthalmol Vis Sci 1980;19:878–885.

88 Muscettola M, Grasso G: Somatostatin and vasoactive intestinal peptide reduce interferon-gamma production by human peripheral blood mononuclear cells. Immunobiology 1990;180:419–430.

89 O'Dorisio MS, Wood CL, O'Dorisio TM: Vasoactive intestinal peptide and neuropeptide modulation of the immune response. J Immunol 1985;135:792s–796s.

90 Ottaway CA: Vasoactive intestinal peptide as a modulator of lymphocyte and immune function. Ann NY Acad Sci 1988;527:486–500.

91 Stanisz AM, Scicchitano R, Bienenstock J: The role of vasoactive intestinal peptide and other neuropeptides in the regulation of the immune response in vitro and in vivo. Ann NY Acad Sci 1988;527:478–485.

92 Tseng J, O'Dorisio MS: Mechanism of vasoactive intestinal peptide-mediated immunoregulation; in Goetzl EJ, Spector NH (eds): Neuroimmune Networks: Physiology and Diseases. New York, Liss, 1989, pp 105–111.

93 Boudard F, Bastide M: Inhibiton of mouse T-cell proliferation by CGRP and VIP: Effects of these neuropeptides on IL-2 production and cAMP synthesis. J Neurosci Res 1991;29:29–41.

94 Ganea D, Sun L: Vasoactive intestinal peptide downregulates the expression of IL-2 but not of INF-γ from stimulated murine T lymphocytes. J Neuroimmunol 1993;47:147–158.

95 Ottaway CA: Selective effects of vasoactive intestinal peptide on the mitogenic response of murine T cells. Immunology 1987;62:291–297.

96 Segura JJ, Guerrero JM, Goberna R, Calvo JR: Characterization of functional receptors for vasoactive intestinal peptide in rat peritoneal macrophages. Regul Pept 1991;33:133–143.

97 Wiik P, Opstad PK, Boyum A: Binding of vasoactive intestinal polypeptide by human blood monocytes: Demonstration of specific binding sites. Regul Pept 1985;12:145–153.

98 Wiik P, Haugen AH, Lovhaug D, Boyum A, Opstad PK: Effect of VIP on the respiratory burst in human monocytes ex vivo during prolonged strain and energy deficiency. Peptides 1989;10:819–823.

99 Wiik P: VIP inhibition of monocyte respiratory burst ex vivo during prolonged strain and energy deficiency. Int J Neurosci 1990;51:195–196.

100 Terenghi G, Polak JM, Ghatei MA, Mulderry PK, Butler JM, Unger WG, Bloom SR: Distribution and origin of calcitonin gene-related peptide immunoreactivity in the sensory innervation of the mammalian eye. J Comp Neurol 1985;233:506–516.

101 Kurz B, Von Gaudecker B, Kranz A, Krisch B, Mentlein R: Calcitonin gene-related peptide and its receptor in the thymus. Peptides 1995;16:1497–1503.

102 Asahina A, Moro O, Hosoi J, Lerner EA, Xu S, Takashima A, Granstein RD: Specific induction of cAMP in Langerhans' cells by calcitonin gene-related peptide: Relevance to functional effects. Proc Natl Acad Sci USA 1995;92:8323–8327.

103 Asahina A, Hosoi J, Biessert S, Stratigos A, Granstein RD: Inhibition of the induction of delayed-type and contact hypersensitivity by calcitonin gene-related peptide. J Immunol 1995;154:3056–3061.

104 Hanesch U, Pfrommer U, Grubb BD, Schaible HG: Acute and chronic phases of unilateral inflammation in rat's ankle are associated with an increase in the proportion of calcitonin gene-related peptide-immunoreactive dorsal root ganglion cells. Eur J Neurosci 1993;5:154–161.

105 Unger WG, Terenghi G, Ghatei MA, Ennis KW, Butler JM, Zhang SQ, Too HP, Polak JM, Bloom SR: Calcitonin gene-related polypeptide as a mediator of the neurogenic ocular injury response. J Ocul Pharmacol 1985;1:189–199.

106 Wahlestedt C, Beding B, Ekman R, Oksala O, Stjernschantz J, Håkanson R: Calcitonin gene-related peptide in the eye: Release by sensory nerve stimulation and effects associated with neurogenic inflammation. Regul Pept 1986;16:107–115.

107 Nong YH, Titus RG, Ribeiro JMC, Remold HG: Peptides encoded by the calcitonin gene inhibit macrophage function. J Immunol 1989;143:45–49.

108 Niizeki H, Alard P, Streilein JW: Calcitonin gene-related peptide is necessary for ultraviolet B-impaired induction of contact hypersensitivity. J Immunol 1997;159:5183–5186.

109 Wang ZY, Link H, Ljungdahl A, Hojeberg B, Link J, He B, Qiao J, Melms A, Olsson T: Induction of interferon-gamma, interleukin-4, and transforming growth factor-beta in rats orally tolerized against experimental autoimmune myasthenia gravis. Cell Immunol 1994;157:353–368.

110 Caspi R, Stiff L, Morawentz R, Miller-Rivero N, Chan C, Wiggert B, Nussenblatt R, Morse H, Rizzo L: Cytokine-dependent modulation of oral tolerance in a murine model of autoimmune uveitis. Ann NY Acad Sci 1996;778:315–324.
111 Chen Y, Kuchroo VK, Inobe JI, Hafler DA, Weiner HL: Regulatory T cell clones induced by oral tolerance: Suppression of autoimmune encephalomyelitis. Science 1994;265:1237–1240.
112 Brauner R, Nonoyama M, Laks H, Drinkwater DC Jr, McCaffery S, Drake T, Berk AJ, Sen L, Wu L: Intracoronary adenovirus-mediated transfer of immunosuppressive cytokine genes prolongs allograft survival. J Thorac Cardiovasc Surg 1997;114:923–933.
113 Croxford JL, Triantaphyllopoulos K, Podhajcer OL, Feldmann M, Baker D, Chernajovsky Y: Cytokine gene therapy in experimental allergic encephalomyelitis by injection of plasmid DNA-cationic liposome complex into the central nervous system. J Immunol 1998;160:5181–5187.
114 Song XY, Gu M, Jin WW, Klinman DM, Wahl SM: Plasmid DNA encoding transforming growth factor-β_1 suppresses chronic disease in a streptococcal cell wall-induced arthritis model. J Clin Invest 1998;101:2615–2621.
115 Wintzen M, Gilchrest BA: Proopiomelanocortin, its derived peptides, and the skin. J Invest Dermatol 1996;106:3–10.
116 Thody AJ, Ridley K, Penny RJ, Chalmers R, Fisher C, Shuster S: MSH peptides are present in mammalian skin. Peptides 1983;4:813–816.

Andrew W. Taylor, Schepens Eye Research Institute, Harvard Medical School,
20 Staniford Street, Boston MA 02114 (USA)
Tel. +1 617 912 7452, Fax +1 617 912 0101, E-Mail awtaylor@vision.eri.harvard.edu

Streilein JW (ed): Immune Response and the Eye.
Chem Immunol. Basel, Karger, 1999, vol 73, pp 90–119

....

Mechanisms of Intraocular Inflammation

M. Teresa Magone, Scott M. Whitcup

National Institutes of Health, National Eye Institute, Bethesda, Md., USA

Introduction

The uvea consists of the choroid, ciliary body, and the iris. Uveitis is a term used to describe the presence of intraocular inflammation, but does not identify the underlying cause or the exact location of disease in the eye. The anatomic site of most intense inflammation serves as the basis for major subdivisions of uveitis: anterior uveitis, if the anterior eye segment is involved; intermediate uveitis, if the area behind the lens, the pars plana, and the ciliary body are affected; and posterior uveitis, if the posterior eye segment is affected. However, intraocular inflammation may be limited to nonuveal tissues, including the retina or sclera. The term uveitis is sometimes applied to these conditions as well, although incorrectly by strict anatomical definition [1].

Intraocular inflammation may have exogenous causes, such as infection or trauma. Most forms of endogenous uveitis are thought to be caused by autoimmunity, characterized by the recognition and destruction of self components by the immune system, described in detail later. The multiple mechanisms involved in intraocular inflammation necessitate the development of several animal models to study pathogenesis and treatment approaches for various forms of the disease. Currently, several animal models parallel to human ocular inflammatory disease are available. These models mimic either autoimmune-mediated diseases, like experimental autoimmune uveitis, or infectious disease, such as the murine toxoplasmosis model [2–4]. In this chapter, we review animal models of uveitis and their relationship to human disease. Importantly we will focus on how these animal models have fostered new understanding of the pathogenesis of uveitis and allowed the development and testing of new therapies for the disease.

Before an inflammatory response in the eye is initiated fully, this organ's unique protective structure and blood flow of this organ must become acces-

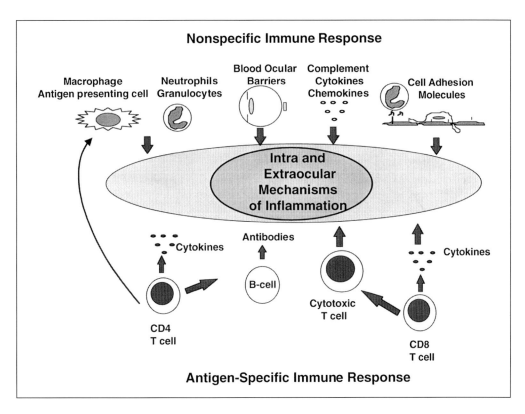

Fig. 1. Components of nonspecific and antigen-specific immune response.

sible for macromolecules and infiltrating cells [5]. The eye's outer surface is covered by the conjunctiva, a thin, well-vascularized, and transparent mucosal layer that serves as an immunological and protective barrier. Inside the eye, both the retina and anterior chamber have a well-regulated vascular network with blood-ocular barriers (BOBs) protecting them from intruding macromolecules. When the BOBs break down, leukocytes infiltrate the eye and release inflammatory mediators [6, 7]. Since the structure of the retina is not only very complex but also lacks the ability to regenerate, intraocular inflammation may lead to permanent damage and visual loss.

As stated in chapter 2, the immune system has two basic ways of responding to intruding antigens. A nonspecific immune response occurs when innate immune cells capture the antigen (fig. 1). This response leads to the elimination of the antigen and the attraction of additional inflammatory cells [8]. A specific immune response occurs when the antigen is processed and presented to specific T cells. Once these T cells are activated, they become effector cells and induce an immune response specific for that particular antigen [9]. In intraocular inflammation infiltrating cells, resident major histocompatibility complex (MHC) class II antigen presenting cells as well as resident mast cells play an important role in disease development [10, 11]. Chapter 9 describes resident ocular cells that participate in ocular inflammation. If inflammation is caused by an infectious organism, immune response may damage surrounding ocular tissue. In autoimmune disease, specific T cells recognize retinal proteins, like soluble antigen (S-Ag) or inter-photoreceptor retinoid-binding protein (IRBP) [12].

This chapter reviews the mechanisms of intraocular inflammation. We will illustrate how our knowledge of these mechanisms was acquired by studying experimental models of intraocular disease. Pursuing the route of an infiltrating cell, we will begin by describing the BOBs, the first obstacles for potential systemic ocular intruders, which leads us to the nonspecific and, finally, the antigen-specific elements of intraocular inflammation.

Nonspecific Immune Response

Blood-Ocular Barriers

The BOBs protect the eye from the influx of macromolecules. Early observations in the literature showed that intravenously applied dyes do not penetrate into the aqueous humor or the vitreous [13–15]. Ashton and Cunha-Vaz [16] demonstrated that histamine infusions did not increase the vascular permeability in the retina. This information pointed toward the presence of a BOB, similar to the blood-brain barrier, which limits permeability of the ocular vessels. Ultrastructural techniques have identified the anatomical basis of the two BOBs: the blood-aqueous barrier (BAB) and blood-retinal barrier (BRB). It is clear now that the tight junctions formed by endothelial and epithelial cells play an essential role in the blood-eye barrier function [17, 18].

The BAB has two components: the epithelial barrier of the nonpigmented and pigmented layers of the ciliary epithelium, and the posterior iris epithelium. These layers restrict flow of protein and cells from vessels into the anterior or posterior chamber (fig. 2). In addition to these anatomical obstacles, diffusion and transport activity into the anterior chamber is pressure-dependent, resembling an osmotic flow model [5, 18].

Figure 3 details the concept of the BRB, which is composed of an inner barrier and an outer barrier. The inner barrier consists of retinal capillaries that have tight junctions of the endothelial cells, a basement membrane, and intramural pericytes that make the vessel impermeable to macromolecules under normal conditions. The outer barrier of the BRB is located at the border

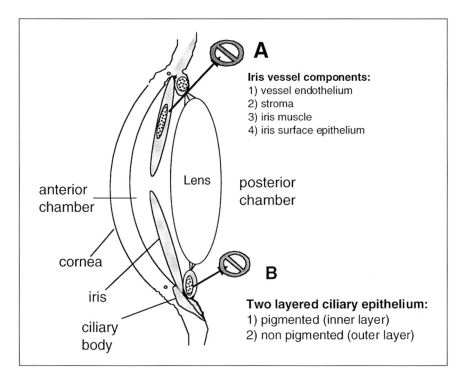

Fig. 2. In the BAB, extravasation of macromolecules from the iris vessels is prevented by four different layers (*A*): the endothelium, the iris stroma, the iris muscle, and the iris surface epithelium. Leakage from the ciliary vessels are kept from extravasation by the two-layered ciliary epithelium consisting of a pigmented and an unpigmented layer (*B*).

between the choriocapillaris, a layer rich in fenestrated vessels, and the retinal pigment epithelium (RPE), a single cell layer in contact with the photoreceptors of the retina [5]. Here, the tight connections between the RPE prevent leakage to the subretinal space and the sensory retina (fig. 3A).

Inflammation causes a breakdown of the BOBs [19]. This condition induces upregulation of cell adhesion molecule expression, and allows cells as well as macromolecules to leak into the vitreous and subretinal space, where cytokine and chemokine production attracts more cells and sustains the inflammatory response (fig. 3B) [7, 19–24]. There are multiple causes for the breakdown of the BOB including infection and trauma.

A model of experimental autoimmune uveitis (EAU) shows that albumin leakage into the peripheral retina starts 8 days after immunization, whereas the central retina is only affected later [25]. This development may be explained by differences in central and peripheral retina blood vessels. The central retina's

---

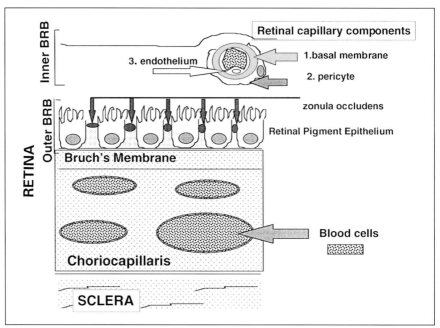

Retinal capillary components

3. endothelium

1.basal membrane

2. pericyte

zonula occludens

Retinal Pigment Epithelium

Bruch's Membrane

Blood cells

Choriocapillaris

SCLERA

Inner BRB

Outer BRB

RETINA

3A

capillary networks are three to four layers, although only one layer in the periphery, which may reduce compensation capacities in the peripheral retina and induce breakdown of the BRB [26, 27]. On the ultrastructural level, the inner BRB at the vascular endothelium seems to be affected first, but tight junctions of the inner and outer BRB are both affected during the inflammatory process. In addition, transendothelial vesicular albumin transport and intraendothelial diapedesis can be detected [7, 25].

Increasing levels of inflammation and the paralleled production of cytokines, chemokines, and cell adhesion molecule upregulation contribute to increased BOB leakage. This process precedes by several days the influx of cells into the eye. Prendergast et al. [28] recently demonstrated that activated S-Ag-specific or concanavalin-A-stimulated T cells from immunized Lewis rats can cross the BOBs after adoptive transfer into naive animals. Antigen-specific T cells have a biphasic infiltration at 24 h and then at 96–120 h after the adoptive transfer of cells, while infiltration of mitogen-activated cells into the retina peaks only at 24 h and then declines steadily.

Cell Adhesion Molecules (CAMs)

CAMs mediate contact between cells, and they interact in a variety of cell signals [29]. They are deeply involved in inflammatory responses and tissue

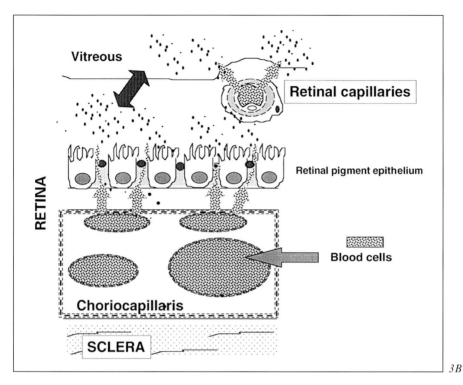

Vitreous

Retinal capillaries

Retinal pigment epithelium

RETINA

Blood cells

Choriocapillaris

SCLERA

3B

Fig. 3. BRB in health and disease. *A* The BRB consists of two parts: the inner BRB of the retinal capillaries, which prevents leakage from the retinal vessels, and the outer BRB, which prevents leakage from the choriocapillaris. *B* During ocular inflammation the barriers break down and macromolecules as well as cells can infiltrate the eye.

repair in response to injury. Several different families of CAMs contribute to leukocyte interaction with the endothelial cells and subsequent transmigration: the selectins, the integrins, the mucins (vascular addressins), and the immuno-globulin superfamily [30–34]. Chemoattractants released by cells in the tissues surrounding the blood vessel diffuse into the vessel and attract and direct cells toward the site of inflammation. CAMs can affect the integrity of the BOB prior to transmigration of inflammatory cells.

This transmigration is a multistep event controlled by the interaction of the cells with several CAMs [35]. The event consists of attachment, rolling, mediated by selectins, arrest, adhesion, and, finally, transendothelial migration of the cells into the tissue, mediated by integrins and members of the immuno-globulin superfamily [36–38].

The selectins are particularly important for leukocyte homing to specific tissues, and initiate the first step, attachment, by forming labile adhesions with the mucins expressed on the vascular endothelium [39]. In animal models of uveitis, E- and P-selectin were shown to be expressed on the vascular endothelium of the ciliary body before the influx of cells into the eye [40–42]. Blockage of CAMs can inhibit development of experimental endotoxin-induced uveitis (EIU) [43, 44]. From studies in selectin knockout mice it was shown that P-selectin is responsible for early neutrophil recruitment [45]. P-selectin also binds to bacterial lipopolysaccharide (LPS) and intravenous administration of LPS resulted in a 5-fold increase in plasma P-selectin in rats [46, 47]. We have previously shown that treatment with monoclonal antibodies to E- and P-selectin inhibited EIU [43]. Similarly, in vivo observations with a scanning laser ophthalmoscope showed reduced rolling and infiltration into the eye after treatment with anti-P-selectin antibodies in EIU [24]. This demonstrates the involvement of the selectins in leukocyte recruitment into the site of inflammation.

This interaction between the leukocyte and the endothelium slows the leukocyte, and it starts rolling along the endothelium. This rolling before onset of experimental uveitis and cellular infiltration into the vitreous has been demonstrated in vivo [24, 48].

The integrin molecules are involved in arrest of the cells. Among the most important is lymphocyte function-associated antigen-1 (LFA-1), which is expressed on all leukocytes (including T cells). LFA-1 binds to its counter-receptor intercellular adhesion molecule (ICAM-1) of the immunoglobulin superfamily, expressed on the vascular endothelium. Prior to the development of acute inflammation, ICAM-1 is expressed at low levels on the ciliary body epithelium, vascular endothelium of the iris and ciliary body, and the cornea [44]. Mast cells, which reside in the eye, play a role in experimental animals' susceptibility to uveitis, can upregulate ICAM-1 and vascular cell adhesion molecule-1, probably through the release of the proinflammatory cytokine tumor necrosis factor-α (TNF-α) [10, 49].

ICAM-1 is upregulated in the eyes of patients with uveitis and in experimental uveitis models [40, 50, 51]. The integrins can be upregulated rapidly during inflammation, and adhesiveness can increase within a few minutes [52]. The cells then arrest, and the actual adhesion between cell and endothelium takes place, enabling transmigration of the leukocyte into the tissue [36].

The role of cell adhesion in cell extravasation and migration offer potential future therapeutic options in the treatment of intraocular inflammation and the associated cellular infiltration [24, 43, 44, 53]. Treatment with monoclonal antibodies to ICAM-1 and LFA-1 may suppress EAU in a manner dependent on dosage and time after immunization [54]. In addition, recent reports show that CAMs also play a role in T-cell activation [55, 56]. These functions offer additional ways to potentially target and decrease T-cell-mediated disease activity present in autoimmune human uveitis.

Recently, the chemokine fractalkine, which is a transmembrane mucin-chemokine hybrid molecule expressed on activated endothelium, and its receptor were identified, which have overlapping functions with CAMs [57, 58]. Fractalkine was shown to mediate capture and integrin-independent adhesion and activation of leukocytes [57, 59]. The presence of leukocyte trafficking regulators which are able to induce cell adhesion and chemotaxis not only sheds new light on leukocyte migration, but it also can become a target for anti-inflammatory agents.

Inflammatory Mediators

While CAMs regulate migration of inflammatory cells into affected tissue, ocular inflammatory disease is mediated through soluble products secreted by participating and recruited inflammatory cells. These products are cytokines, chemokines, complement factors, and cellular enzymes. They initiate the inflammatory response at different levels simultaneously, and exhibit complex interactions, which are still under active investigation. In this section, we describe their functions and roles in intraocular disease.

Complement

There are three ways to complement activation: the classical pathway, the lectin-mediated pathway, and the alternative pathway as reviewed in Janeway and Travers [60]. All result in recruitment of inflammatory cells, opsonization of pathogens, and the destruction of pathogens. As in other tissues, complement is an important comediator in intraocular inflammation [21]. C5a, an anaphylatoxin, is activated by antigen-antibody complexes and when injected into the vitreous induces cellular infiltration [61]. Other complement factors, C3a and C4a, are present in the vitreous of patients with AIDS or bacterial infections [62, 63]. In experimental models, inactivation of plasma complement components inhibited disease in a lens-induced uveitis model, but not in a model of corneal inflammation [64, 65].

Complement, together with chemokines, cytokines, cellular enzymes, and other soluble factors, initiate simultaneous inflammatory response at different levels simultaneously.

Chemokines

Chemokines are chemotactic cytokines involved in cell recruitment and activation during inflammation. They are a group of small proteins with a molar mass of 8–10 kDa, which is still growing as new members are identified. Chemokines can be divided into subgroups depending on the position of the first two cysteines in the amino terminus of the proteins: CXC, CC, and C-x$_3$-C, and C chemokines [58, 66, 67]. The CXC chemokines are primarily chemotactic for neutrophils and for endothelial cells, and interleukin (IL)-8 is the most studied member of this class [68]. In contrast, the CC chemokines are primarily chemotactic for T lymphocytes, macrophages/monocytes, basophils, and eosinophils. RANTES, macrophage inflammatory protein (MIP), and monocyte chemoattractant protein-1 (MCP-1) are the best characterized CC chemokines [60, 68–70]. The C-x$_3$-C chemokine is a recent addition with so far only one identified representative: neurotactin/fractalkine [58]. This chemokine is distinct from other chemokines, because it has cell-adhesive capabilities [59]. It is a membrane-bound glycoprotein with a mucin-like stalk. It can be induced on endothelial cells by inflammatory cytokines and it promotes the adhesion and migration of monocytes and T lymphocytes [57]. The C chemokine subgroup consists of lymphotactin, a chemoattractant for T cells and NK cells [71].

Until now, few chemokines have been investigated in intraocular inflammation, although it is becoming evident that these proteins are crucial in the initial phase of inflammation. IL-8 is produced by lymphocytes, macrophages, fibroblasts, epithelial cells, and vascular endothelial cells. IL-8 attracts mainly PMNs, and its production can be induced by IL-1 and TNF [72, 73]. Intravitreal injection of human IL-8 in rats induces a significant neutrophilic infiltration in the iris, ciliary body, cornea, anterior and posterior chamber 10–24 h after injection [74]. IL-8 was also detected in 45% of vitreous samples of patients with uveitis [75]. In another study, IL-8, MCP-1, and RANTES were elevated in aqueous samples of patients with active anterior uveitis, but undetectable during quiescent phases of disease [76].

MCP-1 is thought to contribute to initial recruitment of inflammatory cells into the anterior chamber in an experimental model of autoimmune encephalomyelitis-associated anterior uveitis [77]. Once activated, T cells migrate in response to the chemokines [78]. The role of MCP-1 and RANTES in initiating cellular infiltration in EAU and EIU are currently under investigation.

Cytokines

During the last decade, a crucial role of cytokines in intraocular inflammation was revealed. These glycoproteins are secreted by inflammatory cells and have autocrine, paracrine, and endocrine functions. Mouse CD4+ T cells are defined as Th1 or Th2 cells by the different cytokines they produce [79–81]. Th1-associated CD4+ T cells are predominant in autoimmune diseases, such as EAU, while Th2 cells accumulate in the conjunctiva of patients with vernal conjunctivitis [82]. Although Th1 and Th2 cells have different functions, they can upregulate and downregulate each other through the cytokines that they produce. For example, IL-10 is a potent inhibitor of IL-12, a Th1-associated cytokine. This inhibition can be synergized by IL-4, a Th2-type cytokine. IL-12 can induce IL-10 production and downregulate itself, as will be described below. However, the constantly increasing knowledge of cytokine-mediated functions demonstrates that those proteins act in a complex interactive network with security nets to avoid exacerbations during an immune response.

IL-1 is mainly produced by macrophages and is considered to be a major proinflammatory cytokine with biologic effects similar to TNF. Different stimuli, such as LPs, TNF, or other cytokines can induce IL-1 production; on the other hand, IL-1 induces the secretion of prostaglandins, tissue-damaging proteases, and cytokines, such as IL-6, and TNF-α [83, 84]. Inflammatory cells can produce receptor antagonists, which downregulate the effects of IL-1 [85].

Experimental studies showed that intravitreal injection of human IL-1 into rabbit eyes induces an acute cellular infiltration of the uvea and retina with PMNs, and subsequently, monocytes [83, 86]. IL-1 receptor antagonists are only protective when injected prior to the cytokine, but ineffective if injected after onset of inflammation. In EIU, the IL-1 receptor antagonist has no effect on disease development [87]. This observation is probably because of involvement of other cytokines in EIU [22]. In addition, inhibition of platelet-activating factor (PAF) through an antagonist, inhibited IL-1-induced inflammation [88].

TNF-α is a mediator of acute inflammatory reactions, especially in response to gram-negative bacteria. As stated previously, the biological activities of TNF-α resemble those of IL-1. TNF-α is secreted by macrophages and is a chemoattractant, upregulating cell adhesion expression on vascular endothelial cells [89, 90]. TNF-α also stimulates mononuclear phagocytes to produce cytokines, including IL-1, IL-6, and itself [90]. Injection of TNF-α into the vitreous induces vascular permeability and cellular infiltration which peaks between 24 and 48 h after injection. This relatively delayed monocytic infiltration may be an indirect effect of other involved mediators. TNF-α is also elevated in the aqueous in EIU in the rat, and, interestingly, neutralization of this cytokine with monoclonal antibodies exacerbated disease [22]. Also, inhibition of TNF-α activity prevents tissue destruction, but not retinal cell infiltration in EAU in the rat [91]. Again, this development suggests a complex interrelationship of this cytokine with other factors of ocular disease.

Another cytokine involved in EIU is IL-6. Intraocular injection of this cytokine induces vascular permeability as well as uveal and retinal infiltration with polymorphonuclear leukocytes. IL-6 can be detected in the aqueous in EIU in rats, and in human uveitis [22, 92]. However, multiple injections in EIU in rats induced desensitization and unresponsiveness [93, 94]. Recently, it was shown that IL-6 knockout mice are able to develop EIU [95]. This indicates that in contrast to the observations in rats, IL-6 does not mediate EIU in mice.

Interferon-γ (IFN-γ) is a central cytokine in autoimmune-mediated uveitis. It is primarily produced by stimulated antigen-specific T cells and skews the immune response towards a Th1 phenotype. Intravitreal injection of this cytokine induced intraocular infiltration into the uvea, the vitreous, and the aqueous humor, consisting mainly of PMNs and monocytes [96]. Low systemic application of IFN-γ induces upregulation of MHC class II molecules on intraocular cells [97].

Recently, through the availability of cytokine-deficient mice, the role of IFN-γ and its close relationship with IL-12 in EAU has been studied. When IL-12 is present, Th1 cells can develop in the absence of IFN-γ [98]. IFN-γ-deficient mice were able to develop EAU, but disease development showed a certain immunodeviation towards a Th-2 phenotype. Interestingly, infiltrating cells in IFN-γ knockout mice had a high granulocytic percentage compared to the monocytic infiltration in wild-type mice [99]. In contrast, IL-12-deficient mice did not develop EAU, and treatment with monoclonal antibodies to IL-12 prevented EAU, which points towards a crucial role of IL-12 in effector T-cell development [100–102]. Surprisingly, exogenous IL-12 treatment can also prevent autoimmune disease, depending on the time point of treatment, as shown in an experimental diabetes model [103]. This paradoxical effect of IL-12 seems to be linked to an induction of IL-10 production, which is an antagonist of IL-12. Anti-IL-10 antibody treatment reversed the protective effect of exogenous IL-12 treatment in collagen-induced arthritis, another Th1-mediated autoimmune disease [104].

IL-10-deficient mice are susceptible to EAU, and exogenous IL-10 treatment in immunized mice had a protective role [105]. Systemic neutralization of IL-10 resulted in elevated disease scores. However, IL-10-deficient mice were also protected from the development of EAU after treatment with exogenous IL-12 [106]. This suggests a disease-limiting, but not an essential role of IL-10 in the development of EAU. In EIU, IL-10 reduced the cellular infiltration into the eye, but had no influence on the protein extravasation into the anterior chamber [107].

Similarly to other models of autoimmunity, exogenous IL-12 treatment in EAU was also protective in susceptible mouse strains immunized with complete Freund's adjuvant (CFA) and *pertussis toxin*, conditions which usually induce high amounts of endogenous IL-12. The observed protective effect of IL-12 treatment in EAU was discussed to be induced by the apoptotic deletion of antigen-specific effector cells in the presence of an excess amount of IL-12 [101]. IL-12 is a major inducer of IFN-γ and the latter is an inducer of nitric oxide synthase (iNOS) and consequently of nitric oxide (NO)

[108–111], and on the other hand, NO can trigger apoptosis [112–114]. In addition, recent experiments with IL-12-, iNOS-, and Bcl2-deficient mice have fortified the theory that IL-12-dependent IFN-γ and NO production trigger the apoptosis of uveitogenic effector cells [106, 115].

Another cytokine, transforming growth factor-β (TGF-β), has been described as an IL-12 antagonist [98]. TGF-β_2 is present in high amounts in the normal aqueous and vitreous, and these levels decrease during inflammation [116–118]. Intravitreal coinjection of LPS and TGF-β_2 in rabbits decreased cellular infiltration into the eye compared to control animals injected with LPS alone [119]. Also, TGF-β production is associated with the induction of protective oral tolerance, and its neutralization can reverse this protection [120]. TGF-β-deficient mice die because of an excessive inflammatory response, which points towards a protective role of this cytokine [121].

Finally, the interaction of the CD40 molecule on the antigen presenting cells (APC) with the CD40 ligand (CD40L) on the T cells was recently described, and its role in autoimmune diseases has been under investigation. This interaction induces costimulation of the B7-molecules and IL-12 release from the APC [122, 123]. The CD40/CD40L interaction is essential for T-cell activation and the induction of autoimmune disease, and blockage of this interaction inhibited disease in different models of autoimmune disease, including EAU [124–129]. Treatment with anti-CD40L antibodies also reduced disease in a delayed treatment group in EAU, which could be potentially useful as a therapeutic approach in human autoimmune uveitis [129].

In summary, although many cytokines play an essential role in autoimmune eye diseases, it seems that IL-12 has a crucial and defining role in the development of effector cells in autoimmune uveoretinitis. The balance of the complex cytokine network, and the timepoint of disease development are potential targets for future intervention and prevention of intraocular inflammation.

Animal Models

Animal models of nonantigen-specific immune reactions mimic ocular inflammation caused by trauma, surgery, or bacterial infection. One of these models, EIU, has been particularly useful to study nonspecific mechanisms of ocular immunity, like cell-adhesion molecule upregulation, cytokine secretion, and cell extravasation [22, 23, 50].

Bacterial Product-Induced Uveitis

EIU is a useful model to study the effects of nonspecific toxic inflammatory products, like endotoxins in the eye. EIU was first described in 1943, when it was discovered that an intravenous injection of endotoxin could induce ocular inflammation in dogs, cats, or rabbits [130]. Later, this method of inducing intraocular inflammation was transferred successfully to Lewis and Columbia-Sherman rats, and, more recently, to C3H/Hen mice [131–133].

Various routes of endotoxin application are possible, such as intraocular, intravenous, intraperitoneal, subcutaneous, or intra-footpad. The latter is the most popular route in mice and rats.

Twenty-four hours after the endotoxin has been deposited into the foot-pad, the animals have ocular disease characterized by miosis, iris hyperemia, breakdown of the BOBs with leakage of protein into the aqueous humor, as well as infiltration of cells into the anterior uvea, anterior chamber, and the vitreous. In mice, the cells infiltrate into the optic nerve head [133]. This cellular infiltration consists of PMNs, monocytes, and T lymphocytes, and is thought to be mediated through cytokines released from activated cells. Endotoxins, like LPS, are inducers of cytokines, oxygen metabolites, prostaglandin E_2, and leukotriene B_4 [134–136]. TNF-α, IL-1, IL-6, and IL-8 are stimulated by endotoxins [72, 93, 137].

The first cytokines that can be detected in the aqueous humor after endotoxin injection are IL-6 and TNF [138]. TNF can have more than inflammatory effects in EIU because, in this model, treatment with neutralizing antibodies to this cytokine exacerbated disease development [22]. CAMs are upregulated in EIU, and, previously, we have shown that monoclonal antibodies against ICAM-1 and LFA-1 can inhibit disease [44, 53]. Also, anti-inflammatory agents, like corticosteroids, can reduce inflammation, which makes this model a good template to study therapeutic approaches of nonspecific intraocular inflammation [139].

Antigen-Specific Immune Response

Autoimmunity

The immune system can discriminate between self and foreign antigen and can be tolerant to self while responding to foreign. This ability can be attributed to elimination of autoreactive cells in the thymus during development (negative selection) [140]. The eye, however, has been considered to be an immunologically privileged organ with expression of ocular proteins exclusively within the intraocular environment [141]. Until recently it was thought that this theoretical sequestration of ocular antigens made auto-immune uveitis possible, because inadvertent exposure of those antigens to the immune system predisposed the host to an immune reaction and subsequently to the development of uveitis. However, the detection of constitutive expression of ocular antigens in the thymus and its relationship to disease resistance in EAU challenges the sequestration theory [142, 143]. It seems that central tolerance is to some extent involved in the development of resistance to organ-specific autoimmune disease [142].

Autoreactive 'intolerant' cells that are not deleted can become activated and induce autoimmune disease [144]. Currently, it is not known what triggers the activation of autoreactive T cells specific for retinal antigens. However, when a foreign antigen that is a molecular mimicry of the retinal self antigen is presented to specific T cells, they become activated and induce disease wherever that antigen is expressed [145–147]. Subsequently, B cells are activated and develop into autoantibody-producing cells [148–150]. The current knowledge on intraocular inflammation has been acquired with the help of experimental animal models of autoimmune diseases. In the next section, we will describe the most important models and briefly discuss their clinical relevance.

Experimental Melanin Protein-Induced Uveitis (EMIU)

This recently developed model affects mainly the anterior segment of the eye, mimicking anterior uveitis in man. EMIU is induced by immunization of Lewis rats with the uveitogenic melanin proteins of bovine or other origin, emulsified in CFA with *pertussis toxin* [151, 152]. Two weeks after immunization, the rats develop anterior uveitis. As in human anterior uveitis, the features of EMIU include hyperemia, pupil constriction, flare, and cells in the aqueous. Histopathologic changes include the presence of exudate and cells in the anterior (fig. 4A) and posterior chambers (fig. 4B). The iris and the ciliary body have mononuclear, as well as polymorphonuclear, infiltration. Although a choroiditis may be present, the retina is not affected. EMIU is thought to be a T-cell-mediated disease. Broekhuyse et al. [151, 153] showed that disease can be transferred adoptively by CD4+ T cells but not by hyperimmune serum. In addition, treatment of the animals with cyclosporine, a T-cell-suppressing drug, can inhibit disease [151]. Idiopathic human anterior uveitis is thought to be autoimmune-mediated, and EMIU is a useful model to study the mechanisms of this disease.

Lens-Induced Uveitis

Clinically, lens-induced uveitis is initiated when the lens capsule is damaged, and large amounts of lens proteins come in contact with the immune system, which then reacts. This reaction can happen, for example, in traumatic intraocular injuries. The resulting inflammatory reaction is thought to be an autoimmune response to those proteins. In the animal models, the lens is punctured artificially after the immunization with the lens protein [154, 155]. Clinically, experimental lens-induced uveitis is characterized by anterior chamber inflammation and flare.

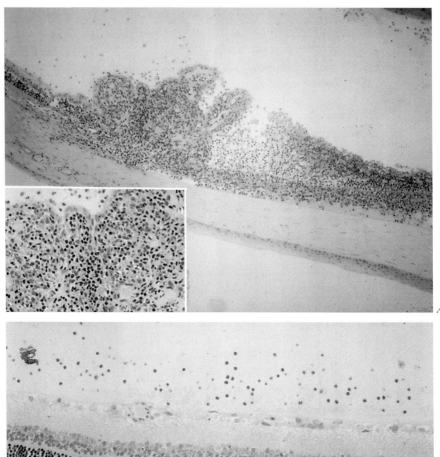

Fig. 4. Microphotograph of histopathology in EMIU. On day 14 after the immunization of the rats a dense cellular infiltration can be observed in the ciliary body and anterior chamber (*A*) (HE, ×100, inset ×400), and in the posterior segment (*B*) (×400). Courtesy of Dr. Chi Chao Chan.

The animal disease is induced by a type III reaction involving antigen antibody complexes and complement [20]. Disease can be transferred into naive animals by passive transfer of serum from sensitized animals into naive animals [156]. In addition, cyclosporine does not inhibit lens-induced uveitis [157], and immunization of rabbits with allogeneic or xenogeneic lens crystallins did not induce cellular immunity towards allogeneic lens antigens [158]. These observations have contributed to the theory of a type III-mediated hypersensitivity reaction.

Recently, a new model of cell-mediated lens-induced uveitis was described [159]. In this model, wild-type FVB/N mice are immunized with hen-egg lysozyme (HEL), a foreign protein emulsified in CFA. Two weeks after priming, the splenocytes from donors are harvested and cultured with HEL in vitro. These stimulated cells are adoptively transferred into a FVBN/ transgenic mouse, which expresses HEL only in the lens. Four days after transfer, these recipients develop lens-induced uveitis with severe cellular infiltration and proteinaceous exudate surrounding the lens in both the anterior and posterior segments of the eye.

Experimental Autoimmune Uveitis

EAU is an important model for autoimmune eye diseases. It represents posterior human uveitis, and new therapeutic approaches can be evaluated with this model that can be monitored clinically through the unique transparent media of the eye. EAU has been induced in a variety of animals, such as mice, rats, guinea pigs, rabbits, and primates [2–4, 160–163]. It is induced by the immunization of susceptible animals with retinal antigens subcutaneously.

The five major uveitogenic retinal antigens are retinal S-Ag, IRBP, rhodopsin, phospoducin, and recoverin [164–167]. S-Ag is a 48-kDa intracellular photoreceptor protein, which is involved in the phototransduction cascade [168]. S-Ag alone does not induce disease; however, it is very uveitopathogenic when adjuvant is added during immunization. This effect can be enhanced by the addition of one simultaneous injection of *pertussis toxin*, but the exact mechanism for this stimulatory effect is still unclear. IRBP is a 148-kDa protein expressed in the interphotoreceptor matrix thought to be involved in vitamin A transport [169]. IRBP is the major soluble protein of the interphotoreceptor matrix of vertebrate retinas and is highly uveitogenic in Lewis rats, mice, monkeys, and rabbits, but not in guinea pigs [4, 170–172]. Rhodopsin is a 40-kDa intracellular protein, which is the pigment of the rod [173]. Recoverin is a 23-kDa calcium-binding protein which is highly uveitogenic in rats, even in very low doses [174, 175]. In addition, recoverin was also identified as a target in a process called cancer-associated retinopathy (CAR) which is thought to be autoimmune-mediated [176–178]. However, a similar clinical disease with

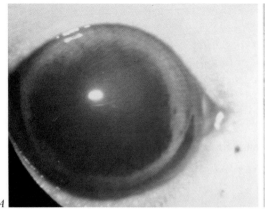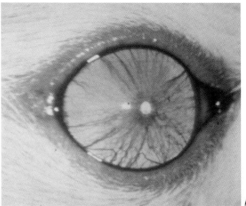

Fig. 5. Clinical appearance of rat EAU. The animals develop dilation of blood vessels in the iris, and inflammatory cells typically infiltrate into the anterior chamber, causing opacity (*A*). Normal rat eye (*B*) EAU.

humoral and also a cellular response to recoverin in the absence of malignancy was recently observed, and this condition was termed recoverin-associated retinopathy [179]. Phosducin is a 33-kDa retinal and pineal phosphoprotein involved in visual phototransduction, which also has mild uveitogenic capacities [165, 166]. IRBP, S-Ag, recoverin, and phosducin are expressed in the retina and the pineal gland. The pineal gland has photoreceptor functions in lower vertebrates, and, although it has evolved to a secretory organ in mammals, S-Ag, IRBP, and recoverin are is still expressed in this organ [20]. Immunization with minimal amounts of these proteins (50 µg), mostly of bovine origin emulsified in adjuvant, causes specific T-cell activation. Those activated cells attack the retinal proteins in the eyes of the experimental animals 10–21 days after immunization, depending on the utilized animal model [180].

EAU is a T-cell-mediated disease and members of the Vβ8+ T-cell subfamily were shown to accumulate in the retina of rats with EAU [181, 182]. This disease can also be induced by adoptive transfer of sensitized lymph node cells, CD4+ T-cell lines, MHC class II-restricted T-cell lines, and in the absence of serum antibodies [183–185]. On the other hand, EAU cannot be induced through the transfer of S-Ag-specific antibodies [186].

Clinically, the animals develop dilation of blood vessels in the iris, synechia (pupil attachment to the lens through deposition of fibrin). In rats, inflammatory cells typically infiltrate into the anterior chamber, causing opacity, and in severe cases, even hyphema (hemorrhage in the anterior chamber) (fig. 5). In the mouse, there is less involvement in the anterior part of the eye, but

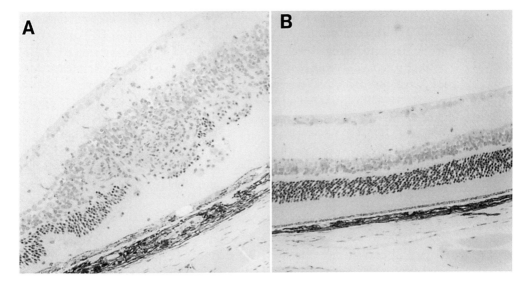

Fig. 6. Microphotograph of the histopathology in EAU in the mouse. Destruction of the retinal structure, and formation of retinal folds can be observed in the eyes of immunized mice (*A*), but not in the normal mouse retina (*B*). HE, ×400.

fundoscopic examination under the microscope reveals vasculitis with perivascular infiltrates, disc edema, and retinal hemorrhages.

Histopathology is graded from 0.5 to 4 and shows infiltration of the photoreceptor layer, retinal folds and granuloma formation, perivasculitis, retinal detachment, and the ultimate result is destruction of the retinal structure in severe cases (fig. 6). T lymphocytes and PMNs are the predominant inflammatory cells involved in the acute phase of rat EAU, but infiltrating macrophages can also be found [183, 187].

Specifically which antigens are involved in human uveitic disease is unclear. In vitro studies show that lymphocytes from patients with uveitis develop lymphoproliferative responses to S-Ag and IRBP [180, 188]. Immunodominant uveitogenic peptides of these antigens may induce disease in animals at doses as low as one tenth of a microgram per animal [189–191]. In addition, inflammatory responses can be induced with synthetic peptides [192].

Genetic susceptibility also plays an important role in the development of disease and in the experimental models MHC, but other factors determine the susceptibility and severity of disease development. Strains with low susceptibility, like the Fischer rats, share parts of the MHC gene products, namely the RT1 gene, with the highly susceptible Lewis rat [193, 194]. This points towards the involvement of other factors in disease development. Also, in the mouse, non-MHC genes seem to determine the severity of disease development [4, 195]. In human uveitic disease, several associations with HLA have been made. Perhaps the most well known are the frequent presence of HLA-B27 positivity in patients with recurrent anterior uveitis and the association between HLA-A29 positivity and birdshot retinochoroidopathy [196–199].

Studies with autoimmune animal models over past decades provide greater understanding of the mechanisms involved in intraocular inflammation. Human uveitic disease, however, is a complex event which involves multiple factors and mechanisms. Future studies need to investigate the exact initiating events of ocular autoimmune disease in order to implement a curative, instead of a therapeutic, intervention.

Ocular Infection – Animal Model

Infectious ocular inflammation models may be induced topically or secondary after systemic infection. We describe here two recently developed models of ocular toxoplasmosis, one induced systemically and the other topically. As in autoimmune diseases, animal models of infectious disease enable the researcher to study different aspects of the disease mechanisms and pathogenesis and to implement potential therapies.

Murine Ocular Toxoplasmosis

Ocular toxoplasmosis is believed to be the most common disease involving the retina of immunocompetent individuals [200]. Although many cases of ocular toxoplasmosis are thought to be congenital, recent studies indicate that a high percentage of patients have acquired disease after birth [201–206]. In a recent model, disease is induced by the intraperitoneal inoculation of C57BL/6 mice with cysts from the ME-49 strain of *toxoplasma gondii*. Two weeks later, the mice develop cysts in the brain and, much less frequently, in the eye [207]. The infiltrating cells in the eye and the brain are mainly CD8 T cells and CD4 T cells, at a ratio of 1:5, as well as macrophages. The cysts and the reaction they induce result in retinal lesions with dense lymphocytic infiltrate, which disrupt the retinal structure (fig. 7). A high upregulation of messenger RNA expression of IFN-γ and TNF-α were also detected in the eyes of infected animals. These cytokines seem to play an essential role in controlling parasite growth in this T-cell-mediated disease; in vivo blockage of the cytokines and/ or of the T cells result in an exacerbation of disease, and treatment with recombinant IFN-γ improved encephalitic disease [207, 208]. Thus, this may contribute to the high incidence rate of toxoplasmosis in immunocompromised patients [209]. This model allows study of the pathogenesis, disease development, and treatment of toxoplasmosis. Another model of acute ocular toxoplasmosis has been developed where the tachyzoites of the PLK strain of

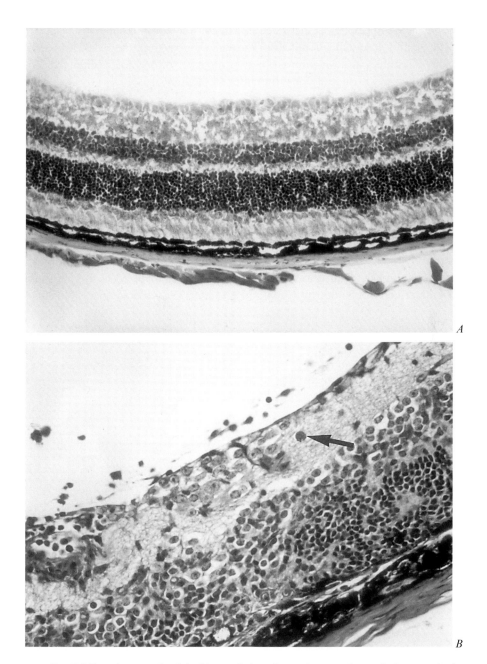

Fig. 7. Microphotograph of the histopathology in murine toxoplasmosis. Intact retinal structure on the day of immunization (*A*), and retinal inflammation and destruction 29 days after immunization (*B*). Cystic infiltrate into the retina can occasionally be observed (arrow). HE, ×400. Courtesy of Dr. Chi Chao Chan.

T. gondii are injected into the vitreous. The intraocular inflammatory response is acute and dose-dependent [210]. Through the injection, the BOBs are artificially disrupted, and the afferent loop of disease pathogenesis is changed, but the model serves to study new therapies for acute disease.

Corneal Transplantation

After the recognition of the donor graft by APC, cytotoxic T cells target and destroy the corneal cells. The resulting inflammation, with the upregulation of CAMs and, ultimately, graft rejection, will be discussed in detail in chapter by Streilein [this volume, pp.186–206].

Ocular Tumor Immunology

Immune responses against intraocular tumors can be cell-mediated and antibody-mediated. The targets for the immune system are either tumor-specific or tumor-associated antigens. The mechanisms involved in this response are described in chapter by Chen and Ksander [this volume, pp. 137–158].

References

1   Nussenblatt RB, Whitcup SM, Palestine AG: Uveitis: Fundamentals and Clinical Practice, ed 2. St Louis, Mosby-Year Book, 1996.
2   Wacker WB, Donoso LA, Kalsow CM, Yankeelov YA, Organisciak DT: Experimental allergic uveitis: Isolation, characterization, and localisation of a soluble uveitopathogenic antigen from bovine retina. J Immunol 1977;119:1949–1958.
3   Nussenblatt RB, Kuwabara T, de Monasterio F, Wacker W: S-antigen uveitis in primates. A new model for human disease. Arch Ophthalmol 1981;99:1090–1092.
4   Caspi R, Roberge F, Chan CC, Wiggert B, Chader GJ, Rozenszajn L, Lando Z, Nussenblatt RB: A new model of autoimmune disease – Experimental autoimmune uveoretinitis induced in mice with two different retinal antigens. J Immunol 1988;140:1490–1495.
5   Cunha-Vaz J: The blood-ocular barriers. Surv Ophthalmol 1979;23:279–294.
6   Dernouchamps JP, Michaels J: Molecular sieve properties of the blood-aqueous barrier in uveitis. Exp Eye Res 1977;25:25–31.
7   Greenwood J, Howes R, Lightman S: The blood-retinal barrier in experimental autoimmune uveoretinitis. Leukocyte interactions and functional damage. Lab Invest 1994;70:39–52.
8   Whitcup SM: The initiating stimuli for uveitis. Eye 1997;11:167–170.
9   Berzofsky JA: Immunodominance in T lymphocyte recognition. Immunol Lett 1988;18:83–92.
10 Li Q, Fujino Y, Caspi RR, Najafian F, Nussenblatt RB, Chan CC: Association between mast cells and the development of experimental autoimmune uveitis in different rat strains. Clin Immunol Immunopathol 1992;65:294–299.
11 Butler TL, McMenamin PG: Resident and infiltrating immune cells in the uveal tract in the early and late stages of experimental autoimmune uveoretinitis. Invest Ophthalmol Vis Sci 1996;37: 2195–2210.
12 Whitcup S, Nussenblatt RB: Immunologic mechanisms of uveitis. Arch Ophthalmol 1997;115: 520–525.
13 Schnaudigel O: Die Vitalfärbung mit Tryptanblau am Auge. Graefes Arch Ophthalmol 1913;86: 93–97.

14   Palm E: On the occurrence in the retina of conditions corresponding to the blood-brain barrier. Acta Ophthalmol 1947;25:29–33.
15   Davson H: Physiology of the Ocular and Cerebrospinal Fluids. London, JAC, 1956.
16   Ashton N, Cunha-Vaz JG: Effect of histamine on the permeability of the ocular vessels. Arch Ophthalmol 1965;73:211–223.
17   Raviola G: The structural basis of the blood-ocular barriers. Exp Eye Res 1977(suppl):27–63.
18   Bill A: The blood-aqueous barrier. Trans Ophthalmol Soc UK 1986;105:149–155.
19   Metrikin DC, Wilson CA, Berkowitz BA, Lam MK, Wood GK, Peshock RM: Measurement of blood-retinal barrier breakdown in endotoxin-induced endophthalmitis. Invest Ophthalmol Vis Sci 1995;36:1361–1370.
20   Gery I, Nussenblatt RB: Immunologic basis of uveitis; in Pepose JS, Holland GN, Wilhelmus KR (eds): Ocular Infection and Immunity. St Louis, Mosby-Year Book, 1996, vol 1, pp 146–147.
21   Cousins SW, Rouse BT: Chemical mediators of ocular disease; in Pepose J, Holland GN, Wilhelmus KR (eds): Ocular Infection and Immunity. St Louis, Mosby, 1995, pp 50–70.
22   De Vos AF: The Role of Cytokines in the Pathogenesis of Endotoxin-Induced Uveitis. Amsterdam, The Royal Netherlands Academy of Arts and Sciences, 1994.
23   Miyamoto K, Ogura Y, Hamada M, Nishiwaki H, Hiroshiba N, Honda Y: In vivo quantification of leukocyte behavior in the retina during endotoxin-induced uveitis. Invest Ophthalmol Vis Sci 1996;37:2708–2715.
24   Miyamoto K, Ogura Y, Hamada M, Nishiwaki H, Hiroshiba N, Tsujikawa A, Mandai M, Suzuma K, Tojo SJ, Honda Y: In vivo neutralization of P-selectin inhibits leukocyte-endothelial interactions in retinal microcirculation during ocular inflammation. Microvasc Res 1998;55:230–240.
25   Luna JD, Derevjanik NL, Mahlow J, Chiu C, Peng B, Tobe T, Campochiaro PA, Vinores SA: Blood-retinal barrier breakdown in experimental autoimmune uveoretinitis: Comparison with vascular endothelial growth factor, tumor necrosis factor-alpha, and interleukin-1-beta-mediated breakdown. J Neurosci Res 1997;49:268–280.
26   Alm A: Ocular circulation; in Moses RA, Hart WJ (eds): Adler's Physiology of the Eye: Clinical Application. St Louis, Mosby, 1991, vol 6, pp 198–201.
27   Sugita A, Hamasaki M, Higashi R: Regional difference in fenestration of choroidal capillaries in Japanese monkey eye. Jpn J Ophthalmol 1982;26:47–52.
28   Prendergast RA, Coskuncan NM, Caspi RR, Sartani G, Tarrant TK, Lutty GA, McLeod DS: T cell traffic and the inflammatory response in experimental autoimmune uveoretinitis. Invest Ophthalmol Vis Sci 1998;39:754–762.
29   Yurochko AD: Adhesion molecules as signal transduction molecules; in Paul LC, Issekutz TB (eds): Adhesion Molecules in Health and Disease, ed 1. New York, Dekker, 1997, pp 155–180.
30   Hynes RO: Integrins: Versability, modulation, and signalling. Cell 1992;69:11–25.
31   Hogg N: Roll, roll, roll your leukocyte gently down the vein. Immunol Today 1992;4:113–115.
32   Hogg N, Landis RC: Adhesion molecules in cell interactions. Curr Opin Immunol 1993;5:383–390.
33   Carlos TM, Harlan JM: Leukocyte-endothelial adhesion molecules. Blood 1994;84:2068–2102.
34   Horton MA: Molecular biology of cell adhesion molecules; in James K, Morris A (eds): Molecular Medical Science Series. Chichester, Wiley, 1996.
35   Wang YF, Calder VL, Greenwood J, Lightman SL: Lymphocyte adhesion to cultured endothelial cells of the blood-retinal barrier. J Neuroimmunol 1993;48:161–168.
36   Springer TA: Traffic signals for lymphocyte recirculation and leukocyte emigration: The multi-step paradigm. Cell 1994;76:301–314.
37   Osborn L: Leukocyte adhesion in inflammation. Cell 1990;62:3–6.
38   Greenwood J, Calder VL: Lymphocyte migration through cultured endothelial cell monolayers derived from the blood-retinal barrier. Immunology 1993;80:401–406.
39   Lasky LA: Selectins: Interpreters of cell-specific carbohydrate information during inflammation. Science 1992;258:964–969.
40   Whitcup SM, Chan CC, Li Q, Nussenblatt RB: Expression of cell adhesion molecules in posterior uveitis. Arch Ophthalmol 1992;110:662–666.
41   Suzuma K, Mandai M, Kogishi J, Tojo SJ, Honda Y, Yoshimura N: Role of P-selectin in endotoxin-induced uveitis. Invest Ophthalmol Vis Sci 1997;38:1610–1618.

Mechanisms of Intraocular Inflammation

42 Suzuma I, Mandai M, Suzuma K, Ishida K, Tojo SJ, Honda Y: Contribution of E-selectin to cellular infiltration during endotoxin-induced uveitis. Invest Ophthalmol Vis Sci 1998;39:1620–1630.

43 Whitcup SM, Kozhich AT, Lobanoff M, Wolitzky BA, Chan CC: Blocking both E-selectin and P-selectin inhibits endotoxin-induced leukocyte infiltration into the eye. Clin Immunol Immunopathol 1997;83:45–52.

44 Whitcup SM, Debarge LR, Rosen H, Nussenblatt RB, Chan CC: Monoclonal antibody against C11b/CD18 inhibits endotoxin-induced uveitis. Invest Ophthalmol Vis Sci 1993;34:673–681.

45 Frenette PS, Wagner DD: Insights into selectin function from knockout mice. Thromb Haemost 1997;78:60–64.

46 Malhotra R, Priest R, Foster MR, Bird MI: P-selectin binds to bacterial lipopolysaccharide. Eur J Immunol 1998;28:983–988.

47 Misugi E, Tojo SJ, Yasuda T, Kurata Y, Morooka S: Increased plasma P-selectin induced by intravenous administration of endotoxin in rats. Biochem Biophys Res Commun 1998;246:414–417.

48 Hamada M, Ogura Y, Miyamoto K, Nishiwaki H, Hiroshiba N, Honda Y: Retinal leukocyte behavior in experimental autoimmune uveoretinitis in rats. Exp Eye Res 1997;65:445–450.

49 Meng H, Tonnesen MG, Marchese MJ, Clark RAF, Bahou WF, Gruber BL: Mast cells are potent regulators of endothelial cell adhesion molecule ICAM-1 and VCAM-1 expression. J Cell Physiol 1995;165:40–53.

50 Whitcup SM, Wakefield D, Li Q, Nussenblatt RB, Chan CC: Endothelial leukocyte adhesion molecule-1 in endotoxin-induced uveitis. Invest Ophthalmol Vis Sci 1992;33:2626–2630.

51 Wakefield D, McCluskey P, Palladinetti P: Distribution of lymphocytes and cell adhesion molecules in iris biopsy specimens from patients with uveitis. Arch Ophthalmol 1992;110:121–125.

52 Diamond MS, Springer TA: The dynamic regulation of integrin adhesiveness. Curr Biol 1994;5:506–517.

53 Whitcup SM, DeBarge LR, Caspi RR, Harning R, Nussenblatt RB, Chan CC: Monoclonal antibodies against ICAM-1 (CD54) and LFA-1 (CD11a/CD18) inhibit experimental autoimmune uveitis. Clin Immunol Immunopathol 1993;67:143–150.

54 Eiichi U, Masaya K, Shun-ichi T, Shigeaki O: Suppression of experimental uveitis with monoclonal antibodies to ICAM-1 and LFA-1. Invest Ophthalmol Vis Sci 1994;35:2626–2631.

55 Yashiro Y, Tai XG, Toyo-oka K, Park CS, Abe R, Hamaoka T, Kobayashi M, Neben S, Fujiwara H: A fundamental difference in the capacity to induce proliferation of naive cells between CD28 and other co-stimulatory molecules. Eur J Immunol 1998;28:926–935.

56 Wulfing C, Sjaastad MD, Davis MM: Visualizing the dynamics of T cell activation: Intracellular adhesion molecule 1 migrates rapidly to the T cell/B cell interface and acts to sustain calcium levels. Proc Natl Acad Sci USA 1998;95:6302–6307.

57 Imai T, Hieshima K, Haskell C, Baba M, Nagira M, Nishimura M, Kakizaki M, Takagi S, Nomiyama H, Schall TJ, Yoshie O: Identification and molecular characterization of fractalkine receptor CX3CR1, which mediates both leukocyte migration and adhesion. Cell 1997;91:521–530.

58 Bazan JF, Bacon KB, Hardiman G, Wang W, Soo K, Rossi D, Greaves DR, Zlotnik A, Schall TJ: A new class of membrane bound chemokine with a Cx_3C motif. Nature 1997;385:640–644.

59 Fong AM, Robinson LA, Steeber DA, Tedder TF, Yoshie O, Imai T, Patel DD: Fractalkine and CX3CR1 mediate a novel mechanism of leukocyte capture, firm adhesion, and activation under physiologic flow. J Exp Med 1998;188:1413–1419.

60 Janeway CAJ, Travers P: Immunobiology. The Immune System in Health and Disease, ed 3. New York, Garland Publishing, 1997.

61 Ben-Zvi A, Rodrigues MM, Gery I, Schiffman E: Induction of ocular inflammation by synthetic mediators. Arch Ophthalmol 1981;99:1436–1444.

62 Mondino BJ, Sidiharo Y, Meyer IJ, Sumner HJ: Inflammatory mediators in the vitreous humor of AIDS patients. Invest Ophthalmol Vis Sci 1990;31:798–804.

63 Mondino BJ, Sidiharo Y, Sumner H: Anaphylatoxin levels in human vitreous humor. Invest Ophthalmol Vis Sci 1988;29:1195–1198.

64 Marak GE, Font RL, Alepa FP, Ward PA: Effects of C3 inactivator factor on the development of experimental lens-induced granulomatous endophthalmitis. Ophthalmic Res 1977;9:416–420.

65 Verhagen C, Breebaart AC, Kijlstra A: The effects of complement depletion on corneal inflammation in rats. Invest Ophthalmol Vis Sci 1992;33:273–279.

66 Hedrick JA, Zlotnik A: Chemokines and lymphocyte biology. Curr Opin Immunol 1996;8:343–347.

67 Howard OMZ, Ben-Baruch A, Oppenheim JJ: Chemokines: Progress toward identifying molecular targets for therapeutic agents. Trends Biotechnol 1996;14:46–51.

68 Bagglioni M, Dewald B, Moser B: Interleukin-8 and related chemotactic cytokines-CXC and CC chemokines. Adv Immunol 1994;55:97–179.

69 Schall TJ: Biology of the RANTES/SIS cytokine family. Cytokine 1991;3:165.

70 Davatelis G, Tekamp-Olson P, Wolpe SD, Hermsen K, Luedke C, Gallegos C, Coit D, Merry-weather J, Cerami A: Cloning and characterization of a cDNA for murine macrophage inflammatory protein, a novel monokine with inflammatory and chemokine properties. J Exp Med 1988;167:1939.

71 Hedrick JA, Saylor V, Figueiroa D, Mizoue L, Xu YM, Menon S, Abrams J, Handel T, Zlotnik A: Lymphotactin is produced by NK cells and attracts both NK cells and T cells in vivo. J Immunol 1997;158:1533–1540.

72 Baggiolini M, Walz A, Kunkel SL: Neutrophil-activating peptide-1/interleukin-8, a novel cytokine that activates neutrophils. J Clin Invest 1989;84:1045–1049.

73 Rolfe MW, Kunkel SL, Standiford TJ, Chensue SW, Allen RM, Evanoff HL, Phan SH, Strieter RM: Pulmonary fibroblast expression of interleukin: A model for alveolar macrophage derived cytokine networking. Am J Respir Cell Mol Biol 1991;5:493–501.

74 Ferrick MR, Thurau SR, Oppenheim MH, Herbort CP, Ni M, Zachariae COC, Matsushima K, Chan CC: Ocular inflammation stimulated by intravitreal interleukin-8 and interleukin-1. Invest Opthalmol Vis Sci 1991;32:1534–1539.

75 de Boer JH, Hack CE, Verhoeven AJ, Baarsma GS, de Jong PT, Rademakers AJ, de Vries-Knoppert WA, Rothova A, Kijlstra A: Chemoattractant and neutrophil degranulation activities related to interleukin-8 in vitreous fluid in uveitis and vitreoretinal disorders. Invest Ophthalmol Vis Sci 1993;34:3376–3385.

76 Verma MJ, Lloyd A, Rager H, Strieter R, Kunkel S, Taub D, Wakefield D: Chemokines in acute anterior uveitis. Curr Eye Res 1997;16:1202–1208.

77 Adamus G, Machnicki M, Amundson D, Adlard K, Offner H: Similar pattern of MCP-1 expression in spinal cords and eyes of Lewis rats with experimental autoimmune encephalomyelitis associated anterior uveitis. J Neurosci Res 1997;50:531–538.

78 Taub DD, Conlon K, Lloyd AR, Oppenheim JJ, Kelvin DJ: Preferential migration of activated CD4+ and CD8+ T cells in response to MIP-1α and MIP-1β. Science 1993;260:355.

79 Mosmann TR, Cherwinski H, Bond MW, Giedlin MA, Coffman RL: Two types of murine helper T cell clones. I. Definition according to profiles of lymphokine activities and secreted proteins. J Immunol 1986;136:2248–2257.

80 Cher DJ, Mosmann TR: Two types of murine helper T cell clones. II. Delayed-type hypersensitivity is mediated by TH1 clones. J Immunol 1987;138:3688–3694.

81 Romagnani S: Lymphokine production by human T cells in disease states. Annu Rev Immunol 1994;12:227–257.

82 Maggi E, Biswas P, Del Prete G, Parronchi P, Macchia D, Simonelli C, Emmi L, De Carli M, Tiri A, Ricci M, Romagnagi S: Accumulation of Th-2-like helper T cells in the conjunctiva of patients with vernal conjunctivitis. J Immunol 1991;146:1169–1174.

83 Kulkarni PS, Mancino M: Studies on intraocular inflammation produced by intravitreal human interleukins in the rabbit. Exp Eye Res 1993;56:275–279.

84 Durum SK, Oppenheim JJ: Macrophage-derived mediators: Interleukin-1, tumor necrosis factor, interleukin-6, interferon and related cytokines; in Paul WE (ed): Fundamental Immunology. New York, Raven Press, 1989.

85 Mazzei GJ, Seckinger PL, Dayer JM, Shaw AR: Purification and characterization of a 26-kDa competitive inhibitor of interleukin-1. Eur J Immunol 1990;20:683–689.

86 Rosenbaum JT, Samples JR, Hefeneider SH, Howes EL: Ocular inflammatory effects of intravitreal IL-1. Arch Ophthalmol 1987;105:1117–1120.

87 Rosenbaum JT, Boney RS: Use of interleukin-1 receptor to inhibit ocular inflammation. Curr Eye Res 1991;10:1137–1139.

88   Rubin RM, Rosenbaum JT: A platelet-activating factor antagonist inhibits interleukin-1-induced inflammation. Biochem Biophys Res Commun 1988;154:429–436.
89   Vassalli P: The pathophysiology of tumor necrosis factors. Annu Rev Immunol 1992;10:411–452.
90   Abbas AK, Lichtman AH, Pober JS: Cytokines; in Abbas AK, Lichtman AH, Pober JS (eds): Cellular and Molecular Immunology. Philadelphia, Saunders, 1994, pp 239–260.
91   Dick AD, Duncan L, Hale G, Waldmann H, Isaacs J: Neutralizing TNF-alpha activity modulates T cell phenotype and function in experimental autoimmune uveoretinitis. J Autoimmun 1998;11: 255–264.
92   Murray PI, Hoekzema R, Van Haren MAC, de Hon FD, Kijlstra A: Aqueous humor interleukin-6 levels in uveitis. Invest Ophthalmol Vis Sci 1990;31:917–920.
93   Hoekzema R, Murray PI, van Haren MAC, Helle M, Kijlstra A: Analysis of interleukin-6 in endotoxin-induced uveitis. Invest Ophthalmol Vis Sci 1991;32:88–95.
94   Hoekzema R, Murray PI, Kijstra A: Cytokines and intraocular inflammation. Curr Eye Res 1990; 9(suppl):207–211.
95   Rosenbaum JT, Kievit P, Han YB, Park JM, Planck SR: Interleukin-6 does not mediate endotoxin-induced uveitis in mice: Studies in gene deletion animals. Invest Ophthalmol Vis Sci 1998;39:64–69.
96   Kusuda M, Gaspari AA, Chan CC, Gery I, Katz SI: Expression of Ia antigen by ocular tissues of mice treated with interferon-γ. Invest Ophthalmol Vis Sci 1989;30:764–768.
97   Cousins SW, Trattler WB, Streilein JW: Immune privilege and suppression of immunogenic inflammation in the anterior chamber. Curr Eye Res 1991;10:287–297.
98   Schmitt E, Rude E, Germann T: The immunostimulatory function of IL-12 in T-helper cell development and its regulation by TGF-beta, IFN-gamma, and IL-4. Chem Immunol 1997;68:70–85.
99   Jones LS, Rizzo LV, Agarwal RK, Tarrant TK, Chan CC, Wiggert B, Caspi RR: IFN-gamma deficient mice develop experimental autoimmune uveitis in the context of a deviant effector response. J Immunol 1997;158:5997–6005.
100 Tarrant TK, Silver PB, Chan CC, Wiggert B, Caspi RR: Endogeneous IL-12 is required for induction and expression of experimental autoimmune uveitis. J Immunol 1998;161:122–127.
101 Caspi RR: IL-12 in autoimmunity. Clin Immunol Immunopathol 1998;88:4–13.
102 Yokoi, H, Kato K, Kezuka T, Sakai J, Usui M, Yagita H, Okumura K: Prevention of experimental autoimmune uveoretinitis by monoclonal antibody to interleukin-12. Eur J Immunol 1997;27: 641–646.
103 O'Hara RMJ, Henderson SL, Nagelin A: Prevention of a Th1 disease by a Th1 cytokine: IL-12 and diabetes in NOD mice. Ann NY Acad Sci 1996;795:241–249.
104 Joosten LAB, Lubberts E, Helsen MMA, Van den Berg WB: Dual role of IL-12 in early and late stages of murine collagen-induced arthritis. J Immunol 1997;159:4094–4102.
105 Rizzo LV, Xu H, Chan CC, Wiggert B, Caspi RR: IL-10 has a protective role in experimental autoimmune uveitis. Int Immunol 1998;10:807–814.
106 Tarrant TK, Silver PB, Wahlsten JL, Rizzo LV, Chan CC, Wiggert B, Caspi RR: Interleukin-12 protects from a Th1-mediated autoimmune disease, experimental autoimmune uveitis, through a mechanism involving IFN-γ, NO and apoptosis. J Exp Med 1999;189:219–230.
107 Hayashi S, Guex-Crosier Y, Delvaux A, Velu T, Roberge FG: Interleukin-10 inhibits inflammatory cells infiltration in endotoxin-induced uveitis. Graefes Arch Clin Exp Ophthalmol 1996;234:633–636.
108 McKnight AJ, Zimmer GJ, Fogelman I, Wolf SF, Abbas AK: Effects of IL-12 on helper T cell-dependent immune responses in vivo. J Immunol 1994;152:2172–2179.
109 Trinchieri G: Interleukin-12 and interferon-gamma. Do they always go together? Am J Pathol 1995; 147:1534–1538.
110 Sanchez-Bueno A, Verkhusha V, Tanaka Y, Takikawa O, Yoshida R: Interferon-gamma-dependent expression of inducible nitric oxide synthase, interleukin-12, and interferon-gamma-inducing factor in macrophages elicited by allografted tumor cells. Biochem Biophys Res Commun 1996;224:555–563.
111 Trinchieri G, Scott P: Interleukin-12: A proinflammatory cytokine with immunoregulatory functions (editorial). Res Immunol 1995;146:423–431.
112 Xie K, Huang S, Wang Y, Beltran PJ, Juang SH, Dong Z, Reed JC, McDonnell TJ, McConkey DJ, Fidler IJ: Bcl-2 protects cells from cytokine-induced nitric-oxide-dependent apoptosis. Cancer Immunol Immunother 1996;43:109–115.

113 Xie K, Wang Y, Huang S, Xu L, Bielenberg D, Salas T, McConkey DJ, Jiang W, Fidler IJ: Nitric oxide-mediated apoptosis of K-1735 melanoma cells is associated with downregulation of Bcl-2. Oncogene 1997;15:771–779.

114 Zettl UK, Mix E, Zielasek J, Stangel M, Hartung HP, Gold R: Apoptosis of myelin-reactive T cells induced by reactive oxygen and nitrogen intermediates in vitro. Cell Immunol 1997;178:1–8.

115 Koblish HK, Hunter CA, Wysocka M, Trinchieri G, Lee WMF: Immune suppression by recombinant interleukin (rIL)-12 involves interferon-gamma induction of nitric oxide synthase 2 (iNOS) activity: Inhibitors of NO generation reveal the extent of rIL-12 vaccine adjuvant effect. J Exp Med 1998; 188:1603–1610.

116 Cousins SW, McCabe MM, Danielpoor D, Streilein JW: Identification of transforming growth factor-β as an immunosuppressive factor in aqueous humor. Invest Ophthalmol Vis Sci 1991;32: 2201–2211.

117 Granstein R, Staszlaski R, Knisely TL, Zeira E, Nazareno R, Latina M, Albert DM: Aqueous humor contains transforming growth factor-β and a small (<3,500 dalton) inhibitor of thymocyte proliferation. J Immunol 1990;144:3021–3026.

118 Jampel H, Roche N, Stark WJ, Roberts AB: Transforming growth factor-β in the aqueous humor. Curr Eye Res 1991;10:963–970.

119 Allen JB, McGahan MC, Ogawa Y, Sellon DC, Clark BD, Fleisher LN: Intravitreal transforming growth factor-beta-2 decreases cellular infiltration in endotoxin-induced ocular inflammation in rabbits. Curr Eye Res 1996;15:95–103.

120 Weiner HL: Oral tolerance: Immune mechanisms and treatment of autoimmune diseases. Immunol Today 1997;18:335–343.

121 Kulkarni AB, Huh CG, Becker D, Geiser A, Lyght M, Flanders KC, Roberts AB, Sporn MB, Ward JM, Karlsson S: Transforming growth factor-beta-1 null mutation in mice causes excessive inflammatory response and early death. Proc Natl Acad Sci USA 1993;90:770–774.

122 Kennedy MK, Picha KS, Fanslow WC, Grabstein KH, Alderson MR, Clifford KN, Chin WA, Mohler KM: CD40/CD40 ligand interactions are required for T cell-dependent production of interleukin-12 by mouse macrophages. Eur J Immunol 1996;26:370–378.

123 Shu U, Kiniwa M, Wu CY, Maliszewski C, Vezzio N, Hakimi J, Gately M, Delespesse G: Activated T cells induce interleukin-12 production by monocytes via CD40-CD40 ligand interaction. Eur J Immunol 1995;25:1125–1128.

124 Grewal IS, Flavell RA: A central role of CD40 ligand in the regulation of CD4+ T cell responses. Immunol Today 1996;17:410–414.

125 Grewal IS, Flavell RS: The role of CD40 ligand in costimulation and T cell activation. Immunol Rev 1996;153:98–100.

126 Durie FH, Fava RA, Foy TM, Aruffo A, Ledbetter JA, Noelle RJ: Prevention of collagen-induced arthritis with an antibody to gp39, the ligand for CD40. Science 1993;261:1328–1330.

127 Gerritse K, Laman JD, Noelle RJ, Aruffo A, Ledbetter JA, Boersma WJA, Claasen E: CD40-CD40 ligand interactions in experimental allergic encephalomyelitis and multiple sclerosis. Proc Natl Acad Sci USA 1996;93:2499–2504.

128 Carayanniotis G, Masters SR, Noelle RJ: Suppression of murine thyroiditis via blockade of the CD40-CD40L interaction. Immunology 1997;90:421–426.

129 Whitcup SM, Chan CC, Gery I, Kalled SL, Wiggert B, Magone T: Anti-CD40 ligand (CD40L) antibody inhibits experimental autoimmune uveitis (abstract). Invest Ophthalmol Vis Sci 1998;39:S886.

130 Ayo C: A toxic ocular reaction. I. New property of Schwartzman toxins. J Immunol 1947;46: 113–132.

131 Rosenbaum JT, McDevitt HO, Guss RB, Egbert PR: Endotoxin-induced uveitis in rats as a model for human disease. Nature 1980;286:611–613.

132 Forrester JV, Worgul BV, Merriam GRJ: Endotoxin-induced uveitis in the rat. Graefes Arch Klin Ophthalmol 1980;213:221–233.

133 Kogiso M, Tanouchi Y, Mimora Y, Nagasama H, Himeno K: Endotoxin-induced uveitis in mice. I. Induction of uveitis and role of T lymphocytes. Jpn J Ophthalmol 1992;36:281–290.

134 Chen TY, Lei MG, Suzuki T, Morrison DC: Lipopolysaccharide receptors and signal transduction pathways in mononuclear phagocytes. Curr Top Microbiol Immunol 1992;181:169–188.

135   Guthrie LA, McPhail LC, Henson PM, Johnston RBJ: Priming of neutrophils for enhanced release of oxygen metabolites. J Exp Med 1984;160:1656–1671.

136   Herbort CP, Okumura A, Mochizuki M: Endotoxin-induced uveitis in the rat: A study of the role of inflammation mediators. Graefes Arch Klin Exp Ophthalmol 1988;226:553–558.

137   Granowitz EV, Santos AA, Poutsiaka DD, Cannon JG, Wilmore DW, Wolff SM, Dinarello CA: Production of interleukin-1 receptor antagonist during experimental endotoxaemia. Lancet 1991; 338:1423–1424.

138   De Vos AF, Van Haren MAC, Verhagen R, Hoekzema R, Kijlstra A: Kinetics of intraocular tumor necrosis factor and interleukin-6 in endotoxin-induced uveitis in the rat. Invest Ophthalmol Vis Sci 1994;35:1100–1106.

139   Chan CC: Effects of anti-inflammins on endotoxin-induced uveitis in rats. Arch Ophthalmol 1991; 109:278–281.

140   Goodnow CC: Balancing immunity and tolerance: Deleting and tuning lymphocyte repertoires. Proc Natl Acad Sci USA 1996;93:2264–2271.

141   Gery I, Streilein JW: Autoimmunity in the eye and its regulation. Curr Opin Immunol 1994;6: 938–945.

142   Egwuagu CE, Charukamnoetkanok P, Gery I: Thymic expression of autoantigens correlates with resistance to autoimmune disease. J Immunol 1997;159:3109–3112.

143   Charukamnoetkanok P, Fukushima A, Whitcup SM, Gery I, Egwuagu CE: Expression of ocular autoantigens in the mouse thymus. Curr Eye Res 1998;17:788–792.

144   Shevach EM: Organ-specific autoimmunity; in Paul WE (ed): Fundamental Immunology, ed 4. Philadelphia, Lippincott-Raven, 1998, p 1089.

145   Singh VK, Kalra HK, Yamaki K, Abe T, Donoso LA, Shinohara T: Molecular mimicry between a uveitopathogenic site of S-antigen and viral peptides – Induction of experimental autoimmune uveitis in Lewis rats. J Immunol 1990;144:1282–1287.

146   Steinman L: A few autoreactive cells in an autoimmune infiltrate control a vast population of nonspecific cells: A tale of smart bombs and the infantry. Proc Natl Acad Sci USA 1996;93: 2253–2256.

147   Singh DP, Kikuchi T, Sigh VK, Shinohara T: A single amino-acid substitution in core residues of S-antigen prevents experimental autoimmune uveitis. J Immunol 1994;152:4699–4705.

148   Takatsu K: Cytokines involved in B-cell differentiation and their sites of action. Proc Soc Exp Biol Med 1997;215:121–133.

149   De Kozak Y: Antibody response in uveitis. Eye 1997;11:194–199.

150   De Kozak Y, Mirshahi M, Boucheix C, Faure JP: Prevention of experimental autoimmune uveoretinitis by active immunization with autoantigen-specific monoclonal antibodies. Eur J Immunol 1987; 17:541–547.

151   Broekhuyse RM, Kuhlmann ED, Winkens HJ: Experimental autoimmune anterior uveitis. I. A new form of experimental uveitis. Induction by a detergent-insoluble intrinsic protein fraction of the retinal pigment epithelium. Exp Eye Res 1991;52:465–474.

152   Chan CC, Hikita N, Dastgheib K, Whitcup SM, Gery I, Nussenblatt RB: Experimental melanin protein-induced uveitis in the Lewis rat. Immunopathologic processes. Ophthalmology 1994;101:1275–1280.

153   Broekhuyse RM, Kuhlmann ED, Winkens HJ: Experimental autoimmune anterior uveitis. II. Dose-dependent induction and adoptive transfer using a melanin-bound antigen of the retinal pigment epithelium. Exp Eye Res 1992;55:401–411.

154   Burky EL: Experimental endophthalmitis phaco-analytica in rabbits. Arch Ophthalmol 1934;12: 536–546.

155   Marak GE, Font RL, Alepa FP: Arthus-type panophthalmitis in rats sensitized to heterologous lens protein. Ophthalmic Res 1977;9:162–170.

156   Marak GE, Font RL, Alepa FP: Experimental lens-induced granulomatous endophthalmitis: Passive transfer with serum. Ophthalmic Res 1976;8:117–120.

157   Palestine AG, Chan CC, Gery I, Nussenblatt RB: The failure of cyclosporin to inhibit granulomatous inflammation in acute Arthus-like panophthalmitis. Immunol Lett 1985;9:235–237.

158   Gery I, Nussenblatt RB, BenEzra D: Dissociation between humoral and cellular immune responses to lens antigens. Invest Ophthalmol Vis Sci 1981;20:235–237.

159   Lai JC, Wawrousek EF, Lee RS, Chan CC, Whitcup SM, Gery I: Intraocular inflammation in transgenic mice expressing a foreign antigen in their lens. Ocul Immunol Inflamm 1995;3:59–62.

160   Iwase K, Fujii Y, Nakashima I, Kato N, Fujino Y, Kawashima H, Mochizuki M: A new method for induction of experimental autoimmune uveoretinitis in mice. Curr Eye Res 1990;9:207–216.

161   De Kozak Y, Sakai J, Thillaye B, Faure JP: S-antigen-induced experimental autoimmune uveoretinitis in rats. Curr Eye Res 1981;1:327–336.

162   Wacker WB, Lipton NM: Experimental allergic uveitis. I. Production in the guinea pig and rabbit by immunization with retina in adjuvant. J Immunol 1968;101:151–156.

163   Wacker WB, Rao NA, Marak GE Jr: Immunopathogenic responses of rabbits to 'S' antigen. I. Phlogistic characteristics associated with antigen source and sensitizing dose. Ophthalmic Res 1981;13:302–311.

164   Gery I, Mochizuki M, Nussenblatt RB: Retinal specific antigens and immunopathogenic processes they provoke; in Osborne NN, Chader GJ (eds): Progress in Retinal Research. New York. Pergamon Press, 1986, vol 5, pp 75–109.

165   Abe T, Satoh N, Nakajima A, Koizumi T, Tamada M, Sakuragi S: Characterization of a potent uveitopathogenic site derived from rat phosducin. Exp Eye Res 1997;65:703–710.

166   Dua HS, Lee RH, Lolley RN, Barrett JA, Abrams M, Forrester JV, Donoso LA: Induction of experimental autoimmune uveitis by the retinal photoreceptor cell protein, phosducin. Curr Eye Res 1992;11(suppl):107–111.

167   Satoh N, Abe T, Nakajima A, Ohkoshi M, Koizumi T, Tamada H, Sakuragi S: Analysis of uveitogenic sites in phosducin molecule. Curr Eye Res 1998;17:677–686.

168   Pfister C, Chabre M, Plouet J, Van Tuyen V, De Kozak Y, Faure JP, Kuehn H: Retinal S antigen identified as the 48K protein regulating light-dependent phosphodiesterase in rods. Science 1985; 228:891–893.

169   Borst DE, Redmond TM, Elser JE, Gonda MA, Wiggert B, Chader GJ, Nickerson JM: Interphotoreceptor retinoid binding protein. Gene characterization, protein repeat structure, and its evolution. J Biol Chem 1989;264:1115–1123.

170   Gery I, Wiggert B, Redmond TM, Kuwabara T, Crawford MA, Vistica BP, Chader GJ: Uveoretinitis and pinealitis induced by immunization with interphotoreceptor retinoid binding protein. Invest Ophthalmol Vis Sci 1986;27:1296–1300.

171   Hirose S, Kuwabara T, Nussenblatt RB, Wiggert B, Redmond TM, Gery I: Uveitis induced in primates by interphotoreceptor retinoid binding protein. Arch Ophthalmol 1986;104:1698–1702.

172   Eisenfeld AJ, Bunt-Milam AH, Saari JC: Uveoretinitis in rabbits following immunization with interphotoreceptor binding protein. Exp Eye Res 1987;44:425–438.

173   Applebury ML, Hargrave PA: Molecular biology of the visual pigments. Vision Res 1986;26: 1881–1895.

174   Adamus G, Ortega H, Witkowska D, Polans A: Recoverin: A potent uveitogen for the induction of photoreceptor degeneration in Lewis rats. Exp Eye Res 1994;59:447–455.

175   Gery I, Chanaud NP III, Anglade E: Recoverin is highly uveitogenic in Lewis rats. Invest Ophthalmol Vis Sci 1994;35:3342–3345.

176   Thirkill CE, Tait RC, Tyler NK, Roth AM, Keltner JL: The cancer-associated retinopathy antigen is a recoverin-like protein. Invest Ophthalmol Vis Sci 1992;33:2768–2772.

177   Adamus G, Guy J, Schmied JL, Arendt A, Hargrave PA: Role of anti-recoverin autoantibodies in cancer-associated retinopathy. Invest Ophthalmol Vis Sci 1993;34:2626–2633.

178   Adamus G, Machnicki M, Elerding H, Sugden B, Blocker YS, Fox DA: Antibodies to recoverin induce apoptosis of photoreceptor and bipolar cells in vivo. J Autoimmun 1998;11:523–533.

179   Whitcup SM, Vistica BP, Milam AH, Nussenblatt RB, Gery I: Recoverin-associated retinopathy: A clinically and immunologically distinctive disease. Am J Ophthalmol 1998;126:230–237.

180   Nussenblatt RB, Gery I: Experimental autoimmune uveitis and its relationship to clinical ocular inflammatory disease. J Autoimmun 1996;9:575–585.

181   Egwuagu CE, Mahdi RM, Nussenblatt RB, Gery I, Caspi RR: Evidence for selective accumulation of V beta 8 + T lymphocytes in experimental autoimmune uveoretinitis induced with two different retinal antigens. J Immunol 1993;151:1627–1636.

182 Egwuagu CE, Bahmanyar S, Mahdi RM, Nussenblatt RB, Gery I, Caspi RR: Predominant usage of V beta 8.3 T cell receptor in a T cell line that induces experimental autoimmune uveoretinitis. Clin Immunol Immunopathol 1992;65:152–160.

183 Mochizuki M, Kuwabara Y, McAllister C, Nussenblatt RB, Gery I: Adoptive Transfer of experimental autoimmune uveoretinitis in rats. Invest Ophthalmol Vis Sci 1985;26:1–9.

184 Caspi RR, Roberge FG, McAllister CG, El Saied M, Kuwabara T, Gery I, Hanna E, Nussenblatt RB: T cell lines mediating experimental autoimmune uveitis. J Immunol 1986;136:928–933.

185 Rizzo LV, Silver PS, Wiggert B, Hakim F, Gazzinelli RT, Chan CC, Caspi RR: Establishment and characterization of a murine CD4+ T cell line and clone that induce experimental autoimmune uveoretinitis in B10. A mice. J Immunol 1996;156:1654–1660.

186 Sakai J: Immune complexes in experimental autoimmune uveo-retinitis. Nippon Ganka Gakkai Zasshi 1983;87:1288–1299.

187 Chan CC, Mochizuki M, Palestine A, BenEzra D, Gery I, Nussenblatt RB: Kinetics of T lymphocyte subsets in eyes of Lewis rats with EAU. Cell Immunol 1985;96:430–434.

188 De Smet MD, Yamamoto JH, Mochizuki M, Gery I, Singh VK, Shinohara T, Wiggert B, Chader GJ, Nussenblatt RB: Cellular immune responses of patients with uveitis to retinal antigens and their fragments. Am J Ophthalmol 1990;110:173–179.

189 Donoso LA, Merryman CF, Sery T, Sanders R, Vrabec T, Fong SL: Human interstitial retinoid-binding protein. A potent uveitopathogenic agent for the induction of experimental autoimmune uveitis. J Immunol 1989;143:79–83.

190 Kotake S, Redmond TM, Wiggert B, Vistica B, Sanui H, Chader GJ, Gery I: Unusual immunologic properties of uveitogenic interphotoreceptor retinoid-binding protein derived peptide R23. Invest Ophthalmol Vis Sci 1991;32:2058–2064.

191 Kotake S, De Smet MD, Wiggert B, Redmond TM, Chader GJ, Gery J: Analysis of the pivotal residues of the immunodominant and highly uveitogenic determinant of interphotoreceptor retinoid-binding protein. J Immunol 1991;146:2995–3001.

192 Sanui H, Redmond TM, Kotake S, Wiggert B, Hu LH, Margalit H, Berzovsky JA, Chader GJ, Gery I: Uveitis and immune responses in primates immunized with IRBP-derived synthetic peptides. Curr Eye Res 1990;9:193–199.

193 Caspi RR, Chan CC, Fujino Y, Oddo S, Najafian B, Bahmanyar S, Heremans H, Wilder RL, Wiggert B: Genetic factors in susceptibility and resistance to experimental autoimmune uveitis. Curr Eye Res 1992;11(suppl):81–86.

194 Caspi RR, Sun B, Agarwal RK, Silver PB, Rizzo LV, Chan CC, Wiggert B, Wilder RL: T cell mechanisms in experimental autoimmune uveoretinitis: Susceptibility is a function of the cytokine response profile. Eye 1997;11:209–212.

195 Caspi RR, Grubbs BG, Chan CC, Chader GJ, Wiggert B: Genetic control of susceptibility to experimental autoimmune uveitis in the mouse model. J Immunol 1992;148:2384–2389.

196 Brewerton DA, Caffrey M, Nicholls A, Walters D, James DC: Acute anterior uveitis and HLA-B27. Lancet 1973;ii:994–996.

197 Nussenblatt RB, Mittal KK, Ryan S, Green WR, Maumenee AE: Birdshot retinochoroidopathy associated with HLA-A29 antigen and immune responsiveness to retinal S-antigen. Am J Ophthalmol 1982;94:147–158.

198 Baarsma GS, Kijlstra A, Oosterhuis JA, Kruit PJ, Rothova A: Association of birdshot retinochoroidopathy and HLA-A29 antigen. Doc Ophthalmol 1986;61:267–269.

199 LeHoang P, Ozdemir N, Benhamou A, Tabary T, Edelson C, Betuel H, Semiglia R, Cohen JH: HLA-A29.2 subtype associated with birdshot retinochoroidopathy. Am J Ophthalmol 1992;113:33–35.

200 Henderly DE, Genstler AJ, Smith RE, Rao NA: Changing patterns of uveitis. Am J Ophthalmol 1987;103:131–136.

201 Silveira Magalhaes CA: Estudo da toxoplasmose ocular na regiao de erechim-RS, Universidade Federal de Sao Paulo, 1997.

202 Glasner PD, Silveira C, Kruszon-Moran D, Martins MC, Burnier MJ, Silveira S, Carmago ME, Nussenblatt RB, Kaslow RA, Belfort RJ: An unusually high prevalence of ocular toxoplasmosis in Southern Brazil. Am J Ophthalmol 1992;114:136–144.

203 Silveira C, Belfort RJ, Burnier MJ, Nussenblatt RB: Acquired toxoplasmic infection as the cause of toxoplasmic retinochoroiditis in families. Am J Ophthalmol 1998;106:362–364.

204 Masur H, Jones TC, Lempert JA, Cherubini TD: Outbreak of toxoplasmosis in a family and documentation of acquired retinochoroiditis. 1978;64:396–402.

205 Montoya JG, Remington JS: Toxoplasmic chorioretinitis in the setting of acute acquired toxoplasmosis. Clin Infect Dis 1996;23:277–282.

206 Burnett AJ, Shortt SG, Isaac-Renton J, King A, Werker D, Bowie WR: Multiple cases of acquired toxoplasmosis retinitis presenting in an outbreak. Ophthalmology 1998;105:1032–1037.

207 Gazzinelli RT, Brezin A, Li Q, Nussenblatt RB, Chan CC: *Toxoplasma gondii*: Acquired ocular toxoplasmosis in the murine model, protective role of TNF-α and IFN-γ. Exp Parasitol 1994;78: 217–229.

208 Suzuki Y, Conley FK, Remington JS: Treatment of toxoplasmic encephalitis in mice with recombinant gamma interferon. Infect Immunol 1990;58:3050–3055.

209 Cachereau-Massin I, Lehoang P, Lantier-Fran M, Zerdoun E, Zazoun L, Rabinet M, Marcel P, Girard B, Katlama C, Leport C, Rozenbaum W, Conland P, Gentilini M: Ocular toxoplasmosis in human immunodeficiency virus-infected patients. Ophthalmology 1991;114:130–135.

210 Hu MS, Schwatzman J, Channon JY, Khan IA, Kasper LH: A novel murine model of acute ocular toxoplasmosis by intracameral inoculation (abstract). Invest Ophthalmol Vis Sci 1998;39:S782.

M. Teresa Magone, National Institutes of Health, National Eye Institute,
Building 10, Room 10B22, 10 Center Drive, MSC 1858, Bethesda, MD 20892 (USA)
Tel. +1 301 594 7429, Fax +1 301 496 7295, E-Mail tmagone@box-t.nih.gov

Scott M. Whitcup, National Institutes of Health, National Eye Institute,
Building 10, Room 10S227, 10 Center Drive, MSC 1863, Bethesda, MD 20892-1863 (USA)
Tel. +1 301 496 9058, Fax +1 301 496 7295, E-Mail scottw@helix.nih.gov

Streilein JW (ed): Immune Response and the Eye.
Chem Immunol. Basel, Karger, 1999, vol 73, pp 120–136

....

Immunopathogenesis of Viral Ocular Infections

Robert L. Hendricks

Department of Ophthalmology,University of Pittsburgh School of Medicine,
The Eye and Ear Institute, Pittsburgh, Pa., USA

Introduction

Immunopathology is a process in which healthy tissue is destroyed by the immune system. However, it is likely that all immune responses destroy some healthy tissue. Therefore, the term typically is used to describe an immune response that causes an unacceptable level of tissue destruction. It is clear that different tissues vary with regard to the degree of tissue destruction they can tolerate. Thus, a response that is considered 'protective' in one tissue may be considered 'immunopathologic' in another. Because of their requirement for absolute clarity, the tissues that comprise the visual axis have a very low tolerance for immunopathology. Yet these tissues must be protected from invasion by pathogens such as viruses. Thus, the ocular tissues present the immune system with a significant regulatory challenge.

The distinction between viral immunity and immunopathology was clearly established nearly two decades ago with studies of the immune response to lymphocytic choriomeningitis virus (LCMV) in mice [reviewed in 1, 2]. Studies revealed that the choriomengitis that developed in immunologically normal mice represented an immunopathological response of T cells of the CD8 subpopulation to LCMV antigens. It is now clear that the tissue destruction associated with many, if not all virus infections is attributable in part to immunopathological responses. Thus, the challenge to viral immunologists is to enhance immune mechanisms that are required for rapid viral clearance, while minimizing immunopathology at sites of infection.

Viral Infections Involving the Eye

A number of viruses are known to cause pathology in the anterior or posterior segment of the eye. I will limit this discussion to a few that are the most frequent causes of eye disease. These include members of the Adenoviridae and the Herpesviridae. The adenoviruses cause eye disease, which can become epidemic. Based on the source of the epidemics and the appearance of the disease, adenovirus ocular disease has been referred to as 'shipyard eye', 'swimming pool conjunctivitis', and 'pinkeye'. The clinical name for the disease is epidemic keratoconjunctivitis (EKC), reflecting the epidemic nature as well as the location of the infection in the cornea and conjunctiva of the eye. EKC epidemics have been attributed to the adenovirus serotypes [3, 4, 7, 8, 19, 37]. Adenovirus ocular infections are typically handled effectively by the host immune system without sequelae. However, following elimination of the virus, subepithelial opacities can develop in the cornea and persist for prolong periods of time. These opacities are thought to result from a delayed-type hypersensitivity response to viral antigens deposited in the cornea during active infection, and can be prevented by aggressive treatment with corticosteroids. However, as is often the case, opacities can return upon withdrawal of steroid treatment, presumably due to persistent viral antigens in the cornea [3].

Several members of the family Herpesviridae are significant causes ocular pathology. Human cytomagalovirus (CMV) is a frequent cause of retinal destruction in patients whose immune system is compromised by cancer chemotherapy, immunosuppressive treatment to prevent transplantation rejection, or the acquired immunodeficiency syndrome (AIDS). Host defense against CMV retinitis appears to be primarily through cell-mediated immune responses involving natural killer (NK) cells and cytotoxic lymphocytes [4–6]. Although the possible involvement of immunopathogenic mechanisms in the retinal degeneration induced by CMV has been suggested, there is no clear supporting evidence.

Varicella-zoster virus (VZV) causes two distinct diseases, Varicella (chickenpox) and herpes zoster (shingles, zona). Ocular complications are rare with Varicella, but more common with herpes zoster [reviewed in 7]. Following a primary infection, VZV establishes a latent infection in sensory ganglia. VZV that has reactivated from latency in the sensory ganglia is thought to be the usual source of virus in herpes zoster. Unlike its close relative herpes simplex virus, VZV reactivates from latency very infrequently, usually once or twice in the lifetime of the host. Reactivation appears to be associated with decreased immunity, and occurs much more frequently in immunologically compromised individuals. Unlike Varicella where eruptions are widely distributed, herpes zoster tends to occur in one or more dermatomes. The dermatomes involved tend to correlate with the areas in which the Varicella exanthems were most dense. Reactivation in the trigeminal ganglion usually occurs in the the the ophthalmic branch, and the periocular area served by that branch is most commonly involved in herpes zoster.

VZV causes several types of ocular disease that are referred to generically as herpes zoster ophthalmicus (HZO). Clinical manifestations of HZO include dermatitis, conjunctivitis, uveitis, retinitis, and secondary glaucoma. Dermatitis typically precedes ocular involvement. Treatment with acyclovir during the early stages of skin eruptions has been shown to significantly reduce the incidence of late ocular manifestations [8]. Two types of lesions occur in the conjunctiva and cornea. Lesions in the epithelial layer are the result of virus replication in and destruction of epithelial cells, whereas lesions that occur in the deeper stromal layer of the cornea are thought to reflect an immunopathologic response to viral antigens. The latter lesions typically respond to treatment with corticosteroids. In complicated cases, tapering of steroids can result in recurrent corneal inflammation with progressive corneal scarring and loss of vision. The reduced incidence of immune lesions with acyclovir treatment may reflect reduced viral antigen deposition in the cornea. Due to the lack of appropriate animal models of VZV disease, little is known about the mechanisms that lead to immune destruction of corneal tissue. However, based on clinical observations it is deemed very likely that the mechanisms involved will parallel those seen in herpes simplex disease, which has been studied in much greater detail (see below). Because of the persistent anesthetic effect of HZO, replacement of scarred corneas through transplantation is usually not an acceptable option [9].

Herpes Simplex Virus (HSV) Ocular Disease

By far the most widely studied viral ocular infection is that caused by HSV. There are two serotypes of HSV. HSV type 2 (HSV-2) is responsible for most genital lesions, but rarely causes ocular disease. HSV-1 is responsible for the majority of oral facial lesions. Most individuals appear to acquire the virus during childhood without clinical manifestations of the infection. The pathology induced by HSV-1 is primarily the result of recurrent disease. During primary infection, the virus colonizes the sensory neurons and establishes a latent infection in the sensory ganglia. Latency refers to a state in which the viral genome is retained in the neurons, but no viral proteins, and therefore no virus particles are produced. In this state, the virus is invisible to the host immune system, and is usually retained in sensory neurons for the life of the individual. However, latency can be perturbed by a variety of poorly defined reactivating stimuli such as stress, hormonal changes, and exposure to ultraviolet radiation. Reactivation leads to production of new viral particles, axonal transport to peripheral tissue and recurrent disease. Immune control of HSV-1 replication and spread in the nervous system is currently an area of intense investigation [10–19].

Although not widely recognized, HSV-1 ocular infections are a common cause of visual morbidity. HSV-1 induces pathology in three areas of the globe: the anterior uveal tract, the retina, and the cornea and conjunctiva. Herpetic uveitis is rare, and little is known of the pathogenesis of the disease. HSV-1 retinitis is also rare, but the consequences can be devastating. HSV-1 retinitis rarely occurs in isolation, but rather in association with encephalitis. Because retinal destruction proceeds rapidly, visual prognosis in individuals who survive the encephalitis is poor. The pathogenesis of HSV-1 retinitis in humans is poorly understood. The available evidence suggests that the retinal destruction may result from a combination of the direct cytopathic effect of the virus on cells of the neural retina, vascular occlusion, and perhaps inflammatory damage. Therapy for HSV-1 retinitis primarily involves systemic antiviral drug treatment. The value of combining antiviral drugs with corticosteroids is controversial.

A mouse model of the HSV-1 retinitis has shed some light on the route by which HSV-1 is transmitted to the retina. Injection of the KOS strain of HSV-1 into the anterior chamber of one eye leads to the development of retinitis in the contralateral eye. Interestingly, the retina of the injected eye is largely spared. Protection of the injected eye is associated with infiltration of CD4+ and CD8+ T lymphocytes [20]. Studies by Atherton and coworkers [21] established that the virus travels from the injected eye to the brain, and thence to the retina of the contralateral eye. Adoptive transfer of T cells from HSV-immune mice can block retinitis in the contralateral eye by controlling virus replication in the brain [22]. The possibility that CD4+ T cells might also contribute to the destruction of the HSV-1-infected contralateral retina was suggested by the observation that CD4+ T-cell depletion reduced the severity of retinitis [23]. The mechanisms by which CD4+ cells might contribute to tissue destruction in the retina have not been defined.

Herpes Simplex Keratitis

HSV-1 infections of the cornea represent the leading infectious cause of blindness in the United States, and a leading cause of blindness worldwide. Epidemiological studies suggest an incidence of about 400,000 new cases of

HSV corneal disease per year in the United States [24]. The majority of these cases involve lesions in the superficial epithelial layer of the cornea. These lesions result from the direct cytopathic effect of the virus, and typically heal without permanent loss of vision. However, about 20% of these individuals go on to develop disease in the deeper stromal layer of the cornea.

There are two forms of stromal disease. The most common form is referred to as disciform keratitis, and is characterized by corneal edema. Edema is thought to result from damage to the corneal endothelium [25], which regulates hydration of the cornea. The pathogenic mechanisms contributing to this disease are not well defined, but animal studies have suggested the possible involvement of immune complex deposition in the cornea [26]. The second type of stromal disease is a necrotizing form of herpes stromal keratitis (HSK). This type of disease leads to scarring of the cornea and progressive loss of vision with each recurrence. HSK often occurs at a time when virus is no longer detectable in the cornea, and its resolution is usually hastened by treatment with corticosteroids. For this reason, HSK has long been suspected of representing an immunopathologic response to viral antigens that are retained following clearance of replicating virus from the cornea. The scarring associated with HSK is a frequent reason for corneal transplantation, which is usually performed between recurrences of active disease. For this reason, the excised tissue is of little use in determining pathogenic mechanisms of the disease.

Immunopathological Mechanisms of HSK as Defined in the Mouse Model

Understanding the pathogenesis of a disease is greatly facilitated by the availability of an appropriate animal model. Studies of HSK have greatly benefited from the availability of several animal models of the disease. The most extensively used models involve HSV-1 infection of the corneas of rabbits and mice. The rabbit offers a well-characterized model with the advantages of a large eye and spontaneous recurrences of viral shedding and disease. The mouse, while lacking spontaneous shedding of virus in the tear film and recurrent corneal disease, does develop a delayed onset corneal inflammation that resembles many of the characteristics of recurrent HSK in humans. Moreover, the wealth of available immunologic reagents in the murine system provides distinct advantages in studying the immunopathological components of HSK.

Any attempt at immunology-based therapy for virus infections must recognize the fact that the tissue destruction that occurs at any site of virus infection results from a combination of viral cytopathology and immunopathology. These two tissue destructive forces presumably maintain a dynamic balance at sites of infection. Reduced host immunity could result in augmented viral cytopathology but reduced immunopathology, whereas heightened host immunity could reduce viral cytopathology but with potentially greater immunopathology. For this reason, identifying and manipulating immunopathogenic mechanisms can be complicated in the presence of an active virus infection. However, the immunopathology associated with primary HSV-1 infection of the mouse cornea is initiated after replicating virus is eliminated. Under these circumstances, one can study immunopathologic mechanisms through manipulation of the immune response without the confounding problem of increased viral cytopathology. Consequently, experimental models of HSK have provided important insights into mechanisms of virus-induced immunopathology.

The cornea possesses certain physical/anatomical characteristics that render it a unique tissue in which to study immunologically regulated inflammatory processes. The cornea is considered to be an immune privileged tissue in part, because it lacks direct access to the immune system. The cornea lacks blood and lymphatic vessels, structures that provide the conduit for transportation of immunologic components into and out of most tissues. The normal cornea also lacks professional antigen presenting cells (APCs) such as dendritic cells and macrophages that are resident in most other tissues. However, all of this immune apparatus is present in the limbus, a tissue that constitutes a zone between the cornea and surrounding conjunctiva. During the course of inflammation, the cornea becomes vascularized and Langerhans' cells migrate into the central cornea. Moreover, early in the inflammatory process, leukocytes extravasate from blood vessels in the limbus and migrate towards the center of the cornea. Because the normal cornea is transparent, one can qualitatively and quantitatively observe the development of these inflammatory processes, and determine how they are influenced by various immunological manipulations. The accessibility of cornea and its relative sequestration from the immune system also facilitates local immunologic manipulations without confounding systemic effects. Thus, the infected cornea offers a unique opportunity to study the T-cell effector functions that regulate inflammation.

In the mouse models of HSK, the cornea is abraded (usually with a sterile needle) immediately before or simultaneously with the topical application of a virus suspension. Within 2 days of infection, lesions with a characteristic dendritic morphology develop as a result of virus replication in and destruction of corneal epithelial cells. Fibroblasts in the corneal stroma underlying the site of the lesion are also infected, and appear to undergo apoptotic cell death [27]. The duration of virus replication in the cornea varies with the dose of virus, the strain of virus, and the strain of mice. However, in most systems, replicating virus it eliminated from the cornea within 4–7 days of infection. During the period of virus replication, the cornea is infiltrated by neutrophils and mononuclear cells, which extravasate from limbal vessels and then migrate towards the center of the cornea. The available evidence suggests that neutrophils and NK cells contribute to the control of virus replication in the cornea [28–30].

Following elimination of replicating virus, the cornea appears normal by both clinical and histological criteria. However, around 8–10 days after infection some of the previously infected corneas develop HSK. The incidence of HSK depends on the mouse strain and virus strain used. In the model used in our laboratory, 60–90% of the corneas of A/J or BALB/c mice develop HSK after corneal infection with 1×10^5 PFU of the RE strain of HSV-1. In the initial stages of HSK, leukocytes extravasate from limbal vessels and migrate into the center of the cornea. Gradually, blood vessels grow into the central cornea from the limbus, and serve as a continued source of leukocytes. Following corneal infection with most strains of HSV-1, the infiltrate is dominated by neutrophils but smaller numbers of T lymphocytes and a scattering of plasma cells are also present.

Much of our current knowledge of the regulation of this inflammatory process traces to a seminal observation by Metcalf et al. [31] that the inflammation does not develop in T-cell-deficient, athymic nude mice. Subsequent studies established that nude mice could be rendered susceptible to HSK through adoptive transfer of T cells from euthymic mice [32]. In addition, with most strains of HSV-1 the chronic inflammation was found to be regulated by the CD4 subpopulation of T lymphocytes [32–35]. An exception to this rule was the observation that corneal infection with the KOS strain of HSV-1 led to a predominantly mononuclear infiltrate in which CD8 cells represented the major infiltrating T-lymphocyte subpopulation, and played an essential role in the inflammatory process [35]. Despite this one exception, which will be discussed further below, corneal infection with most strains of HSV-1 leads to an inflammatory infiltrate that is dominated by neutrophils and CD4+ T lymphocytes.

CD4+ T lymphocytes regulate neutrophilic infiltration into HSV-1-infected corneas through the elaboration of cytokines. A role of Th1-type cytokines in regulating this inflammatory process was established in studies in which monoclonal antibodies were used to neutralize cytokine functions in vivo [36]. Neutralization of the Th1 cytokines interferon-γ (IFN-γ) and interleukin (IL)-2 markedly diminished chronic inflammation in the HSV-1-infected cornea. In contrast, neutralization of the Th2 cytokine IL-4 did not alter the inflammatory process. The authors concluded that neutrophilic infiltration into the HSV-1-infected cornea resulted from production of Th1 cytokines by CD4 T lymphocytes in the cornea. A similar conclusion was reached in a second study in which a reverse transcriptase-polymerase chain reaction (RT-PCR) assay was used to demonstrate the presence in the HSV-1-infected cornea of mRNA coding for Th1 but not Th2 cytokines [37]. Although a role for Th1 cytokines in HSK is well documented, one cannot rule out the involvement of Th2 cytokines under certain circumstances. For instance, in one study a Th2 T-cell line and a Th2 T-cell clone reportedly exacerbated HSK in both HSK-susceptible and HSK-resistant mouse strains [38]. The preferential production of Th1 cytokines in the HSV-1-infected cornea might reflect the manner in which HSV antigens are presented to infiltrating CD4+ T cells as discussed below.

Control by IL-2 and IFN-γ of neutrophil accumulation in HSV-1-infected corneas is exerted at three levels. Studies by Tang and Hendricks [39] demonstrated that IFN-γ regulated neutrophilic extravasation into the perivascular space in the peripheral cornea. Mice exhibiting a moderate level of corneal inflammation following HSV-1 infection were treated systemically with monoclonal antibodies to IFN-γ. Within 24–48 h of antibody treatment, neutrophil extravasation from blood vessels in the peripheral cornea was markedly reduced. Reduced neutrophilic extravasation was associated with a significant reduction in CD31 (PECAM-1) expression on vascular endothelium. These results provided the first in vivo demonstration that PECAM-1 expression on vascular endothelium can be regulated by IFN-γ, and that neutrophils lose PECAM-1 expression during the process of extravasation. The second level at which neutrophilic infiltration is regulated involves the directed migration of extravasated neutrophils from the peripheral to the central cornea. Both IL-2 and IFN-γ are necessary for the establishment of a chemotactic gradient for neutrophils in the infected cornea [28]. The third level at which neutrophil accumulation in the infected cornea is regulated is through their activation and retention at the inflammatory site. IL-2 neutralization caused neutrophils that were present in the inflamed cornea to rapidly undergo apoptosis [38]. In addition to establishing mechanisms by which cytokines regulate inflammation, these studies demonstrated the feasibility of treating active HSK through modulation of cytokine function.

Several groups are currently investigating the role of chemokines in regulating neutrophilic infiltration of the HSV-1-infected cornea. Su et al. [40] used an RT-PCR assay to demonstrate the sequential production of a variety of chemokines in the infected cornea. A different pattern of chemokines appear to be produced early after infection during the period of HSV-1 replication, and later during the T-lymphocyte-regulated chronic inflammation. For instance, mRNA for the monocyte chemoattractant protein (MCP-1) was upregulated during the course of virus replication but declined at the onset of T-cell-mediated chronic inflammation. In contrast, mRNA for the CC chemokine macrophage inflammatory protein (MIP-1α) was not expressed during the period of virus replication, but was upregulated in the infected cornea at the onset of chronic inflammation. In agreement with these findings was the observation of Chen et al. [28] that HSV-1 infection induces two temporally separated neutrophil chemotactic gradients in the mouse cornea: an early, transient, T-cell-independent gradient; and a later, chronic, T-cell-dependent gradient. Recently, Tumpey et al. [41] demonstrated that treatment of mice with IL-10 prevented the expression of MIP-1α and chronic inflammation in HSV-1-infected corneas. Moreover, mice with targeted disruption of the MIP-1α gene were resistant to development of chronic inflammation following HSV-1 corneal infection [42]. These studies suggest that the CC chemokine MIP-1α plays a necessary role in regulating the persistent infiltration of neutrophils into the HSV-1-infected cornea. The previous demonstration of a necessary role for IL-2 in establishing a chemotactic gradient in the infected cornea would suggest that MIP-1α production might be regulated by IL-2. This chronic neutrophilic infiltration appears to be responsible for the destruction of the corneal architecture that leads to corneal scarring and loss of vision [29].

Antigen Presentation in the HSV-1-Infected Cornea

The fact that chronic neutrophilic infiltration of the cornea is regulated by CD4+ T lymphocytes and Th1 cytokines suggested a sequence of events in which CD4+ T lymphocytes infiltrate the infected cornea and are activated by viral antigens presented on the surface of APCs. Although the normal cornea lacks APCs that are capable of presenting antigens to CD4+ T lymphocytes, Langerhans' cells rapidly migrate into the central cornea following HSV-1 infection. Two types of studies established an important role for Langerhans' cells in HSK. One approach [43, 44] compared the severity of HSK in normal corneas and those with preexisting Langerhans' cells (due to trauma or corneal dystrophy). The presence of Langerhans' cells in the cornea at the time of HSV-1 infection resulted in more severe HSK. In a second approach, one cornea of each mouse was depleted of Langerhans' cells by exposure to UV-B light, and then both corneas were infected with HSV-1. Inflammation developed normally in the nonirradiated cornea, but failed to develop in the companion eye that was depleted of Langerhans' cells. These studies provided the first clear demonstration of an essential role for Langerhans' cells in the effector phase of an immunopathological T-lymphocyte response induced by a viral infection.

Another interesting observation of this study was the fact that virus strains can vary in their capacity to induce Langerhans' cell infiltration into the cornea. As noted above, the KOS-321 strain of HSV-1 induced a unique form of immunopathology in the cornea. CD8+ rather than CD4+ T lymphocytes preferentially infiltrated the KOS-321-infected corneas, and depletion of CD8+ T cells reduced the incidence and severity of disease. When compared to other HSV-1 strains, KOS-321 was less efficient at inducing Langerhans' cell migration into the cornea. Depletion of Langerhans' cells from the cornea did not influence the incidence or severity of HSK induced by corneal infection with the KOS-321 strain. Moreover, KOS-321 HSV-1 infection of corneas that were previously infiltrated with Langerhans' cells resulted in neutrophil and CD4+ T lymphocyte accumulation in the infected cornea. Thus, the density of Langerhans' cells in the cornea at the time of T-cell infiltration seems to influence the type of inflammation that develops in the HSV-1-infected cornea. A heavy density of Langerhans' cells appears to result in preferential activation and accumulation of CD4+ T lymphocytes resulting in a predominantly neutrophilic infiltrate. In contrast, a low density of Langerhans' cells appears to favor CD8+ T-cell activation resulting in a predominantly mononuclear leukocyte infiltration.

Recent studies using in vivo treatment with CTLA-4Ig [45] or monoclonal antibodies to B7-1 and B-2 [46] established a requirement for B7 costimulation in this immunopathological process induced by HSV-1 corneal infection. The latter study established that B7 costimulation is required at certain inflammatory sites. Moreover, an association was noted between the proportion of corneas exhibiting elevated numbers of B7-1+ Langerhans' cells and the incidence of chronic inflammation in this model. Thus, expression of the B7-1 costimulatory molecule on corneal Langerhans' cells appears to be an important predisposing factor for the development of chronic inflammation following herpes simplex virus corneal infection. The requirement for costimulation of effector T lymphocytes is controversial. It has been suggested that the microenvironment in which an immune response takes place might influence the requirement for costimulation of effector T cells [47]. Such factors as the presence of proinflammatory cytokines and a high density of antigen within the tissue might mitigate the need for costimulation of effector T cells. In this experimental model, replicating HSV-1 is typically cleared from the infected cornea 2–6 days before the onset of HSK. Based on both clinical and histologic criteria, the cornea appears normal at the time of HSK onset. Based on these observations, one would predict that the cornea would contain low levels of proinflammatory cytokines and a low density of viral antigens at the time of HSK onset. Under these conditions, costimulation of infiltrating CD4+ T lymphocytes might be essential for the induction of Th1 cytokine production and the initiation of inflammation in the cornea.

Does HSV-1 Trigger an Autoimmune Response in the Cornea?

For two decades, immunologists have studied the mechanisms by which T lymphocytes regulate inflammation in the HSV-1-infected cornea. However, to date no one has identified specific viral antigens that induce the immunopathology. This gap in our knowledge is attributable at least in part to the difficulty of generating HSV-reactive T-cell clones in strains of mice that are susceptible to HSK. Moreover, a number of provocative observations have caused many investigators to question whether viral antigens are actually involved in the induction of HSK. Some investigators have observed that T lymphocytes obtained from HSV-1-infected and noninfected mice are equally effective in adoptively transferring HSK susceptibility to BALB/c athymic nude (nu/nu) mice and severe combined immunodeficiency (SCID) mice [pers. unpubl. observ. and 48]. Moreover, mice can be protected from HSK by in vivo depletion of CD4+ and CD8+ T lymphocytes. However, when T-lymphocyte depletion was discontinued 30 days after corneal infection, the mice promptly developed HSK [49]. The corneas of these mice were free of replicating virus or immunohistochemically detectable HSV-1 antigens for at least 3 weeks at the time of HSK onset. These observations tend to reinforce previous speculation that HSK represents an autoimmune response to corneal tissue.

More direct support for this concept came from recent studies of BALB/c congenic strains that exhibit dramatically different susceptibility to HSK [50]. The susceptible C.AL-20 strain expresses the Igh^d allotype whereas the resistant C.B-17 strain expresses the Igh^b allotype. C.AL-20 mice were rendered resistant to HSK when tolerized to IgG2a^b. Moreover, susceptibility to HSK could be adoptively transferred to T-cell-deficient BALB/c nu/nu mice with CD4+ T cells from C.AL-20 mice that were immunized with HSV-1 or with IgG2a^b. HSK susceptibility could not be adoptively transferred with naive T cells or T cells from Igh^e-immunized C.AL-20 mice. Furthermore, two IgG2a^b-reactive T-cell clones, C1-6 and C1-15, could adoptively transfer susceptibility to HSK to BALB/c nu/nu mice. The C1-6 and C1-15 T-cell clones could be stimulated in vitro with an extract from normal cornea. Subsequent studies [51] established that the C1-6 and C1-15 clones could also be stimulated in vitro by an epitope from the HSV-1 UL6 coat protein. The implication of these studies is that HSV-1 infection of the cornea exposes a normally sequestered corneal epitope to the immune system. Autoaggressive CD4+ T cells reactive to this epitope then infiltrate the cornea and mediate corneal destruction. Expression of a cross-reactive epitope by HSV-1 may enhance this autoimmune response through molecular mimicry. Mice that express a cross-reactive epitope in their IgG2ab molecules are tolerant to the epitope, and thus resistant to HSK.

This interesting model demonstrates a mechanism by which host genotype can influence susceptibility to virus-induced immunopathology. They also underpin the potential importance of autoreactivity in viral disease. It is possible, however, that some of the observations in these studies may be unique to the model employed. For instance, naïve T cells from C.AL-20 mice could not transfer HSK susceptibility to BALB/c nu/nu mice. In contrast, naïve T cells from euthymic BALB/c mice are as effective as HSV-immune T cells at transferring HSK susceptibility to BALB/c nu/nu mice [pers. unpubl. observ.]. Moreover, CD4+ T cells from C.B-17 mice that are tolerant to Igh[b] epitopes can adoptively transfer HSK susceptibility to BALB/c SCID mice [48]. This latter observation established that the HSK-resistant C.B-17 mice possess effector cells that can mediate HSK in an appropriate host. Thus, systemic tolerance to cross-reactive corneal antigens cannot explain the resistance of C.B-17 mice to HSK. The reason for these apparently discordant results requires clarification. Another observation that is seemingly at odds with the results of Cantor and coworkers [51, 52] is that T-cell lines and clones that are reactive to an epitope on HSV-1 glycoprotein D can render C.B-17 mice susceptible to HSK [38]. Again, it is difficult to reconcile this observation with the proposal that the resistance of C.B-17 mice to HSK is due to tolerance to an epitope that is shared by IgG2a[b], a corneal protein, and the HSV-1 UL6 protein.

In yet another interesting twist to this complicated story, Rouse and coworkers [53] recently reported that HSK susceptibility could be adoptively transferred to SCID mice with CD4+ T cells bearing a transgenic TCR specific for an OVA peptide and lacking detectable reactivity to HSV antigens. In these studies it appeared that HSK could develop in the absence of T-cell recognition of HSV antigens. However, the likelihood that T cells with such a limited TCR repertoire (all expressing the OVA-specific TCR) would react to corneal antigens also seems somewhat remote. The authors suggest that bystander activation of CD4+ T cells resulting from exposure to cytokines in the infected cornea might contribute to HSK. Cytokines clearly are produced in the cornea during the course of HSV-1 replication [54]. Moreover, the SCID mice that received TCR transgenic T cells failed to control HSV replication, and their corneas contained replicating virus at the onset of HSK. Thus, the corneas of these mice might have contained sufficiently high concentrations of cytokines to activate cytokine production by infiltrating CD4+ T cells in the absence of cognate antigen recognition. However, in immunologically normal mice, HSK is initiated 4–30 days after replicating virus is eliminated from the cornea [49]. The possibility that a 'cytokine storm' activates T lymphocytes that infiltrate a clinically quiescent cornea seems much less likely. Moreover, the notion of bystander activation by cytokines seems to be incompatible with the requirement of Langerhans' cells and B7 costimulatory molecule expression in the infected cornea for the development of HSK. Thus, the relative contribution of HSV-reactive, autoaggressive, and bystander-activated CD4+ T cells to the immunopathology that is induced in the cornea by HSV-1 infection remains unresolved.

Conclusion

It emerges from the above discussion that HSK represents a very complex immunopathological process. The genotype of the host and the virus can qualitatively and quantitatively influence the nature of the inflammatory process that occurs in the infected cornea. Moreover, even when genetically identical inbred mice are infected with the same virus preparation, only a portion of the infected corneas develop HSK. Attempts to associate the development of HSK with quantitative or qualitative differences in the systemic immune response to HSV-1 antigens have failed to reveal any significant associations [46]. Clearly factors within the microenvironment of the infected cornea are crucial to the outcome of HSV-1 infection. Factors such as cytokine and chemokine production, expression of adhesion molecules and antigen presentation all appear to contribute significantly to HSK susceptibility. Our working model of immunopathology in HSV-1-infected corneas is illustrated in figure 1.

Despite the complexity of the disease process, it appears that individually modulating certain components of the immunopathological process can dramatically reduce inflammation in the infected cornea. Neutralizing the Th1 cytokines IFN-γ or IL-2, inhibiting production of the chemokine MIP-1α, and blocking B7 costimulation can each dramatically inhibit the development of inflammation in the infected cornea. It is particularly encouraging to note the therapeutic value of some of these treatments. For instance, neutralizing IL-2 or IFN-γ in mice with established HSK dramatically, and in many cases completely reversed the inflammatory process 24–48 h after a single treatment [39, 55]. Thus, approaches designed to modify cytokine and APC function within the microenvironment of the HSV-1-infected cornea may have therapeutic value in treating HSK. Indeed, treatment of the infected cornea with IL-10 [56], or with plasmids containing the gene encoding IL-10 [57], can dramatically reduce the severity of HSK in mice.

Another potentially useful approach to modulating HSK is through tolerization of certain aspects of the immune response to HSV-1. For instance, injection of HSV-1 into the anterior chamber of the eye induces a deviant form of immunity referred to as anterior chamber-associated immune deviation (ACAID) [58]. Preferential inhibition of CD4+ T-cell functions such as delayed-type hypersensitivity and production of Th1 cytokines characterize ACAID [59]. Induction

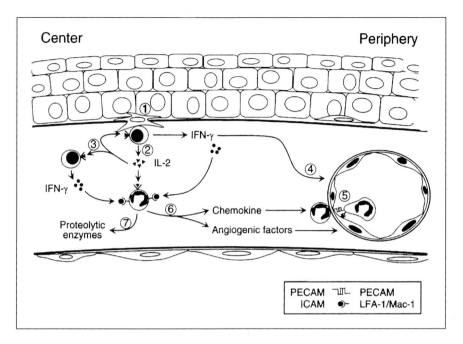

Center   Periphery

PECAM ┐Ⴎᴸ PECAM
ICAM ●ー LFA-1/Mac-1

Fig. 1. Proposed mechanisms by which CD4+ T lymphocytes regulate neutrophilic infiltration and destruction of the HSV-1-infected cornea: (1) Infiltrating CD4+ T lymphocytes are activated by HSV and/or self antigens that are presented by Langerhans' cells. Costimulation by the B7-1 and B7-2 costimulatory molecules is required. (2) The activated CD4+ T lymphocytes produce IL-2. (3) The IL-2 acts in an autocrine or paracrine fashion to maintain IFN-γ production. (4) IFN-γ upregulates PECAM-1 expression on the vascular endothelium. (5) An interaction of PECAM-1 on the neutrophils and vascular endothelium facilitates transendothelial migration of circulating neutrophils into the infected cornea. (6) IL-2 and IFN-γ indirectly contribute to the establishment of a chemotactic/haptotactic gradient for neutrophils within the cornea. MIP-1α appears to be an essential chemokine. Its source in the infected cornea is not known, but could be the activated neutrophils. (7) IL-2 and IFN-γ activate neutrophils, protecting them from apoptotic death and augmenting their exocytosis of collagenases and other proteolytic enzymes that contribute to the destruction of the corneal architecture. [Reprinted from 38, with permission.]

of ACAID to HSV antigens at the time of HSV-1 corneal infection protects the cornea from HSK, without rendering mice susceptible to disseminated disease [60]. Because of the relative immune privilege of the cornea, approaches to tolerance induction such as oral tolerance might be more effective at inhibiting immunopathology in the cornea [61, 62]. Since it is now clear that tolerance can be induced in the face of an active immune response, such approaches might prove useful in preventing recurrent HSK. Indeed the eye might prove to be the most amenable tissue for immunology-based therapy.

References

1 Doherty PC, Allan W, Eichelberger M, Carding SR: Roles of alpha beta and gamma delta T cell subsets in viral immunity. Annu Rev Immunol 1992;10:123–151.
2 Doherty PC, Allan JE, Lynch F, Ceredig R: Dissection of an inflammatory process induced by CD8+ T cells. Immunol Today 1990;11:55–59.
3 Gordon YJ, Aoki K, Kinchington PR: Adenovirus keratoconjunctivitis; in Pepose JS, Holland GN, Wilhelmus KR (eds): Ocular Infection and Immunity. St Louis, Mosby Year Book, 1998, pp 877–894.
4 Bigger JE, Thomas CA, Atherton SS: NK cell modulation of murine cytomegalovirus retinitis. J Immunol 1998;160:5826–5831.
5 Shanley JD: In vivo administration of monoclonal antibody to the NK 1.1 antigen of natural killer cells: Effect on acute murine cytomegalovirus infection. J Med Virol 1990;30:58–60.
6 Quinnan GV, Ennis FA: Cell-mediated immunity in cytomegalovirus infections – A review. Comp Immunol Microbiol Infect Dis 1980;3:283–290.
7 Pavan-Langston D, Dunkel EC: Varicella-zoster virus diseases: Anterior segment of the eye; in Pepose JS, Holland GN, Wilhelmus KR (eds): Ocular Infection and Immunity. St Louis, Mosby Year Book, 1996, pp 933–957.
8 Hoang-Xuan T, Buchi ER, Herbort CP, Denis J, Frot P, Thenault S, Pouliquen Y: Oral acyclovir for herpes zoster ophthalmicus. Ophthalmology 1992;99:1062–1070.
9 Mackensen G, Sundmacher R, Witschel H: Late wound complications after circular keratotomy for zoster keratitis. Cornea 1984;3:95–98.
10 Cantin EM, Hinton DR, Chen J, Openshaw H: Gamma interferon expression during acute and latent nervous system infection by herpes simplex virus type 1. J Virol 1995;69:4898–4905.
11 Gebhardt BM, Hill JM: Cellular neuroimmunologic responses to ocular herpes simplex virus infection. J Neuroimmunol 1992;28:227–236.
12 Gesser RM, Valyi-Nagy T, Fraser NW: Restricted herpes simplex virus type 1 gene expression within sensory neurons in the absence of functional B and T lymphocytes. Virology 1994;200: 791–795.
13 Ghiasi H, Cai S, Nesburn AB, Wechsler SL: Vaccination with herpes simplex virus type 1 glycoprotein K impairs clearance of virus from the trigeminal ganglia resulting in chronic infection. Virology 1996;224:330–333.
14 Goldsmith K, Chen W, Johnson DC, Hendricks RL: Infected cell protein (ICP)47 enhances herpes simplex virus neurovirulence by blocking the CD8+ T cell response. J Exp Med 1998;187:341–348.
15 Halford WP, Gebhardt BM, Carr DJJ: Persistent cytokine expression in trigeminal ganglion latently infected with herpes simplex virus type 1. J Immunol 1996;157:3542–3549.
16 Liu T, Tang Q, Hendricks RL: Inflammatory infiltration of the trigeminal ganglion after herpes simplex virus type 1 corneal infection. J Virol 1996;70:264–271.
17 Sciammas R, Kodukula P, Tang Q, Hendricks RL, Bluestone JA: T cell receptor-γ/δ cells protect mice from herpes simplex virus type 1-induced lethal encephalitis. J Exp Med 1997;185:1969–1975.
18 Shimeld C, Whiteland JL, Williams NA, Easty D, Hill TJ: Reactivation of herpes simplex virus type 1 in the mouse trigeminal ganglion: An in vivo study of virus antigen and immune cell infiltration. J Gen Virol 1996;77:2583–2590.
19 Simmons A, Tscharke DC: Anti-CD8 impairs clearance of herpes simplex virus from the nervous system: Implications for the fate of virally infected neurons. J Exp Med 1992;175:1337–1344.
20 Azumi A, Atherton SS: Sparing of the ipsilateral retina after anterior chamber inoculation of HSV-1: Requirement for either CD4+ or CD8+ T cells. Invest Ophthalmol Vis Sci 1994;35: 3251–3259.
21 Matsubara S, Atherton SS: Spread of HSV-1 to the suprachiasmatic nuclei and retina in T cell depleted BALB/c mice. J Neuroimmunol 1997;80:165–171.
22 Zhao M, Atherton SS: Immune effector cell (IEC)-mediated protection from HSV-1 retinitis occurs in the brain. J Neuroimmunol 1997;75:51–58.
23 Azumi A, Cousins SW, Kanter MY, Atherton SS: Modulation of murine herpes simplex virus type 1 retinitis in the uninoculated eye by CD4+ T lymphocytes. Invest Ophthalmol Vis Sci 1994;35: 54–63.

24 Liesegang TJ, Melton LJ, Daly PJ, Ilstrup DM: Epidemiology of ocular herpes simplex. Incidence in Rochester, MN, 1950 through 1982. Arch Ophthalmol 1989;107:1155–1159.

25 Sundmacher R: Clinical aspects of herpetic eye diseases. Curr Eye Res 1987;6:183–188.

26 Meyers-Elliott RH, Chitjian PA: Immunopathogenesis of corneal inflammation in herpes simplex virus stromal keratitis: Role of the polymorphonuclear leukocyte. Invest Ophthalmol Vis Sci 1981; 20:784–798.

27 Wilson SE, Pedroza L, Beuerman R, Hill JM: Herpes simplex virus type-1 infection of corneal epithelial cells induces apoptosis of the underlying keratocytes. Exp Eye Res 1997;64:775–779.

28 Chen W, Tang Q, Hendricks RL: Ex vivo model of leukocyte migration into herpes simplex virus-infected mouse corneas. J Leukoc Biol 1996;60:167–173.

29 Thomas J, Gangappa S, Kanangat S, Rouse BT: On the essential involvement of neutrophils in the immunopathologic disease: Herpetic stromal keratitis. J Immunol 1997;158:1383–1391.

30 Tumpey TM, Chen SH, Oakes JE, Lausch RN: Neutrophil-mediated suppression of virus replication after herpes simplex virus type 1 infection of the murine cornea. J Virol 1996;70:898–904.

31 Metcalf JF, Hamilton DS, Reichert RW: Herpetic keratitis in athymic (nude) mice. Infect Immun 1979;26:1164–1171.

32 Russell RG, Nasisse MP, Larsen HS, Rouse BT: Role of T-lymphocytes in the pathogenesis of herpetic stromal keratitis. Invest Ophthalmol Vis Sci 1984;25:938–944.

33 Newell CK, Sendele D, Rouse BT: Effects of CD4+ and CD8+ T-lymphocyte depletion on the induction and expression of herpes simplex stromal keratitis. Reg Immunool 1989;2:366–369.

34 Newell CK, Martin S, Sendele D, Mercadal CM, Rouse BT: Herpes simplex virus-induced stromal keratitis: Role of T-lymphocyte subsets in immunopathology. J Virol 1989;63:769–775.

35 Hendricks RL, Tumpey TM: Contribution of virus and immune factors to herpes simplex virus type 1 induced corneal pathology. Invest Ophthalmol Vis Sci 1990;31:1929–1939.

36 Hendricks RL, Tumpey TM, Finnegan A: IFN-gamma and IL-2 are protective in the skin but pathologic in the corneas of HSV-1-infected mice. J Immunol 1992;149:3023–3028.

37 Niemialtowski MG, Rouse BT: Predominance of Th1 cells in ocular tissues during herpetic stromal keratitis. J Immunol 1992;149:3035–3039.

38 Jayaraman S, Heiligenhaus A, Rodriguez A, Soukiasian S, Dorf ME, Foster CS: Exacerbation of murine herpes simplex virus-mediated stromal keratitis by Th2 type T cells. J Immunol 1993;151: 5777–5789.

39 Tang Q, Hendricks RL: IFN-gamma regulates PECAM-1 expression and neutrophil infiltration into herpes simplex virus-infected mouse corneas. J Exp Med 1996;184:1435–1447.

40 Su YH, Oakes JE, Lausch RN: Ocular avirulence of a herpes simplex virus type 1 strain is associated with heightened sensitivity to alpha/beta interferon. J Virol 1990;64:2187–2192.

41 Tumpey TM, Cheng H, Yan XT, Oaks JE, Lausch RN: Chemokine synthesis in the HSV-1-infected cornea and its suppression by interleukin-10. J Leukoc Biol 1998;63:486–492.

42 Tumpey TM, Cheng H, Cook DN, Smithies O, Oaks JE, Lausch RN: Absence of macrophage inflammatory protein-1α prevents the development of blinding herpes stromal keratitis. J Virol 1998; 72:3705–3710.

43 Jager MJ: Corneal Langerhans' cells and ocular immunology. Reg Immunol 1992;4:186–195.

44 Jager MJ, Bradley D, Atherton SS, Streilein JW: Presence of Langerhans' cells in the central cornea linked to the development of ocular herpes in mice. Exp Eye Res 1992;54:835–841.

45 Gangappa S, Manickan E, Rouse BT: Control of herpetic stromal keratitis using CTLA4Ig fusion protein. Clin Immunol Immunopathol 1998;86:88–94.

46 Chen H, Hendricks RL: B7 costimulatory requirements of T cells at an inflammatory site. J Immunol 1998;160:5045–5052.

47 Gause WC, Mitro V, Via CS, Linsley P, Urban J Jr, Greenwald RJ: Do effector and memory T helper cells also need B7 ligand costimulatory signals? J Immunol 1997;159:1055–1058.

48 Thomas J, Rouse BT: Immunopathology of herpetic stromal keratitis: Discordance in CD4+ T cell function between euthymic host and reconstituted SCID recipients. J Immunol 1998;160: 3965–3970.

49 Hendricks RL, Tumpey TM: Concurrent regeneration of T lymphocytes and susceptibility to HSV-1 corneal stromal disease. Curr Eye Res 1991;10:47–53.

50   Avery AC, Zhao ZS, Rodriguez A, Bikoff EK, Soheilian M, Foster CS, Cantor H: Resistance to herpes stromal keratitis conferred by an IgG2a-derived peptide. Nature 1995;376:431–433.
51   Zhao ZS, Granucci F, Yeh L, Schaffer PA, Cantor H: Molecular mimicry by herpes simplex virus-type 1: Autoimmune disease after viral infection. Science 1998;279:1344–1347.
52   Akova YA, Dutt J, Rodriguez A, Jabbur N, Foster CS: The role of Igh-1 disparate congenic mouse T lymphocytes in the pathogenesis of herpetic stromal keratitis. Curr Eye Res 1993;12:1093–1101.
53   Gangappa S, Babu JS, Thomas J, Daheshia M, Rouse BT: Virus-induced immunoinflammatory lesions in the absence of viral antigen recognition. J Immunol 1998;161:4289–4300.
54   Staats HF, Lausch RN: Cytokine expression in vivo during murine herpetic stromal keratitis. J Immunol 1993;151:277–283.
55   Tang Q, Chen W, Hendricks RL: Proinflammatory functions of IL-2 in herpes simplex virus corneal infection. J Immunol 1997;158:1275–1283.
56   Tumpey TM, Elner VM, Chen SH, Oakes JE, Lausch RN: Interleukin-10 treatment can suppress stromal keratitis induced by herpes simplex virus type 1. J Immunol 1994;153:2258–2265.
57   Daheshia M, Kuklin N, Kanangat S, Manickan E, Rouse BT: Suppression of ongoing ocular inflammatory disease by topical administration of plasmid DNA encoding IL-10. J Immunol 1997; 159:1945–1952.
58   Whittum JA, Niederkorn JY, McCulley JP, Streilein JW: Intracameral inoculation of herpes simplex virus type I induces anterior chamber associated immune deviation. Curr Eye Res 1983;2:691–697.
59   Streilein JW: Immune regulation and the eye: A dangerous compromise. FASEB J 1987;1:199–208.
60   Ksander BR, Hendricks RL: Cell-mediated immune tolerance to HSV-1 antigens associated with reduced susceptibility to HSV-1 corneal lesions. Invest Ophthalmol Vis Sci 1987;28:1986–1993.
61   Ma D, Mellon J, Niederkorn JY: Conditions affecting enhanced corneal allograft survival by oral immunization. Invest Ophthalmol Vis Sci 1998;39:1835–1846.
62   Ma D, Li XY, Mellon J, Niederkorn JY: Immunologic phenotype of hosts orally immunized with corneal alloantigens. Invest Ophthalmol Vis Sci 1998;39:744–753.

Robert L. Hendricks, PhD, Department of Ophthalmology,
University of Pittsburgh School of Medicine, The Eye and Ear Institute,
203 Lothrop Street, Pittsburgh, PA 15213 (USA)
Tel. +1 412 647 5754, Fax +1 412 647 5880, E-Mail hendricksrr@msx.upmc.edu

Streilein JW (ed): Immune Response and the Eye.
Chem Immunol. Basel, Karger, 1999, vol 73, pp 137–158

....

Immune Privilege, Tumors, and the Eye

Peter W. Chen, Bruce R. Ksander

Schepens Eye Research Institute and Department of Ophthalmology,
Harvard Medical School, Boston, Mass., USA

Introduction

During the past decade, conclusive evidence has shown that spontaneous human tumors express antigens. This important finding presents a confounding situation; although tumors present antigens that can be recognized by immune effector cells, they fail to induce antitumor immunity that prevents tumor progression. Moreover, current clinical trials of immunotherapies directed against tumor antigens indicate these antigens are not highly immunogenic, since the clinical response of these therapies has fallen far short of expectations. In order to improve the design of these treatments so they successfully eliminate tumors, we need to better understand the mechanisms that tumors use to escape immune detection and elimination.

Immune privileged sites are highly effective at preventing immune-mediated elimination of cells expressing foreign antigens. Our laboratory and others have proposed that tumors establish their own immune privileged environment and therefore, tumors possess the ability to transform a nonprivileged site into an immune privileged site. However, how tumors achieve privilege is incompletely understood at this time. Extensive studies, some described in other chapters of this book, have been conducted to determine how the eye establishes immune privilege. We predict the eye and spontaneous tumors share common pathways used to establish immune privilege. Moreover, studies of ocular immune privilege indicate that privilege can be terminated, suggesting there are methods of preventing immune privilege within the eye that may be useful in terminating privilege within tumors. In the absence of immune privilege, the effectiveness of cancer immunotherapies may be increased dramatically.

Tumors as Immune Privileged Sites and Privileged Tissues

The historical definition of an immune privileged site is an anatomical site where transplanted foreign tissue survives for an extended period of time in an immunocompetent host. Therefore, in order for tumors to qualify as an immune privileged site, they must satisfy two criteria. First, they must express antigens that can be recognized as foreign. Second, tumors must survive in a host capable of responding to the tumor antigens. In 1974, Robert North [1] first proposed that tumors were immune privileged sites. In his experiments, he used an animal model to compare the survival of *Listeria* injected into a nonprivileged site, the hind footpad, with the survival of a similar injection of *Listeria* into a progressively growing tumor in the contralateral hind footpad. Surprisingly, the *Listeria* survived within the tumor site, but was rapidly rejected from the normal footpad. North proposed that macrophages infiltrating into the tumor environment were altered and unable to eliminate *Listeria* within the tumor site. However, North's idea that tumors were immune privileged sites was not widely accepted. This was probably due to the fact that, in 1974, it was still controversial whether spontaneous human tumors expressed tumor antigens. Therefore, the privileged environment within a tumor would be a moot point if tumors failed to express any foreign antigens. In the past decade, two discoveries have revived the idea that tumors create an immune privileged environment. By far the most important discovery was the identification of genes that encode tumor antigens and the characterization of T cells that recognize these antigens [2]. This confirmed that tumors expressed antigens that the immune system could potentially recognize. The second discovery directly connected tumors with immune privileged sites. In 1995, it was first reported that Fas ligand was constitutively expressed only on tissues within immune privileged sites and the expression of this apoptosis-inducing molecule was an important feature of immune privilege [3]. This was followed by the discovery that some spontaneous human tumors also expressed Fas ligand constitutively and it was proposed that tumors also use Fas ligand to establish immune privilege [4]. Together, these recent discoveries have revived the concept that at least some tumors possess the ability to establish and maintain an immune privileged environment.

Privileged sites are identified by transplantation experiments in which the survival of the transplant in the 'privileged' site must be longer than the survival of the same graft in a 'nonprivileged' site. Typically, grafts were placed into the subcutaneous tissues of the skin as the nonprivileged site. Therefore, the traditional concept of immune privilege was always related to an anatomical site (eye, brain, testis, and the maternal-fetal interface). However, more recently, the concept of immune privilege has evolved to include immune privileged 'tissues' [5]. These 'privileged tissues' possess the ability to survive when transplanted into a foreign host regardless of which anatomical site the graft is placed. In other words, these 'privileged tissues' possess the ability to create their own immune privileged site. This concept started with the experiments of Bellgrau et al. [6], who demonstrated foreign Sertoli cell grafts survived when placed into the kidney capsule of allogeneic mice.

Although the topic of immune privileged tissues is discussed in detail in another chapter of this issue, this raises the question of whether spontaneous human tumors are either immune privileged sites, privileged tissues, or both.

It would be highly advantageous for a tumor cell to possess properties of a 'privileged tissue' since it would allow a mobile metastatic tumor cell to escape immune destruction regardless of which organ it invaded. However, we predict that if tumors become privileged tissues, this only occurs late in disease development. We feel it is more likely that tumors first acquire the properties of an immune privileged site during formation of the primary tumor. However, since immune privilege is maintained by multiple mechanisms, it is likely that tumors gradually acquire the individual properties of a privileged site through time. It is unclear exactly when during disease progression tumors acquire immune privilege. If the purpose of immune privilege is to mask an immune response against tumor antigens, it is likely the appearance of immune privilege in tumors coincides with the expression of tumor antigens. We predict that sometime after the initial stages of malignant transformation, tumor antigens are expressed as an unavoidable consequence of the activation or mutation of genes controlling cellular proliferation. Continued success of the tumor now depends on acquiring the ability to establish an immune privileged environment. The more antigenic a tumor becomes, the more dependent it will be on acquiring the characteristics of an immune privileged site. A tumor that expresses no antigens would not be dependent upon establishing immune privilege. By contrast, highly antigenic tumors would have to quickly develop privilege or risk immune elimination. Since tumors establish privilege in order to escape immune recognition of tumor antigens, it is important to understand the properties of antigens expressed by tumors. The following section will briefly describe different types of tumor antigens.

Tumor Antigens

Identification of Tumor Antigens

Originally, tumor antigens were identified by generating antibodies against tumor cells [7]. However, analysis of the immunoprecipitates from these antibodies demonstrated that their specificity for tumor cells was relatively poor, and resulted in the coprecipitation of proteins found on normal cells. Current techniques used to identify antigens demonstrate a much higher level of specificity for isolating tumor-specific antigens. One common method uses chromatography to purify and fractionate peptides eluted from MHC class I molecules. Fractions are then tested to determine if proteins contained in the specific fractions sensitize target cells for lysis by a panel of antigen-specific cytotoxic T lymphocytes [8, 9]. Other methods used to identify tumor antigens involve insertion of tumor cell DNA libraries into target cells that express MHC class I and screening the transfected cells for their ability to stimulate CTL proliferation [10]. Tumor antigen genes are then isolated, cloned, and sequenced from transfected cells that successfully stimulate CTL proliferation. These approaches have been used recently to identify a large number of tumor antigens that serve as potential targets for immunotherapy. Although tumors originating from a variety of organs and tissues express tumor antigens, the majority of tumor antigens identified to date are found on skin melanomas and can be classified according to their pattern of expression.

Tumor Differentiation Antigens

Differentiation antigens genes are transcribed in tumor cells and normal pigmented cells (skin melanocytes, retinal pigment epithelial cells, and choroidal melanocytes) but are not transcribed by normal unpigmented cells. While normal pigmented melanocytes and tumor cells express identical differentiation antigen genes, unique tumor antigens are generated from post-translational modification of the translated proteins. Peptide sequences of the differentiation tumor antigens Tyrosinase [11–14], MART-1 [15, 16], and gp100 [17, 18], exhibit post-translational modifications which alters the binding characteristics of antigen peptides to class I, resulting in presentation of the tumor peptides by class I molecules.

Expression of differentiation tumor antigens also results from alternative transcription of differentiation antigen genes. Two tumor antigens produced by this method are TRP-1 [19] and TRP-2 [20]. Genes for these antigens contain multiple overlapping open reading frame, and tumor antigens are produced when an alternate reading frame is transcribed. Because differentiation tumor antigens genes are transcribed by normal pigmented cells and tumor cells, there are some concerns that immunotherapy against tumors that express differentiation antigens will induce autoimmune responses against normal melanocytes and pigmented cells in the retina. Clinical trials using immunotherapies that target differentiation antigens to treat patients with metastatic skin melanoma have demonstrated that vitiligo is associated with an antitumor response, but there have been no reported side effects in the retina [21].

Tumor Antigens Generated by Mutations

Since mutations occur frequently in tumor cells, genes encoding mutant proteins may produce new tumor antigens. Screening melanoma cell cDNA libraries with T-cell clones has led to the identification of a number of tumor antigens in this category, including β-catenin, cyclin-dependent kinase-4 (CDK-4), and MUM-1 [22–24]. In nonmalignant cells, these genes encode proteins that regulate cell adhesion, cell cycling, and the initiation of apoptosis. Mutations of these genes promote tumor survival by increasing cellular proliferation and migration. However, the undesirable side effect for the tumor cell is the expression of mutated peptide antigens on the cell surface. For example, CDK-4 controls cell cycle progression, but a point mutation in the CDK-4 gene in melanomas generates a protein that inhibits CDK-4 binding to its inhibitor, p16, resulting in uncontrolled tumor cell growth. In addition, the mutation also results in the expression of a unique tumor antigen presented on the cell surface by HLA class I molecules.

Overexpression of Normal Antigens

CTL clones from melanoma patients have also identified antigens expressed on both normal and tumor cells that are produced by nonmutated genes. The HER2/Neu protein, which is expressed in breast and ovarian cancer, is an example of this type of tumor antigen [25]. Although this antigen is expressed on normal cells, they are not lysed by CTL because they express only very low levels of HER2/Neu. By contrast, tumor cells express significantly higher levels of HER2/Neu and are consequently recognized and lysed by CTL. Recently, the first example of this type of antigen on skin melanoma cells was identified. The PRAME (Preferentially Expressed Antigen of MElanoma) antigen is expressed at high levels on skin melanoma cells and also on a wide variety of other types of tumors, but is only expressed at low levels on normal cells [26].

Tumor-Specific Antigens

Boon and coworkers [27, 28] identified a family of 12 genes located on the X chromosome of metastatic skin melanoma cells that encode tumor-specific antigens. These antigens are recognized by CD8 cytotoxic T cells, and are known as the MAGE (Melanoma Antigen GEne) genes. These genes are unusual since they are present in all normal cells, but only transcriptionally active in tumor cells and the testis. While both primary and metastatic cutaneous melanoma cells express MAGE antigens, they are not detected in a variety of normal cells including cutaneous melanocytes, lymphocytes, muscle cells, skin fibroblasts, and kidney cells. The only exception is the testis, specifically, the spermatogonia and spermatocytes [29]. However, these cells are unlikely to be recognized by MAGE-specific CTL since they express little or no MHC class I. Recently, other genes have been identified that encode MAGE-like tumor-specific antigens expressed in tumors and testis, and include the LAGE-1/NY-ESO-1, and GAGE genes [30, 31].

Tumor Antigens due to Abnormal Intron Transcription

Errors in the excision of introns from exon-intron pairs also generate tumor antigens. Recently, a novel tumor-specific antigen derived from N-ace-tylglucosaminyltransferase-V (Gn-T-V) was identified by screening a cDNA library from melanoma cells with HLA-A2-specific CTL clones [32]. Normally, the Gn-T-V protein is involved in the synthesis of oligosaccharides and is expressed by all normal and malignant cells. However, a unique Gn-T-V peptide is produced in melanoma cells from incomplete splicing of an intron-exon pair revealing part of an intron sequence. This unique Gn-T-V peptide is recognized by specific CTL. Further studies demonstrate that this antigen is frequently expressed on melanomas, but not expressed in normal tissues.

Tumor Escape Mechanisms

The idea that tumors evade immune elimination is not novel. Many laboratories have identified different methods used by tumors to escape immune effector cells. We would like to know what role immune privilege plays in these tumor escape mechanisms: Is immune privilege within the eye similar to immune privilege within tumors? Are the same mechanisms used to establish immune privilege in these sites? And, does the study of ocular immune privilege suggest an approach to terminate immune privilege that can be used to increase the effectiveness of immunotherapies? In order to address these questions, we will first compare and contrast tumor escape mechanisms with ocular immune privilege. The following sections will describe how tumors, (a) prevent induction of immunity by secretion of immunosuppressive factors, (b) prevent tumor antigen recognition by altering antigen processing and presentation, and (c) escape following active immunization of cancer patients. These are summarized in table 1.

Preventing Induction of Immunity by Secretion of
Immunosuppressive Factors

Several immunosuppressive cytokines and factors are known to prevent monocytes, macrophage, and dendritic cells from becoming fully functional antigen presenting cells by inhibiting antigen processing and presentation.

Table 1. Tumor escape mechanisms

Immunosuppressive environment
    Interleukin-10
    Transforming growth factor-β
    Vascular endothelial growth factor

Reduced or eliminated class I expression

Inhibition of antigen processing pathway
    Loss of LMP
    Loss of TAP

Inhibition of tumor infiltrating antigen-presenting cells

Deviant immune effector cells
    Inhibit in situ activation of CTL
    Inhibition of NK cells

Loss of tumor antigen gene transcription

A number of these factors are produced by tumor cells and are described below.

Interleukin-10 (IL-10)

IL-10 is an immunosuppressive cytokine that inhibits antigen presenting cells from effectively presenting tumor antigens. IL-10 is secreted by a variety of tumors including head and neck, melanoma, and non-small cell lung tumors [33–35]. Granstein and coworkers [36] examined the role of IL-10 in inhibiting primary and secondary antitumor immune responses. A primary immune response was observed when naïve mice were immunized with tumor antigen-pulsed Langerhans' cells. However, only Langerhans' cells that were first activated with GM-CSF in vitro successfully primed naïve mice. Repeated immunization with activated Langerhans' cells induced antitumor immunity that protected mice from a challenge of live tumor cells in the flank. By contrast, IL-10-treated Langerhans' cells neither primed, nor produced protective immunity. Langerhans' cells were only inhibited if IL-10 was delivered before activation by GM-CSF. If Langerhans' cells were treated with GM-CSF *prior* to IL-10 exposure, the inhibitory effect of IL-10 was lost, and Langerhans' cells primed the mice effectively.

IL-10 also inhibited a secondary immune response against tumor antigens presented by Langerhans' cells. If mice were first primed against tumor antigens, a secondary response was observed by injecting tumor antigen-pulsed Langerhans' cells in the hind footpad and measuring DH. If the Langerhans' cells used to elicit the secondary immune response were treated with IL-10, they were unable to induce DH. Thus, these studies demonstrate that IL-10 can block antigen presentation by Langerhans' cells to primed specific T cells. Together, these studies indicate IL-10 can inhibit antigen presentation to either naïve, or primed T cells. However, IL-10 is effective only during a critical window prior to activation of Langerhans' cells.

Transforming Growth Factor-β (TGF-β)

TGF-β exists in 3 isoforms and controls cell growth and differentiation by inhibiting activation, and proliferation of cells that mediate antitumor immunity [37]. TFG-β was first purified and cloned from a human glioblastoma cell line [38]. In addition to glioblastomas, head and neck tumors, skin melanoma, and ovarian adenocarcinomas also secrete various isoforms of TGF-β [39–42]. Takeuchi et al. [43] has recently demonstrated that TGF-β prevents the afferent phase of the immune response by blocking antigen-presenting cells from activating antigen-specific T cells. Ovalbumin peptide (OVA)-pulsed peritoneal exudate cells (PEC) cultured with TGF-β fail to activate OVA peptide-specific T cells. RT-PCR analysis of mRNA from TGF-β-treated PEC demonstrates that culturing PEC with TGF-β upregulates transcription of TGF-β genes, inducing autocrine secretion of TGF-β by PEC. In addition, culturing PEC pulsed with OVA peptide and TGF-β downregulates transcription of the IL-12 genes. While these studies clearly demonstrate that TGF-β directly blocks the ability of APC to activate specific T cells, TGF-β has recently been shown to also *indirectly* block APC function by stimulating the secretion of vascular endothelial growth factor (VEGF) [44]. The role of VEGF in inhibiting APC will be discussed in the next section.

Vascular Endothelial Growth Factor

VEGF is an angiogenic factor that is produced when endothelial cells undergo hypoxic stress. In addition, VEGF induces neovessel formation that increases the local blood supply [45]. Abnormal production of VEGF is evident in a number of diseases including inflammatory bowel syndrome, diabetic retinopathy, and corneal neovascularization [46–48]. VEGF is secreted by almost all tumor cells and is responsible for establishing neovascularization of tumor tissue, which is essential for the survival and progression.

While VEGF is best known for its angiogenic properties, it also downregulates APC presentation of antigens by blocking phagocytosis. Gabrilovich et al. [49] demonstrated that dextran beads are readily phagocytized by dendritic cells stimulated with GM-CSF. By contrast, VEGF inhibited phagocytosis of dextran beads by stimulated dendritic cells. Dendritic cell phagocytosis was also inhibited by tumor cell supernatants, which was removed by treating tumor supernatants with neutralizing antibodies against VEGF. Further studies to determine the mechanism by which VEGF blocks phagocytosis revealed that VEGF prevents maturation of dendritic cells. Esterase is a marker found on mature dendritic cells. However, VEGF-treated dendritic cells failed to express the esterase marker, indicating that the dendritic cells were at an immature stage of development. Interestingly, FACS analysis using CD34 antibody, a marker for DC, demonstrated that both esterase-positive and esterase-negative staining dendritic cells proliferate in the presence of VEGF. Therefore, dendritic cells that migrate into the tumor environment and are exposed to VEGF continue to proliferate, but fail to differentiate into mature dendritic cells capable of phagocytizing and presenting tumor antigens. Electrophoretic mobility shift assays performed by Oyama et al. [50] demonstrated the failure of dendritic cells to mature was caused by VEGF binding to its receptor, Flt-1, on immature dendritic cells, which inhibited activation of NFκB. Inhibition of NFκB in turn suppressed the production of GM-CSF, which blocked dendritic cell maturation.

Preventing Tumor Antigen Recognition by Altering Antigen Processing and Presentation

Proper assembly of HLA class I molecules is essential for presentation of antigens to effector cells. The proteasomes LMP2 and LMP7 are required to generate peptides within the cytoplasm from endogenous proteins, which are transported across the endoplasmic reticulum by the peptide transporter molecules TAP1 and TAP2. Final assembly of HLA class I molecules requires proper expression of HLA class I heavy chain components and β_2-microglobulin [51]. Downregulation of HLA class I molecules is one method commonly used by tumors to escape elimination. The mechanisms of HLA class I downregulation will be discussed below.

Downregulation of HLA Class I Genes

Low HLA class I expression by tumor cells has generally been attributed to downregulation of class I heavy chain gene transcription. Genetic instability greatly increases the opportunity for tumors to downregulate class I expression by loss of HLA class I loci. A high frequency of metastatic tumors that are highly aneuploid experience chromosomal deletions or translocations resulting in a complete loss of either two or three of the HLA class I loci [52]. By contrast, only a limited number of tumors lose a single HLA class I locus. Incubation of melanoma cells that are HLA-B-negative with IFN-γ upregulates HLA-B expression, demonstrating the loss of HLA-B is due to downregulation of transcription and not gene mutations. One mechanism used to inhibit HLA-B gene transcription is the overexpression of the *myc* oncogene, which prevents NFκB binding to the HLA-B class I enhancer region, thus blocking HLA-B gene transcription [53].

The most frequent mechanism to downregulate HLA class I in primary and metastatic tumors is the deletion of one or more class I alleles. Allelic class I downregulation occurs from a number of genetic mutations ranging from the complete loss of specific class I heavy chain genes on chromosome 6, to partial loss of the HLA gene [54, 55]. HLA genes have multiple promoter regions that are selectively used for transcribing RNA for specific HLA alleles. Sequencing of DNA from cervical carcinomas demonstrates that HLA-A24, HLA-A74 and HLA-B15 allele expression were lost due to a point mutation in the HLA promoter region responsible for the transcription of these genes [56].

Downregulation of β_2-Microglobulin Expression

A high frequency of tumors from breast, colon, lung, and kidney cancer patients downregulate expression of class I molecules by loss of β_2-micro-globulin [57, 58]. Cloning and sequencing of the β_2-microglobulin gene from primary and metastatic melanomas demonstrates the failure to synthesize β_2-microglobulin results from deletion of either the β_2-microglobulin gene or the β_2-microglobulin gene promoter sequence [59]. In addition, sequencing the RNA from class I-negative tumors indicates that frameshift mutations occur within the β_2-microglobulin gene, resulting in the transcription of truncated β_2-microglobulin molecules that are unable to associate with class I heavy chain [60].

Loss of Accessory Molecules

In most instances, MHC class I expression in tumor cells can be restored by upregulating expression of either class I heavy chain or β_2-microglobulin. This was confirmed in experiments where the expression of class I heavy chain and β_2-microglobulin was restored in tumor cells by transfection with vectors containing class I heavy chain and β_2-microglobulin genes. However, some transfected tumors *still* failed to express class I, suggesting that defects in antigen processing and transport may be responsible for class I downregulation [61]. Restifo et al. [62] have demonstrated by Northern blot analysis that some class I-negative tumor cells transcribe low or nondetectable levels of RNA from both LMP and TAP genes. Downregulation of both LMP and TAP genes was not due to mutations in these respective genes, but resulted from an unknown inhibitory signal that blocked LMP and TAP gene transcription. LMP and TAP transcription was upregulated in tumor cells treated with IFN-γ. IFN-γ treatment of tumor cells restored their ability to present endogenous tumor antigens that were successfully recognized by specific CTL.

Fas Ligand (FasL) and Tumor Escape

FasL is a trimer that is expressed on a limited number of nonlymphoid tissues and is specifically bound by cells expressing the Fas receptor. When Fas receptor-positive cells engage FasL, a signal transduction cascade is initiated from the Fas receptor that results in apoptosis. Interest in FasL increased when it was discovered that FasL was expressed constitutively only on tissues within immune privileged sites (testis, eye, brain, and maternal fetal interface) [3, 6, 63, 64]. Data from several laboratories supported the concept that constitutive expression of FasL helps to maintain immune privilege by eliminating Fas receptor-positive lymphocytes that encounter FasL. Experiments by Griffith et al. [3] indicate that FasL is expressed within the eyes of mice on corneal epithelium and endothelium, iris and ciliary body cells, and within the retina. After this discovery, it was reported that adenocarcinomas [4], metastatic skin melanomas [65], and certain leukemias and lymphomas [66] all constitutively express FasL. Moreover, these tumors were shown to induce apoptosis in Fas-positive lymphocytes, indicating this may be a tumor escape mechanism. Since FasL was not expressed on normal tissues, it appeared that at some time during tumor development, transcription of the FasL gene was triggered. However, more recent experiments have cast a shadow over the role of FasL in tumor escape from immune effector cells. In an effort to demonstrate FasL could create an immune privileged environment, several laboratories expressed FasL by gene transfer in immunogenic tumor cell lines. To their surprise, FasL-positive tumor cells were rejected at an accelerated rate compared with FasL-negative tumors [67]! Tumor rejection was mediated by neutrophils, and subsequent experiments demonstrated that FasL activated Fas-positive neutrophils to become cytolytic and lyse tumor cells. In spite of these data, FasL appears to have the opposite effect within the eye and testis. We will discuss a possible explanation of these conflicting data when we compare immune privilege within the eye with privilege within tumors.

Tumor Escape Following Active Immunization of Cancer Patients

The tumor escape mechanisms described above were all identified among tumor samples from patients with progressive disease. It is unclear what role, if any, the immune response plays in the development of these escape mechanisms, since it is difficult to detect evidence that immune effector cells control tumor growth in these patients. By contrast, the recent clinical trials of immunotherapies for cancer patients have provided an opportunity to examine tumor escape in patients that possess tumor-specific cytotoxic T cells generated from active immunization against tumor antigens. In vitro studies have demonstrated that specific CTL induce tumor escape mutants by applying selective pressure. The ability to eliminate a certain number of tumor cells is dependent upon how many CTL are present. If enough CTL are added to a culture to eliminate 90% of the tumor cells, 10% of the tumor cells will survive. If these tumor cells are allowed to proliferate, they can again be subjected to another round of CTL lysis. If repeated cycles of this selective T-cell pressure are applied, escape mutants eventually appear that are resistant to CTL lysis [68]. This in vitro method was used to successfully generate tumor escape mutants that evade lysis by CTL. Selective T-cell pressure may also generate tumor escape mutants in patients receiving immunotherapy. If treatment causes only a transient reduction in the tumor burden, recurring tumor cells may have acquired an escape mutant phenotype.

Loss of Tumor Antigen Expression

Tumors escape specific T-cell-mediated immunity not only by downregulating class I gene transcription, but also by downregulating genes that encode tumor antigens. Maeurer et al. [69] observed that a metastatic skin melanoma patient treated by surgical resection and high-dose IL-2 therapy experienced disease remission that coincided with the appearance of CTL that recognized MART-1 presented by HLA-A2 class I. Unfortunately, this patient developed recurrent metastatic tumors 6 years later, which were not lysed by MART-1-specific CTL. Interestingly, the recurrent tumor cells no longer transcribed the MART-1 gene, as no MART-1 mRNA was detected by RT-PCR. Moreover, immunostaining of cells with anti-TAP1 antibody indicated that TAP1 was no longer expressed, resulting in a loss of class I expression. Transfection of the TAP1 and MART-1 genes into the recurrent tumor cells restored recognition and lysis by MART-1-specific CTL. While the mechanism that prevented transcription of the MART-1 gene was not determined, these results clearly indicate that tumors can evade antitumor immunity by downregulating transcription of tumor antigen genes. These data also imply that this escape mechanism develops in patients following immunization that results in activation of tumor-specific CTL.

Killer Inhibitory Receptors (KIR) Expressed on T Cells

Selective downregulation of specific class I alleles has the advantage of: (a) preventing lysis by specific T cells, and (b) preventing lysis by NK cells. The latter is achieved because NK cells express KIR which bind to class I molecules and prevent NK cell lysis. Therefore, if tumor cells lost all surface class I molecules, they would become targets for NK cells. Bakker et al. [70] have recently demonstrated that artificial expression of KIR receptors on T cells could be used to block CTL lysis. A CTL clone that lysed tumor cells expressing the gp100 tumor antigen presented by HLA-A2 class I was transfected with the KIR gene that binds HLA-A2. CTL that expressed KIR were no longer able to lyse gp100-positive tumor cells, indicating that, if KIR are expressed on T cells, they can effectively block tumor cell killing by specific CTL.

While the study described above demonstrates KIR are capable of inhibiting CTL, KIR expression on T cells was artificially induced in vitro. Ikeda et al. [26] have recently demonstrated that T cells can be induced to express KIR in a cancer patient following active immunization against tumor antigens. A metastatic skin melanoma patient received a prolonged immunotherapeutic treatment for over 8 years. The patient initially had a metastatic tumor resected and IL-2 therapy. A tumor cell line was established from this tissue (MEL.A) that was used several years later as an autologous tumor cell vaccine. Following these treatments, 29 different CTL clones were isolated from the peripheral blood lymphocytes of the patient. These CTL recognized different tumor antigens on MEL.A presented by either A, B, or C class I loci. All of these CTL clones effectively lysed MEL.A tumor cells. However, 4 years after starting the tumor cell vaccine treatment, the patient developed a metastatic tumor nodule in the small bowel. This tumor was resected and a cell line established (MEL.B). MEL.B tumor cells were *not* lysed by any of the CTL clones that lysed MEL.A. This was because MEL.B lost expression of *all* class I, except a single allele (HLA-A24). They were able to generate a CTL clone specific for a new tumor antigen (PRAME) presented by HLA-A24 on MEL.B. Surprisingly, these CTL failed to recognize and lyse MEL.A even though the tumor cells expressed both HLA-24 and the PRAME tumor antigen. The reason for this was that CTL specific for PRAME expressed a KIR that recognized HLA-Cw7, which was expressed on MEL.A but not on MEL.B. Therefore, CTL failed to recognize and lyse MEL.A because the KIR was triggered by HLA-Cw7. Since MEL.B did not express HLA-Cw7, the KIR was not triggered and the CTL lysed the tumor cells.

Normally, KIR are found exclusively on NK cells. This is the first example of a patient possessing T cells that express KIR that blocked a response against a tumor antigen. It is unclear what the relationship is between the immunotherapy, tumor progression, and the expression of KIR in this patient. However, it would be a powerful escape mechanism from specific T cells if tumors could induce expression of KIR on T cells. It is interesting to note that immune privileged sites have been reported to alter T-cell receptor expression. A mouse with transgenic T cells specific for H-2K^b class I was used to follow the fate of these T cells when the mouse was pregnant with a fetus expressing H-2K^b class I. Surprisingly, the reactive T cells displayed transient tolerance and failed to reject H-2K^b-positive tumor grafts during pregnancy [71]. The tolerance coincided with a reduction in T-cell receptor expression. T-cell tolerance was terminated after pregnancy.

Table 2. Characteristics of ocular immune privilege

Blood-tissue barrier

Deficient afferent lymphatics

Reduced or impaired class I and class II expression

Deviant immune effector cells
   Inhibition of DH and CTL effectors
   Inhibition of NK cells
   Altered antibody production

Unconventional antigen-presenting cells

Unique immunosuppressive environment
   Transforming growth factor-β
   α-Melanocyte-stimulating hormone
   Vasoactive intestinal peptide
   Calcitonin gene-related peptide
   Migration inhibitory factor

These data demonstrate immune privileged sites can alter T-cell responses through changes in the T-cell receptor.

These last two studies provide examples of how selective T-cell pressure drives the development of escape mutant tumor cells in cancer patients receiving immunotherapy. In vitro models that use specific CTL to generate escape mutants are established when inefficient effector T cells eliminate some, but not all tumor cells. When residual tumor cells are allowed to proliferate for a significant length of time, escape mutants develop. Therefore, an effective escape mechanism of tumors would be to establish an immune privileged environment that slows tumor rejection. If this reduces the killing efficiency of effector T cells, it may change an antitumor T-cell response into a T-cell response that promotes long-term tumor growth by applying selective T-cell pressure that promotes development of escape mutant tumor cells.

Comparing Immune Privilege within the Eye and Tumors

In an effort to determine if tumors escape immune-mediated elimination by utilizing some, or all of the mechanisms used within the eye to establish immune privilege, the following section will compare tumor escape mechanisms with ocular immune privilege. Other chapters in this issue describe ocular immune privilege in great detail. Therefore, only the major components will be highlighted here. The characteristics of ocular immune privilege are summarized in table 2.

Ocular Immune Privilege

The goal of ocular immune privilege is to prevent nonspecific inflammation within the eye that may threaten vision. The eye prevents inflammation by: (a) inhibiting the proliferation, differentiation, and maturation of specific effector T cells (CD4$^+$ T cells and CD8$^+$ T cells), (b) inhibiting nonspecific NK effector cells, and (c) deleting Fas-positive lymphocytes that infiltrate the eye.

Inhibition of these immune effector functions is achieved by (a) induction of splenic regulatory T cells that prevent development of DH and CTL (ACAID), (b) soluble factors in aqueous humor (migration inhibitory factor (MIF) and TGF-β) that inhibits NK cells; (c) soluble factors in aqueous humor (TGF-β, α-melanocyte-stimulating hormone (α-MSH), vasoactive intestinal peptide (VIP), and calcitonin gene-related protein (CGRP)) that also inhibit proliferation and cytokine secretion by primed T cells, and (d) constitutive expression of FasL on ocular tissues induces apoptosis among Fas-positive infiltrating lymphocytes. Splenic immune-regulating T cells are induced by unconventional APC that are produced when ocular infiltrating APC are exposed to soluble factors within aqueous humor. When these APC migrate via the blood vasculature to the spleen, they are unable to activate T cells in a conventional manner. Therefore, soluble factors within the local microenvironment of the eye are critical in maintaining immune privilege and participate in regulating both afferent and efferent phases of the immune response by: (a) inhibiting infiltrating APC, and (b) inhibiting infiltrating T cells and NK cells.

Ocular tissues also display reduced expression of MHC class I and class II which is likely to play an important role in masking recognition of antigens by specific T cells. However, currently little is known about effector T-cell recognition of antigens presented by ocular tissue. Several physical characteristics of the eye help to maintain the unique environment and therefore are important in maintaining privilege. The eye has: (a) blood-tissue barriers, (b) deficient efferent lymphatic pathways, and (c) direct drainage pathways to the spleen via the blood vasculature.

In conclusion, immune privilege within the eye is maintained by multiple and overlapping mechanisms. For this reason, it has been difficult to determine what specific mechanisms are required to establish ocular immune privilege. In other words, it is unclear at this time how to 'construct' an artificial immune privileged site at a nonprivileged anatomical site. This is important within tumors since tumors may possess some, but not all the features of immune privilege.

Immune Privilege within Tumors

Like the eye, tumors establish immune privilege by creating an immunosuppressive environment around the tumor. As described in previous sections, the ability of tumors to secrete immunosuppressive cytokines inhibits the processing and presentation of tumor antigens, thus preventing the induction of antitumor immune responses. In addition, the immune privileged environment of tumors also prevents the proliferation and maturation of precursor effector T cells. In skin melanoma, Itoh et al. [72] isolated primary and metastatic melanoma samples containing populations of tumor-infiltrating lymphocytes (TIL). However, TIL were not activated and expressed surface markers that identified them as immature precursor cytotoxic T cells. When TIL were isolated from the tumor and placed in culture with IL-2, precursor TIL were induced to differentiate into cytolytic T cells that killed autologous tumor cells. These results indicate that lymphocytes that infiltrate into tumors are exposed to immunosuppressive factors that arrest their development. It is interesting to note the ocular microenvironment also prevents the terminal differentiation of precursor cytotoxic T cells that infiltrate into the eye [73].

Other types of tumors besides melanomas create an immunosuppressive environment that inhibits infiltrating lymphocytes. Studies by Yano et al. [74] demonstrate that TIL isolated from lung adenocarcinomas proliferate in response to exogenous IL-2, but cannot produce IFN-γ or kill autologous tumor cells. These data suggest that different types of tumors may create unique environments that inhibit TIL by different mechanisms.

The immune privileged environment of tumors also suppresses activation of nonspecific effector cells. Tumors often exhibit downregulation of MHC class I to escape tumor-specific T-cell elimination. However, this leaves tumor cells vulnerable to attack by NK cells. Therefore, it is not surprising that tumors have devised methods to suppress the activation of NK cells. Aparicio-Pages et al. [75] reported that NK cells were found within and surrounding tumor nodules in patients with gastric carcinomas of the esophagus and stomach. When NK cells were recovered from the tumor site and stimulated with IFN-γ, in vitro, NK cytolytic activity was detected, but at significantly lower levels than normal controls. Although it is unclear if MIF is responsible for inhibiting NK activity within these tumors, these results indicate the environment within tumors and the eye share the ability to inhibit infiltrating NK cells.

The loss of MHC class I and class II expression plays a major role in the establishment of tumor escape mutants since MHC molecules present antigens that are targets for tumor-specific effector cells. In fact, almost all tumors demonstrate a high frequency of MHC downregulation that is the result of either (a) loss of heavy chain or β_2-microglobulin assembly, or (b) defects in the processing and presentation of tumor peptides. In most cases, loss of class I expression does not necessarily mean that all class I alleles are absent. In fact, complete loss of class I expression may induce NK-mediated killing of class I-negative tumor cells. Therefore, expression of class I molecules that are not presenting relevant tumor antigen peptides allows tumors to escape NK killing through interaction of class I molecules with the inhibitory receptors expressed by NK. It is unclear at this time if expression of class I alleles are altered on ocular tissue, or whether there are any defects in antigen processing and presentation (such as mutations in LMP or TAP) on cells within the eye. However, melanomas that develop within the ocular environment have a very high frequency of tumors that downregulate specific class I alleles. It will be interesting to determine if inhibition of specific class I alleles on uveal melanomas is the result of the surrounding ocular environment.

While the eye and some tumors express FasL constitutively, it remains controversial whether FasL is immunoprotective or immunodestructive. Within the eye, FasL appears to be immunoprotective. By contrast, several laboratories have reported an immunodestructive role for FasL on tumor cells. One possible explanation of these contradictory results was provided by Nabel and coworkers [76], who observed that FasL-positive tumors injected into the flank, a nonprivileged site, were rapidly rejected. Tumor rejection was due to FasL activation of neutrophil cytolytic activity. Surprisingly, these same tumors were not rejected from the anterior chamber of the eye. A soluble factor within aqueous humor, primarily TGF-β, was found to block FasL-mediated activation of neutrophils. Therefore, the local environment may determine whether FasL is immunoprotective or immunodestructive. Tumors that express FasL and create an environment similar to the eye may experience a protective effect due to FasL. By contrast, tumors that express FasL that fail to create an ocular environment may experience a destructive effect due to FasL.

In addition to sharing immune privilege mechanisms with the eye, tumors also possess unique mechanisms that enable progressively growing tumors to escape immune elimination. Probably the most important of these mechanisms is the ability of tumors to inhibit transcription of tumor antigen genes. Since this escape mechanism probably does *not* result from the surrounding tumor environment, but results from mutations that develop during selective T-cell pressure, it is unlikely to occur within the eye. The eye inhibits most specific T-cell responses, therefore, it is hard to envision how there could be selective T-cell pressure within the eye.

Summary: Two decades ago, Robert North proposed that tumors escape antitumor immune responses by establishing an immune privileged environment. Although the mechanisms tumors used to establish immune privilege were not largely known at the time, it was suspected that tumors secreted immunosuppressive factors that blocked protective immunity. Extensive studies of how immune privilege is established within the eye supports the general concept that privilege is dependent upon creating a unique microenvironment that contains a variety of immunosuppressive factors. A comparison of immune

Table 3. Similarities between immune privilege within the eye and tumors

Mechanism	Eye	Tumors
Blood-tissue barrier	+	–
Deficient afferent lymphatics	+	–
Reduced class I expression	+	+
Deviant immune effector cells	+	+
Inhibition of infiltrating APC	+	+
Fas ligand expressed constitutively	+	+
Unique immunosuppressive environment	+	+
Loss of antigen gene transcription	–	+
Inhibition of antigen processing pathways	–	+

privilege within the eye and tumors reveals that, in general, both use similar mechanisms to evade the immune system (table 3). The major exception is that tumors develop escape mutants that shut off transcription of tumor antigen genes. Since the eye and tumors share common pathways to create immune privilege, it seems reasonable to expect that methods used to terminate immune privilege in the eye will be successful in terminating privilege within tumors. The development of effective cancer immunotherapies is likely to be dependent upon terminating or limiting the ability of tumors to create a privileged environment. Therefore, we believe the study of ocular immune privilege has great potential for providing important insights into how to develop successful anticancer immunotherapies.

Acknowledgments

Supported by USPHS grants EY08122 and EY09294.

References

1   Spitalny GL, North RJ: Subversion of host defense mechanisms by malignant tumors: An established tumor as a privileged site for bacterial growth. J Exp Med 1977;145:1264–1277.
2   Lethe B, Van den Eynde B, Corradin G, Boon T: Mouse tumor rejection antigen P815A and P815B: Two epitopes carried by a single peptide. Eur J Immunol 1992;22:2283–2288.
3   Griffith TS, Brunner T, Fletcher SM, Green DR, Ferguson TA: Fas ligand-induced apoptosis as a mechanism of immune privilege. Science 1995;270:1189–1192.
4   O'Connell J, O'Sullivan GC, Collins JK, Shanahan F: The Fas counterattack: Fas-mediated T cell killing by colon cancer cells expressing Fas ligand. J Exp Med 1996;184:1075–1082.
5   Streilein JW: Unraveling immune privilege. Science 1995;270:1189–1192.

6   Bellgrau D, Gold D, Selawry H, Moore J, Franzusoff A, Duke RC: A role for CD95 ligand in preventing graft rejection. Nature 1995;377:630–632.

7   Parker GA, Rosenberg SA: Serologic identification of multiple tumor-associated antigens on murine sarcomas. J Natl Cancer Inst 1997;58:1303–1309.

8   Cox AL, Skipper J, Chen Y, Henderson RA, Darrow TL, Shabanowitz J, Engelhard VH, Hunt DF, Slingluff CL Jr: Identification of a peptide recognized by five melanoma specific human cytolytic T cell lines. Science 1994;264:716–719.

9   Celis E, Tsai V, Crimi C, DeMars R, Wentworth PA, Chesnut RW, Grey HM, Sette A, Serra HM: Induction of anti-tumor cytotoxic T lymphocytes in normal humans using primary cultures and synthetic peptide epitopes. Proc Natl Acad Sci USA 1994;91:2105–2109.

10   Kawakami Y, Eliyahu S, Delgado CH, Robbins PF, Sakaguchi K, Appella E, Yannelli JR, Adema GJ, Miki T, Rosenberg SA: Identification of a human melanoma antigen recognized by tumor infiltrating lymphocytes associated with in vivo tumor rejection. Proc Natl Acad Sci USA 1994; 191:6458–6452.

11   Brichard V, Van Pel A, Wolfel T, Wolfel C, De Plaen E, Lethe B, Coulie P, Boon T: The tyrosinase gene codes for an antigen recognized by autologous cytolytic T lymphocytes on HLA-A2 melanomas. J Exp Med 1993;178:489–495.

12   Kang XQ, Kawakami Y, el-Gamil M, Wang R, Sakaguchi K, Yannelli JR, Appella E, Rosenberg SA, Robbins PF: Identification of a tyrosinase epitope recognized by HLA-A24 restricted tumor-infiltrating lymphocytes. J Immunol 1995;155:1343–1348.

13   Brichard VG, Herman JK, Van Pel A, Wildmann C, Gaugler B, Wolfel T, Boon T, Lethe B: A tyrosinase nonapeptide presented by HLA-B44 is recognized on a human melanoma by autologous cytolytic T lymphocytes. Eur J Immunol 1996;26:224–230.

14   Skipper J, Hendrickson RC, Gulden PH, Brichard V, Van Pel A, Chen Y, Shabanowitz J, Wolfel T, Slingluff CL Jr, Boon T, Hunt DF, Engelhard VH: An HLA-A2-restricted tyrosinase antigen on melanoma cells results in post-translational modification and suggests a novel pathway for processing of membrane proteins. J Exp Med 1996;183:527–534.

15   Kawakami Y, Eliyahu S, Delgado CH, Robbins PF, Rivoltini L, Topalian SL, Miki T, Rosenberg SA: Cloning of the gene coding for a differentiation antigen recognized by autologous T cells infiltrating into tumor. Proc Natl Acad Sci USA 1994;91:3515–3519.

16   Kawakami Y, Eliyahu S, Sakaguchi K, Robbins PF, Rivoltini L, Yannelli JR, Appella E, Rosenberg SA: Identification of the immunodominant peptides of the MART-1 human melanoma antigen recognized by the majority of HLA-A2-restricted tumor infiltrating lymphocytes. J Exp Med 1994; 180:347–352.

17   Bakker A, Scherures M, Tafazzul G, de Boer AJ, Kawakami Y, Adema GJ, Figdor CG: Identification of a novel peptide derived from the melanocyte-specific gp100 antigen as the dominant epitope recognized by a HLA-A2.1-restricted anti-melanoma CTL line. Int J Cancer 1995;63:97–102.

18   Kawakami Y, Eliyahu S, Jennings C, Sakaguchi K, Kang X, Southwood S, Robbins PF, Sette A, Appella E, Rosenberg SA: Recognition of multiple epitopes in the human melanoma antigen gp100 associated with in vivo tumor regression. J Immunol 1995;154:3961–3968.

19   Wang RF, Robbins PF, Kawakami Y, Kang XQ, Rosenberg SA: Identification of a gene encoding a melanoma tumor antigen recognized by HLA-31-restricted tumor infiltrating lymphocytes. J Exp Med 1995;181:799–804.

20   Wang RF, Parkhurst M, Kawakami Y, Robbins PF, Rosenberg SA: Utilization of an alternative open reading frame of a normal gene in generating a novel human cancer antigen. J Exp Med 1996;183:1131–1140.

21   Rosenberg SA, White DE: Vitiligo in patients with melanoma: Normal tissue antigens can be targets of cancer immunotherapy. J Immunother 1996;19:81–84.

22   Robbins PF, el-Garmil M, Li YF, Kawakami Y, Loftus D, Appella E, Rosenberg SA: A mutated β-catenin gene encodes a melanoma-specific antigen recognized by tumor infiltrating lymphocytes. J Exp Med 1996;183:1185–1192.

23   Wolfel T, Hauer M, Scheider J, Serrano M, Wolfel C, Klehmann-Hieb E, De Plaen E, Hankeln T, Meyer zum Buschenfelde KH, Beach D: A p16INK4a-insensitive CDK4 mutant targeted by cytolytic T lymphocytes in a human melanoma. Science 1995;269:1281–1284.

24   Coulie PG, Lehmann F, Lethe B, Herman J, Lurquin C, Andrawiss M, Boon T: A mutated intron sequence codes for an antigenic peptide recognized by cytolytic T lymphocytes on a human melanoma. Proc Natl Acad Sci USA 1995;92:7976–7980.

25   Fisk B, Blevins TL, Wharton JT, Ioannides CG: Identification of an immunodominant of HER-2/neu proto-oncogene recognized by ovarian tumor-specific cytotoxic T lymphocytes. J Exp Med 1995;181:2109–2117.

26   Ikeda H, Lethe B, Lehmann F, van Baren N, Baurain JF, de Smet C, Chambost H, Vitale M, Moretta A, Boon T, Coulie PG: Characterization of an antigen that is recognized on a melanoma showing partial HLA loss by CTL expressing an NK inhibitory receptor. Immunity 1997;6:199–208.

27   De Plaen E, Arden K, Traversari C, Gaforio JJ, Szikora JP, De Smet C, Brasseur F, van der Bruggen P, Lethe B, Lurquin C, Boon T: Structure, chromosomal location and expression of twelve genes of the MAGE family. Immunogenetics 1994;40:360–369.

28   Van der Bruggen P, Traversari C, Chomez P, Lurquin C, De Plaen E, Van den Eynde B, Knuth A, Boon T: A gene encoding an antigen recognized by cytolytic T lymphocytes on a human melanoma. Science 1991;254:1643–1647.

29   Takahashi K, Shichijo S, Noguchi M, Hirohata M, Itoh K: Identification of MAGE-1 and MAGE-4 proteins in spermatogonia and primary spermatocytes of testis. Cancer Res 1995;55: 3478–3482

30   Lethe B, Lucas S, Michaux L, De Smet C, Godelaine D, Serrano A, De Plaen E, Boon T: LAGE-1, a new gene with tumor specificity. Int J Cancer 1998;76:903–908.

31   Van den Eynde B, Peeters O, De Backer O, Gaugler B, Lucas S, Boon T: A new family of genes coding for an antigen recognized by autologous cytolytic T lymphocytes on a human melanoma. J Exp Med 1995;182:689–698.

32   Guilloux Y, Lucas S, Brichard VG, Van Pel A, Viret C, De Plaen E, Brasseur F, Lethe B, Jotereau F, Boon T: A peptide recognized by human cytolytic T lymphocytes on HLA-A2 melanomas is encoded by an intron sequence of the N-acetylglucosaminyltransferase V gene. J Exp Med 1996; 183:1173–1183.

33   Sato T, McCue P, Masuoka K, Salwen S, Lattime EC, Mastrangelo MJ, Berd D: Interleukin-10 production by human melanoma. Clin Cancer Res 1996;2:1383–1390.

34   Huang M, Wang J, Lee P, Sharma S, Mao JT, Meissner H, Uyemura K, Modlin R, Wollman J, Dubinett SM: Human non-small cell lung cancer cells express a type 2 cytokine pattern. Cancer Res 1995;55:3847–3853.

35   Young MR, Wright MA, Lozano Y, Matthews JP, Benefield J, Prechel MM: Mechanisms of immune suppression in patients with head and neck cancer: Influence on the immune infiltrate of the cancer. Int J Cancer 1996;67:333–338.

36   Beissert S, Ullrich SE, Hosoi J, Granstein RD: Supernatants from UVB radiation-exposed keratinocytes inhibit Langerhans cell presentation of tumor-associated antigens via IL-10 content. J Leukoc Biol 1995;58:234–240.

37   Ranges GE, Figari IS, Espevik T, Palladino MA Jr: Inhibition of cytotoxic T cell development by transforming growth factor-beta and reversal by recombinant tumor necrosis factor-alpha. J Exp Med 1987;166:991–998.

38   Kuppner MC, Hamou MF, Bodmer S, Fontana A, de Tribolet N: The glioblastoma-derived T-cell suppressor factor/transforming growth factor-beta-2 inhibits the generation of lymphokine-activated killer cells. Int J Cancer 1988;42:562–567.

39   Rodeck U, Melber K, Kath R, Menssen HD, Varello M, Atkinson B, Herlyn M: Constitutive expression of multiple growth factor genes by melanoma cells but not normal melanocytes. J Invest Dermatol 1991;97:20–26.

40   Bartlett JM, Langdon SP, Scott WN, Love SB, Miller EP, Katsaros D, Smyth JF, Miller WR: Transforming growth factor-beta isoform expression in human ovarian tumours. Eur J Cancer 1997; 33:2397–2403.

41   Gomella LG, Sargent ER, Wade TP, Anglard P, Linehan WM, Kasid A: Expression of transforming growth factor-alpha in normal human adult kidney and enhanced expression of transforming growth factors-alpha and -beta-1 in renal cell carcinoma. Cancer Res 1989;49:6972–6975.

Chen/Ksander

42 Vitolo D, Kanbour A, Johnson JT, Herberman RB, Whiteside TL: In situ hybridisation for cytokine gene transcripts in the solid tumour microenvironment. Eur J Cancer 1993;29A:371–377.

43 Takeuchi M, Kosiewicz MM, Alard P, Streilein JW: On the mechanisms by which transforming growth factor-beta-2 alters antigen-presenting abilities of macrophages on T cell activation. Eur J Immunol 1997;27:1648–1656.

44 Koochekpour S, Merzak A, Pilkington GJ: Vascular endothelial growth factor production is stimulated by gangliosides and TGF-beta isoforms in human glioma cells in vitro. Cancer Lett 1996; 102:209–215.

45 Ferrara N, Houck KA, Jakeman LB, Winer J, Leung DW: The vascular endothelial growth factor family of polypeptides. J Cell Biochem 1991;47:211–218.

46 Beck PL, Podolsky DK: Growth factors in inflammatory bowel disease. Inflamm Bowel Dis 1999; 5:44–60.

47 Boulton M, Foreman D, Williams G, McLeod D: VEGF localisation in diabetic retinopathy. Br J Ophthalmol 1998;82:561–568.

48 Amano S, Rohan R, Kuroki M, Tolentino M, Adamis AP: Requirement for vascular endothelial growth factor in wound- and inflammation-related corneal neovascularization. Invest Ophthal Vis Sci 1998;39:18–22.

49 Gabrilovich DI, Chen HL, Girgis KR, Cunningham HT, Meny GM, Nadaf S, Kavanaugh D, Carbone DP: Production of vascular endothelial growth factor by human tumors inhibits the functional maturation of dendritic cells. Nat Med 1996;2:1096–1103.

50 Oyama T, Ran S, Ishida T, Nadaf S, Kerr L, Carbone DP, Gabrilovich DI: Vascular endothelial growth factor affects dendritic cell maturation through the inhibition of nuclear factor-kappa B activation in hemopoietic progenitor cells. J Immunol 1998;160:1224–1232.

51 York IA, Rock KL: Antigen processing and presentation by the class I major histocompatibility complex. Annu Rev Immunol 1996;14:369–396.

52 Marincola FM, Shamamian P, Alexander RB, Gnarra JR, Turetskaya RL, Nedospasov SA, Simonis TB, Taubenberger JK, Yannelli J, Mixon A: Loss of HLA haplotype and B locus down-regulation in melanoma cell lines. J Immunol 1994;153:1225–1237.

53 Versteeg R, Kruse-Wolters KM, Plomp AC, van Leeuwen A, Stam NJ, Ploegh HL, Ruiter DJ, Schrier PI: Suppression of class I human histocompatibility leukocyte antigen by c-myc is locus specific. J Exp Med 1989;170:621–635.

54 Maeurer MJ, Gollin S, Storkus WJ, Swaney W, Karbach J, Martin D, Castelli C, Salter R, Knuth A, Lotze MT: Tumor escape from immune recognition: Loss of HLA-A2 melanoma cell surface expression is associated with a complex rearrangement of the short arm of chromosome 6. Clin Cancer Res 1996;2:641–652.

55 Lassam N, Jay G: Suppression of MHC class I RNA in highly oncogenic cells occurs at the level of transcription initiation. J Immunol 1989;143:3792–3797.

56 Laforet M, Froelich N, Parissiadis A, Bausinger H, Pfeiffer B, Tongio MM: An intronic mutation responsible for a low level of expression of an HLA-A24 allele in cervical carcinoma. Tissue Antigens 1997;50:340–346.

57 Gattoni-Celli S, Kirsch K, Timpane R, Isselbacher KJ: Beta-2-microglobulin gene is mutated in a human colon cancer cell line (HCT) deficient in the expression of HLA class I antigens on the cell surface. Cancer Res 1992;52:1201–1204.

58 Chen HL, Gabrilovich D, Virmani A, Ratnani I, Girgis KR, Nadaf-Rahrov S, Fernandez-Vina M, Carbone DP: Structural and functional analysis of beta-2-microglobulin abnormalities in human lung and breast cancer. Int J Cancer 1996;67:756–763.

59 Hicklin DJ, Wang Z, Arienti F, Rivoltini L, Parmiani G, Ferrone S: Beta-2-microglobulin mutations, HLA class I antigen loss, and tumor progression in melanoma. J Clin Invest 1998;101:2720–2729.

60 Wang Z, Cao Y, Albino AP, Zeff RA, Houghton A, Ferrone S: Lack of HLA class I antigen expression by melanoma cells SK-MEL-33 caused by a reading frameshift in beta-2-microglobulin messenger RNA. J Clin Invest 1993;91:684–692.

61 Weis JH, Seidman JG: The expression of major histocompatibility antigens under metallothionein gene promoter control. J Immunol 1985;134:1999–2003.

Immune Privilege, Tumors, and the Eye   157

62 Restifo NP, Esquivel F, Kawakami Y, Yewdell JW, Mule JJ, Rosenberg SA, Bennink JR: Identification of human cancers deficient in antigen processing. J Exp Med 1993;177:265–272.

63 Saas P, Walker PR, Hahne M, Quiquerez AL, Schnuriger V, Perrin G, French L, Van Meir EG, de Tribolet N, Tschopp J, Dietrich PY: Fas ligand expression by astrocytoma in vivo: Maintaining immune privilege in the brain? J Clin Invest 1997;99:1173–1178.

64 Hunt JS, Vassmer D, Ferguson TA, Miller L: Fas ligand is positioned in mouse uterus and placenta to prevent trafficking of activated leukocytes between the mother and the conceptus. J Immunol 1997;158:4122–4128.

65 Hahne M, Rimoldi D, Schroter M, Romero P, Schreier M, French LE, Schneider P, Bornand T, Fontana A, Lienard D, Cerottini J, Tschopp J: Melanoma cell expression of Fas(Apo-1/CD95) ligand: Implications for tumor immune escape. Science 1996;274:1363–1366

66 Tanaka M, Suda T, Haze K, Nakamura N, Sato K, Kimura F, Motoyoshi K, Mizuki M, Tagawa S, Ohga S, Hatake K, Drummond AH, Nagata S: Fas ligand in human serum. Nat Med 1996;2: 317–322.

67 Seino K, Kayagaki N, Tsukada N, Fukao K, Yagita H, Okumura K: Transplantation of CD95 ligand-expressing grafts: Influence of transplantation site and difficulty in protecting allo- and xenografts. Transplantation 1997;64:1050–1054.

68 Boon T, Van Snick J, Van Pel A, Uyttenhove C, Marchand M: Immunogenic variants obtained by mutagenesis of mouse mastocytoma P815. II. T lymphocyte-mediated cytolysis. J Exp Med 1980; 152:1184–1193.

69 Maeurer MJ, Gollin SM, Martin D, Swaney W, Bryant J, Castelli C, Robbins P, Parmiani G, Storkus WJ, Lotze MT: Tumor escape from immune recognition: Lethal recurrent melanoma in a patient associated with downregulation of the peptide transporter protein TAP-1 and loss of expression of the immunodominant MART-1/Melan-A antigen. J Clin Invest 1996;98:1633–1641.

70 Bakker AB, Phillips JH, Figdor CG, Lanier LL: Killer cell inhibitory receptors for MHC class I molecules regulate lysis of melanoma cells mediated by NK cells, gamma delta T cells, and antigen-specific CTL. J Immunol 1998;160:5239–5245.

71 Tafuri A, Alferink J, Moller P, Hammerling GJ, Arnold B: T cell awareness of paternal alloantigens during pregnancy. Science 1995;270:630–633.

72 Itoh K, Platsoucas CD, Balch CM: Autologous tumor-specific cytotoxic T lymphocytes in the infiltrate of human metastatic melanomas. Activation by interleukin-2 and autologous tumor cells, and involvement of the T cell receptor. J Exp Med 1988;168:1419–1441.

73 Ksander BR, Streilein JW: Failure of infiltrating precursor cytotoxic T cells to acquire direct cytotoxic function in immunologically privileged sites. J Immunol 1990;145:2057–2063.

74 Yano T, Yasumoto K, Togami M, Ishida T, Kimura G, Sugimachi K, Nomoto K: Properties of recombinant interleukin-2-cultured tumor-infiltrating lymphocytes in human lung cancer. Int J Cancer 1989;43:619–623.

75 Aparicio-Pages NM, Verspaget HW, Pena SA, Lamers CB: Impaired local natural killer cell activity in human colorectal carcinomas. Cancer Immunol Immunother 1989;28:301–304.

76 Chen JJ, Sun Y, Nabel GJ: Regulation of the proinflammatory effects of Fas ligand (CD95L). Science 1998;282:1714–1717.

Peter W. Chen, Schepens Eye Research Institute, Harvard Medical School,
20 Staniford St., Boston, MA 02114 (USA)
Tel. +1 617 912 7444, Fax +1 617 912 0113, E-Mail pwchen@vision.eri.harvard.edu

Bruce Ksander, Schepens Eye Research Institute, Harvard Medical School,
20 Staniford St., Boston, MA 02114 (USA)
Tel. +1 617 912 7443, Fax +1 617 912 0115, E-Mail ksander@vision.eri.harvard.edu

Streilein JW (ed): Immune Response and the Eye.
Chem Immunol. Basel, Karger, 1999, vol 73, pp 159–185

....

Immunopathogenic Mechanisms in Intraocular Inflammation

John V. Forrester[a], *Paul G. McMenamin*[b]

[a] Department of Ophthalmology, University of Aberdeen, UK and
[b] Department of Ophthalmology, University of Western Australia, Nedlands, W.A., Australia

Introduction – What Is Uveitis?

The uveal tract, comprising the iris, ciliary body and choroid, represents the lymphovascular organ of the eye, i.e. in addition to providing most of the blood supply to the intraocular structures, it acts as the conduit for immune cells, particularly lymphocytes, to enter the eye. Consequently, the uveal tract is almost always involved in any form of inflammation within the eye irrespective of which tissue or cell becomes the target of attack, and clinically many of these conditions manifest as one form or other of 'uveitis', even though the uveal tract itself may not be the primary focus. Therefore, what was previously considered to represent a specific clinical entity, i.e. uveitis, is probably a misnomer unless antigens within the uvea are the direct target of the inflammatory process. A better term for the condition is intraocular inflammation (IOI) [1].

This conceptual shift in thinking about IOI has resulted from the pioneering work of Waldon Wacker [2, 3], who showed that in contrast to the repeated failures of uveal antigens to demonstrate uveitogenicity, retinal antigens were powerfully uveitogenic and could induce different clinical forms of the disease which depended on coincident factors (see below). Since then, numerous experimental models using different antigens from the eye have been produced [4–8], all of which initiate some form of IOI (uveitis) in which the common features are intraocular inflammatory cells, vascular dilatation and engorgement, inflammatory infiltrates visible for instance as nodules on the iris or granulomas in the choroid, and oedema of sight-regulating tissues such as the retina or cornea [9, 10]. These clinico-pathological features occur in most forms of IOI to some degree and are the hallmarks of 'uveitis' [11, 12].

Therefore, in considering immunopathogenic mechanisms in uveitis in which antigens, either foreign or self, represent the initial element in the process of inflammation, it is probably more useful to consider what is the likely specific target tissue or cell within the eye, rather than concentrate on the uveal tract even though this tissue may appear to be most markedly involved with inflammatory components. It is of course possible that cells or structures within the uveal tract itself will be the target, e.g. melanocytes in Vogt-Koyanagi-Harada disease [13, 14] or endothelial cells in systemic vasculitis [15] but selective involvement of the uveal tract in IOI is relatively uncommon.

This chapter deals with how general pathogenic mechanisms involved in IOI are modified under certain conditions.

Causes of IOI

There are many causes of IOI. Clinically they are subdivided into infectious or noninfectious causes [1] and experimentally into inducible by foreign or self antigens [7, 16]. In general, there is considerable overlap in the phenotypic manifestations, both clinically and pathologically, of clinical and experimental IOI [9] and it is likely that similar tissue-destroying processes are at play.

Infectious IOI can be caused by any class of micro-organism including bacteria, mycobacteria, viruses, parasites and even some indeterminate micro-organisms such as rickettsiae. Typical causes of infectious IOI include *Toxoplasma gondii, Toxocara canis,* cytomegalovirus (CMV) in AIDS patients, *Borrelia burgdorferi* in endemic areas and *Mycobacterium tuberculosis* in third world populations. However, in a majority of cases a direct infectious cause for IOI cannot be found on clinical examination or laboratory testing and such cases, even when associated with a systemic disease such as generalized vasculitis or sarcoidosis, are considered to be immune-mediated if not auto-immune.

Experimentally, models of infectious IOI have been developed and mimic closely the clinical disease [16, 17]. However, based on the premise that most clinical forms of IOI cannot be linked with micro-organisms and are therefore likely to be induced by self antigens, experimentalists have set about demonstrating that ocular autoantigens could induce IOI [see above, ref. to W.B. Wacker]. The clinical paradigm, par excellence, for these studies was sympathetic ophthalmia, a rare form of IOI in which the fellow eye develops IOI 6–12 weeks following penetrating injury of the first eye [18]. This clinical condition has been considered a classic example of organ-specific autoimmune disease and the causative autoantigen(s) have been sought for many years. Several ocular antigens have now been shown to induce IOI (see below) and many attempts have been made to show that patients with IOI demonstrate immune reactivity to such antigens either by elevated levels of circulating antibodies or by evidence of cell-mediated immunity to the antigens [19–25]. The published data remain contradictory. In studies of mixed groups of patients with IOI, the results have generally been nonsupportive of a role for autoimmunity to ocular autoantigens [21–23]. However, some groups of patients such as those with birdshot retinochoroidopathy, have been shown to possess lymphocyte responsiveness to retinal antigens such as S antigen [21–24]. Indeed, some believe that the evidence for autoimmunity to retinal antigens is sufficiently strong in certain individuals with IOI that this test is used as one of the main entry criteria to an ongoing study of mucosal tolerance therapy using large oral doses of retinal antigens [26].

Clinically, IOI or uveitis induced by foreign antigens is distinguished from direct intraocular infection by, for instance, invading bacterial micro-organisms postsurgically or as part of metastatic infection. In such circumstances the condition is termed endophthalmitis and is caused by direct tissue-destroying lytic enzymes released by the micro-organisms [1]. In contrast, the much more common nonendophthalmitic forms of 'infectious' IOI often have a considerable acquired immunological component. For instance, *T. gondii* invades the tissues including the retina and brain but does not cause inflammation until the life-cycle of the organism is over and an overwhelming reaction to the foreign antigen ensues, much of it mediated by lymphocytes and macrophages [27, 28]. In the choroid, where ready access of such cells is possible, the inflammatory response can be intense. However, in the retina, where cells infiltrating the tissues must cross the blood-retinal barrier, the inflammatory response is considerably less intense [29, 30] (fig. 1, 2). Similarly, CMV directly infects neural cells and proliferates within the tissues where it induces a cytotoxic T-cell response, thereby inducing associated 'bystander' damage to the tissues [31]. However, CMV also invades the endothelial cells and its primary mode of damage may be via a microvasculopathy [32], including intravascular coagulation events [33] which promotes leukocyte adhesion, trapping and invasion of the tissue [34].

Where no direct infectious cause of the IOI can be found, an infectious aetiology may nevertheless be frequently implicated. Typical of many forms of IOI is a history of generalized infection such as a flu-like illness with lymphadenopathy or an episode of gastroenteritis which is followed several

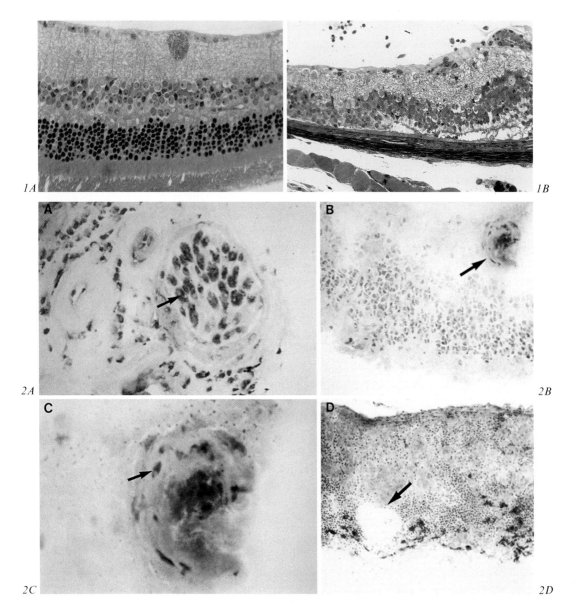

Fig. 1. A Light micrograph of retina in mouse model of congenital ocular toxoplasmosis showing toxoplasma cyst in normal retina. B A second specimen from mouse model of congenital ocular toxoplasmosis showing intense inflammation in the absence of identifiable cysts.

Fig. 2. Photomicrographs of a case of human toxoplasmosis showing: A intact toxoplasma cyst in the retina with minimal inflammation; B partially degenerate cyst (arrow) in the retina also with minimal inflammation; C higher power view of B (arrow), and D massively thickened choroid with inflammatory cell infiltration and presumed site of previous cyst represented by a lytic space (arrow). Orig. Magn.: A ×420; B ×75; C ×420; D ×75.

weeks to months later by IOI, affecting either the anterior or posterior segment, for instance with a multifocal choroiditis (fig. 3). How such infections 'cause' the IOI is unclear as is the relationship of this type of IOI to the 'autoimmune' form of IOI in which there is no history of previous infection but in whom a subclinical infection may have occurred. Possible mechanisms include molecular mimicry and bystander damage (see below).

Pathology of IOI

The two major forms of IOI are anterior segment intraocular inflammation (ASII) (anterior uveitis) and posterior segment intraocular inflammation (PSII) (posterior uveitis) both of which are clinically and pathogenetically distinct [12]. In some cases combined anterior and posterior segment intraocular inflammation may occur (CAPSII) (panuveitis) [1] and usually represents progression in severity of one or other primary form. ASII and PSII occur in infectious and noninfectious forms.

Pathological studies of clinical forms of IOI have been infrequent due to obvious difficulties in obtaining biopsy material and the fact that most postmortem material which has been obtained is mostly end-stage disease. Consequently, most of the informative pathological material at least with regard to cellular mechanisms has come from experimental models.

Clinical ASII

ASII may be acute or chronic, recurrent, and unilateral or bilateral, sometimes alternating. Infectious causes of ASII may be obvious such as secondary to herpes simplex keratitis but usually it is difficult to differentiate infectious from noninfectious. The most common form of ASII is a self-limiting recurrent iritis or iridocyclitis, associated with HLA-B27 in about 50% cases and often linked to spondyloarthropathies [35]. An association with gram-negative bacteria has long been suspected but not proven [36].

Infectious

Diagnostic aqueous taps in cases of ASII show a mixed population of inflammatory cells but no reports of positive culture for micro-organisms have been made except in cases of endophthalmitis (see above). Extensive searches for evidence of infection in recurrent ASII have proved negative [37] even using sensitive techniques such as antibody testing and PCR, for example for herpes viruses [38].

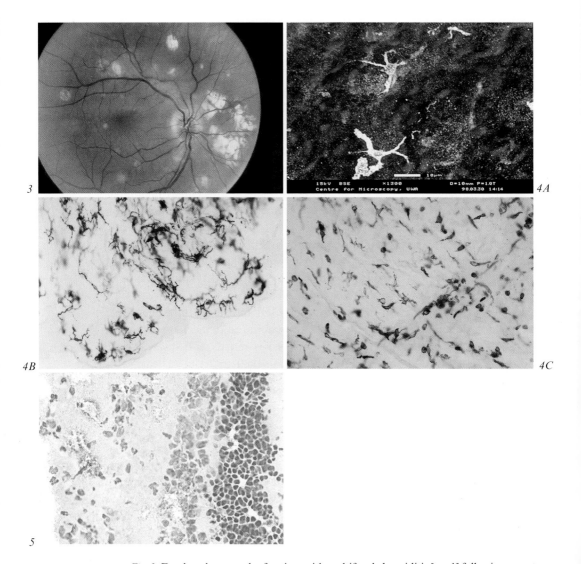

Fig. 3. Fundus photograph of patient with multifocal choroiditis [see 1] following recent Epstein-Barr virus infection.

Fig. 4. Dendritic cells (DC) in the rat uveal tract. *A* Iris whole mounts stained with anti-MHC class II (OX6) monoclonal antibody (mAB) and visualized with streptavidin-gold/silver enhancement. The iris is viewed from the anterior aspect using environmental scanning electron microscopy in backscatter detector mode. Only labelled cells on the iris surface are identifiable. *B* Immunoperoxidase on DC in the ciliary processes (whole mount, OX6 mAb). *C* DC in choroid whole mount. Orig. magn.: *B, C* × 150.

Fig. 5. Immunohistochemistry of the mouse model of IRBP peptide-induced EAU showing expression of MIP-1α distributed on vessels in the inner retina. Orig. magn.: × 140.

Noninfectious

As indicated above, most cases of ASII prove negative on testing for infectious agents. Accordingly, analysis of the cellular infiltrate has been performed to determine whether different forms of ASII may have different cellular mechanisms. Recent studies have shown that the cellular infiltrate in acute ASII is predominantly CD4 + T cells while patients with Fuch's heterochromic cyclitis, a low-grade form of anterior uveitis with minimal tissue damage, have a higher proportion of CD8 + T cells in their aqueous [39].

Further recent studies investigating the mechanism of recurrence in patients with ASII have shown that high levels of functional sFas and sFasL occur in patients with ASII and may represent a means whereby the inflammation is rapidly controlled [Dick et al., submitted].

Few studies of tissue biopsies have been performed in ASII. Cases of sarcoidosis have shown the typical noncaseating granulomas while clinical patterns of ASII vasculitis have been differentiated from pigment epitheliitis on iris fluorescein angiograms [40]. A series of iris biopsies revealed differential expression of various adhesion molecules on iris biopsies from patients with ASII, taken during surgery for the complications of the disease [41].

In general, most studies have shown a pattern of inflammation which comprised cellular infiltration of the tissues and fluids with activated T cells and macrophages, minimal infiltration with B cells, iris granulomas in some cases with upregulation of adhesion molecule expression, (peri)vasculitis of the iris vessels and oedema and infiltration of the tissues.

Clinical PSII

Clinical pathological studies of active PSII have also been infrequent for similar reasons as with ASII. Most studies have been performed on injured eyes removed during development of, or where there is a high risk of, sympathetic ophthalmia [18, 42]. The subject has been reviewed in detail elsewhere and only a brief summary is given here.

Infectious PSII

Pathological studies of toxoplasma choroiditis have been reported showing the presence of tachyzoites in the tissues in the absence of significant inflammation and extensive inflammation when the organism is no longer viable (see fig. 1, 2). In addition, case reports of infectious PSII in conditions such as CMV and other infections have shown the value of diagnostic biopsy [43].

In most of these conditions, extensive tissue destruction has been found usually representing the fact that the tissue has been obtained at an advanced stage of the disease and consequently many secondary phenomena have occurred in the tissues. Such material therefore is useful mostly for diagnostic purposes rather than unravelling the pathogenetic mechanism of disease induction.

Noninfectious PSII

Histology of eyes with noninfectious PSII reveals four characteristic features: typical multifocal chorioretinal infiltrates best seen in cases of sympathetic ophthalmia; inflammatory retinal (peri)vasculitis for example in sarcoidosis; retinal oedema especially at the macula and subretinal oedema with exudative detachment in severe cases such as Vogt-Koyanagi-Harada disease [9], and cellular infiltration into the vitreous. These features characterize many forms of noninfectious PSII and probably also some infectious forms of PSII and generally reflect the limited set of responses within the posterior segment of the eye in response to an inflammatory insult.

Immunological studies of PSII have been rarely reported. In general, inflammatory cells in the vitreous comprise a mixed population of lymphocytes and macrophages while immunohistological studies of chorioretinal microgranulomata reveal typical accumulations of activated macrophages strongly expressing CD68+ in the centre of the lesions with mixed CD4+ and CD8+ T cells in the surrounding tissues. High levels of MHC class II expression can be found in these cells, many of which have a dendritiform appearance. Similar findings have been observed in recently reported cases of Behçet's disease [44].

In some forms of chronic PSII characterized by extensive subretinal fibrosis, large numbers of B cells have been found indicating that a late, profibrotic healing stage of the disease can also have deleterious consequences for retinal architecture and sight. Extensive signs of apoptosis appeared to be associated with the pathological changes [45]. In addition, low-grade forms of PSII such as the histoplasmosis-like syndrome which is characterized by short-lived inflammatory lesions leaving chorioretinal scars and foci of subretinal neovascularization [46] also represents a late 'healing' stage of PSII in which a low level immune/inflammatory response persists. The condition has a direct counterpart in the experimental model of late stage autoimmune uveoretinitis (see below) and chemokines induced by inflammatory cells may be actively involved in the neovascular process. Indirectly, an immunological basis to many of these forms of PSII, including the subretinal neovascularization response, can be inferred from their positive response to immunosuppressive drugs [47].

Experimental ASII

Several models of experimental ASII have been developed, some of which are based on an infectious aetiology of ASII such as endotoxin-induced uveitis and others which are based on autoimmunity to ocular antigens.

Infectious

Since gram-negative bacteria are frequently considered to underlie the pathogenesis of several types of recurrent ASII, despite the lack of firm evidence, experimental models of the disease using intraocular injections of endotoxin (endotoxin-induced uveitis, EIU) have been developed [48]. This produced a reproducible form of EIU which also has a sympathetic component to the disease in that the noninjected fellow eye also developed disease. However, it was quickly realized that systemic intramuscular or intradermal injections of endotoxin were capable of inducing EIU and this has become the standard model [49, 50]. In many ways it is similar to clinical ASII but unlike clinical disease it does not induce lasting tissue damage. Instead, inflammatory cells appear to traffic through the tissues leaving the intraocular structures intact.

More recently, a model of ASII induced directly with gram-negative bacteria has been described and appears not to be linked with HLA-B27 [16].

Noninfectious

In the search for experimental models of ASII which were more representative of the clinical disease than those models which involved retinal antigens, two groups investigated antigens associated with melanin and showed that an antigen bound to melanin granules induced an inflammatory disease which was restricted to the anterior segment [5, 51]. The model is known as experimental melanin-protein-induced uveitis (EMIU) or experimental autoimmune anterior uveitis (EAAU) and produces a mild to moderate inflammatory infiltration of macrophages and lymphocytes located predominantly at the ciliary body vessels with infiltration into the aqueous humour. Interestingly the disease can be induced without adjuvant somewhat like EIU although with a different time scale [52]. Minimal infiltration appears to occur in the choroid although some foci of inflammatory cells can be detected in eyes with severe inflammation. EAAU differs from photoreceptor antigen-induced ocular inflammation in that there is a lack of retinitis and pinealitis.

Table 1. Retinal antigens and uveitogenic peptides

Retinal antigen	Uveitogenic epitopes, n
Retinal S antigen	>6
Interphotoreceptor retinol-binding protein	4 (×4 repeats)
Rhodopsin	1
Recoverin	1
Phosducin	1

Experimental PSII

Infectious

Specific models of infectious PSII have been developed including toxoplasmosis and *Onchocerca* [17, 53]. Models of toxoplasmosis have utilized live organisms and the inflammatory process appears to mimic the clinical disease well. This model appears to be extremely useful for studying mechanisms of tissue damage in toxoplasmosis [54]. Experimental models of onchocercal disease have been developed using the parasite antigen rather than the live organism and in this model the disease is very low grade involving infiltration of the choroid layer only but associated with some retinal microglial activation, perhaps nonspecifically [53]. In this model, the authors suggest that there is a significant overlap with ocular antigens, particularly an antigen in the retinal pigment epithelium with which they believe there is significant homology and thus they invoke a molecular mimicry mechanism for this model (see below).

Noninfectious

By far the most commonly utilized experimental models of IOI are those involving retinal antigens and on the basis of their extreme evolutionary structural conservation, these antigens are assumed to behave like autoantigens. The disease they induce is termed experimental autoimmune uveoretinitis (EAU) and in this respect, they resemble many other models of presumptive autoimmune diseases such as experimental autoimmune encephalomyelitis (EAE) and collagen-induced arthritis [15, 55–57].

Several antigens have now been described (table 1) and many of the uveitogenic epitopes are also known, amounting now to over 50. The pathology of EAU induced by each of these antigens shows some specific features for each of the antigens but remarkably single antigens, especially the originally described antigen (S antigen), can induce a range of retinal pathologies which resemble many different forms of clinical PSII depending on factors such as dose of antigen used, species of animal, degree of immunocompetence, type of adjuvant used, etc. [9]. Accordingly it has been suggested that many of the clinical forms of PSII represent specific points in the spectrum of pathologic manifestations induced by retinal antigens and although this is not confirmation of the involvement of autoantigens in noninfectious PSII, it indicates mechanisms whereby such processes may occur.

For the moment at least, the great value of these models has been the opportunity to investigate how noninfectious PSII may develop and to provide models for the development of therapeutic strategies.

How Is IOI Induced?

It seems difficult to envisage how the infectious models of IOI can be reconciled with the immune-mediated or autoimmune models despite the fact that an infectious aetiology for clinical IOI is suspected in many cases on the basis of clinical findings, and that the ocular manifestations appear identical in both cases. For instance, many forms of multifocal choroiditis are classified as 'idiopathic' which in effect usually means that the clinician believes there is an immunological if not a frankly autoimmune basis, to the disease. In some of these instances, immune responsiveness to human retinal antigens or their peptides can be demonstrated [19, 20, 24]. In contrast, very similar multifocal choroiditis can be found for instance during acute viral illness when the condition is very likely to be induced by viral or other antigens (see fig. 3). Similarly the ocular histoplasmosis syndrome which is widely believed to be induced by infection with *Histoplasma capsulatum* in the USA [58] has an identical counterpart in Europe and elsewhere for which no evidence of infection from any organism can be found [59].

It is necessary therefore to develop a working hypothesis which incorporates these ideas. Clearly, truly infectious models of PSII in which the organism can be detected in the tissues, such as toxoplasmosis and CMV retinitis, can be explained on the basis of direct immune responses to the organisms locally within the tissues, even if there is a significant acquired immunological response to the foreign antigen plus an additional component of immune responsiveness to ocular autoantigens released in the process of tissue damage.

More difficult to explain is how clinical or subclinical infections, distant either in space or time to the development of the apparently isolated ocular inflammation, can be responsible for the induction of the disease. Indeed this question is more general since it applies to all autoimmune diseases including conditions such as rheumatoid arthritis and multiple sclerosis to name but two.

For many years, an 'infectious' aetiology has been proposed for autoimmune diseases [see 55] and recently the notion of molecular mimicry has been in vogue [60]. However, there are several other possible mechanisms.

Autoimmune disease occurs when there is a breakdown in mechanisms of tolerance and previously tolerated antigens are recognized as 'dangerous' [61] and become targets to be eliminated. From a pathological viewpoint, the process of antigen elimination is likely to be the same whether the antigen is a foreign antigen, a transplanted antigen or a self antigen. Most of the differences in each of these immune responses are quantitative rather than qualitative. Thus most organ-specific autoimmune diseases are mediated via CD4 + Th1 cells [56] although some models of chronic disease can be mediated in their chronic phase by Th2 cells. Similarly, autoimmune-mediated diseases which target cell-associated antigens and utilize CD8 + cytotoxic T cells, require CD4 + T cells to initiate tissue damage [62], otherwise a tolerogenic state is induced.

The mechanism of tolerance breakdown and induction of autoimmune disease are the same as those of any immunogenic response, i.e. it involves antigen uptake by antigen presenting cells and presentation of that antigen to CD4 + T cells in the context of pro-inflammatory cytokines. Why should antigens which normally induce a tolerogenic signal when constitutively sampled, suddenly change to inducing an immunogenic signal? Several factors are important here. These include antigen avidity, antigen dose, the cytokine microenvironment, genetic predisposition and T-cell receptor 'promiscuity' [see 63].

It is generally recognized that autoimmunity occurs due to a breakdown or alteration in the mechanisms by which regulatory controls over autoreactive T and B cells are sustained in the periphery. Normally the numbers of randomly-generated autoreactive cells are low and prevention of clonal expansion of such cells is an active process, currently thought to be mediated by regulatory T cells. Several mechanisms have been proposed whereby clonal expansion of autoreactive T cells might occur including concepts as diverse as molecular mimicry which centres on antigen specificity and polyclonal activation in which clonal expansion of autoreactive lymphocytes is seen as a stochastic process.

Substantial circumstantial evidence exists to show that autoimmune diseases may be initiated or aggravated by infection. How this might occur is not clear but molecular mimicry, which proposes that homology between self and foreign antigens underpins autoimmune responses, has been suggested as one mechanism. Although the T-cell receptor displays a high degree of specificity in its interaction with the peptide-MHC complex, the level of specificity is orders of magnitude less than that of the B-cell receptor (antigen-antibody interactions) and in fact the T-cell receptor shows considerable degrees of promiscuity, i.e. it can interact to a greater or less degree with a range of peptide-MHC complexes [63]. The range of peptides that can bind a single T-cell receptor is relatively limited and such peptides are considered to have 'homology' and to show cross-reactivity. However, the source of such peptides can be very diverse and several peptides from micro-organisms have been shown to be homologous to autoantigenic peptides [64]. Many examples exist, for instance rheumatic fever and streptococcal infection, gram-negative infection and ulcerative colitis and most recently in molecular mimicry models of diabetes induced by coxsackie B infection [65]. It has even been suggested that some forms of clinical posterior uveitis may have a similar pathogenetic basis [66].

Examples of IOI induced by mechanisms of molecular mimicry are difficult to demonstrate but cross-reaction between HLA-B27 and retinal antigens have been found [67]. In addition, patients with pars planitis have been identified in which a 36-kD protein with homology to yeast nucleopore complex have been identified [68, 69]. Patients with Behçet's disease also appear to have immunity to a 60-kD heat-shock protein (HSP) which has homology with similar micro-organismal HSPs and appears to involve γδ T cells [70].

The notion that polyclonal activation of lymphocytes may be implicated in autoimmune disease induction is based on evidence that some bacterial components can activate B and T cells with several clonal specificities simultaneously and not through conventional receptor mechanisms. The need for antigenic specificity dictated by the molecular mimicry model can thus be circumvented. Polyclonal activation of B cells by bacterial or viral products is well known to induce autoantibody production in a T-cell-independent fashion [71] but most of these antibodies are nonpathogenic and of the low affinity IgM isotype, at least when they are produced in the absence of T-cell help. Polyclonal activation of T cells also may occur for instance by binding superantigens (Sag) [72, 73]. Sag are molecules which can activate T cells by directly binding the T-cell receptor at regions outwith the conventional peptide-binding groove. Examples include such molecules as staphylococcal A (M protein) which has in fact been shown to have some degree of homology to certain retinal antigens such as retinal S antigen [74]. Up to 10% of T cells can be stimulated nonspecifically by superantigen infection and at least some of these T cells will be autoreactive T cells which may then go on to induce autoimmune disease by targeting the original tissue antigens.

By either of these mechanisms, prodromal infection in intraocular inflammatory disease can aberrantly lead to systemic activation of autoreactive T cells in sufficient numbers which allow them to traffic to the eye. Once at the tissues site, several other factors must come into play to permit local antigen presentation and T-cell proliferation, finally inducing tissue damage either through cytotoxic T cells or through macrophage activation. However, according to this model, signs of systemic T-cell activation should still be present when the patient presents with active IOI.

Experimental Models

Experimental models of uveitis also depend on systemic activation of antigen-specific T cells in this case usually induced by immunization of the animals with antigen in the presence of adjuvant. Here, a local inflammatory reaction induced at the site of inoculation leads to antigen uptake by professional antigen presenting cells (APCs) which then traffic to the regional lymph node where they activate naive T cells. Antigen-specific T cells then re-circulate and traffic to the tissues. Interestingly, experimental models of molecular mimicry and superantigen exist, including models of experimental autoimmune uveoretinitis, in which for instance peptides from *Escherichia coli*, streptococcus A and yeast organisms appear to have sequence homology to retinal antigens and to possess uveitogenicity [74, 75]. A further recent example demonstrating the specificity of the autoantigen for the disease has recently been shown using HSV-1 to induce 'autoimmune' keratitis. It was found that mutant viruses lacking the specific antigenic epitope to which the autoreactive T cells responded, also failed to induce the corneal disease [76].

Evidence for Systemic Activation of T Cells in Uveitis

If the above concepts are plausible, i.e. that IOI is a systemic disease manifested by inflammatory activity in the eye, they require evidence of systemic activation of T cells both experimentally and clinically and preferably antigen-specific T-cell activation. Some evidence for the latter has been found in Behçet's disease [77] and in idiopathic uveitis [78, 79] while evidence for non-antigen-specific T-cell activation in patients with uveitis has been demonstrated on several occasions [see, for instance, 80]. Experimentally, interferon-γ locally or systemically produced, is associated with activation of both the early cellular infiltrate and later effector cells, indicating a Th1 polarization of the T-cell response [81].

Mechanisms of Tissue Damage in IOI

APCs in the Eye
Systemically activated autoreactive T cells, induced either by autoantigens or cross-reactive foreign antigens, thus enter the tissues and react on contact with antigen. This process requires APCs with access to the respective organ-specific antigens. Under normal circumstances, professional APCs are absent from the retina but extensive networks of dendritic cells and macrophages

reside in the iris, ciliary body and choroid [82–84] (fig. 4). Dendritic cells in particular, like dendritic cells elsewhere, have the potential to traffic to the regional lymph nodes and spleen, and to present ocular antigens to autoreactive T cells in the lymph nodes, now known to be available to intraocular antigens [85]. Normally this response to the T-cell/APC interaction leads to a tolerogenic response and clonal expansion of autoreactive T cells does not occur. However, if the T cells have been activated by prior exposure to cross-reactive antigen they may interact directly with antigen-loaded APCs in the tissues and undergo proliferation and cytokine production.

Several mechanisms within the eye exist to inhibit this response (see below) and similar if less complete inhibitory mechanisms occur generally in many tissues. However, failure of this regulatory mechanism, also known as by-stander suppression, may permit initiation of the disease at the target site. Thus, it is possible for patients to have raised levels of potentially autoreactive T cells within their pool of circulating lymphocytes but to fail to demonstrate organ-specific disease until local regulatory controls are breached, either at the level simply of access of leukocytes to the tissue or by virtue of absence of such factors as co-stimulation.

Role of Innate Immunity

As indicated above, APCs are normally excluded from the tissue sites which contain most of the potent ocular autoantigens, i.e. cornea, lens, retina and retinal pigment epithelium. There is likely to be some degree of APC exposure to intraocular antigens such as retinal S antigens during physiological processes such as rod outer segment phagocytosis [86] and the normal presence of low levels of serum antibodies to retinal antigens [22] indicates that sustained low levels of immunoreactivity occur. However, as indicated above, induction of immunity rather than tolerance to such antigens depends on factors such as antigen dose. Thus it is likely that autoimmune diseases are initiated by nonspecific inflammatory damage such as that induced by a focal viral infection of the retinal pigment epithelium, or NK cell or mast cell release of pro-inflammatory cytokines through unrelated systemic illness, causing sufficient local activation of antigen-loaded APCs to activate randomly circulating auto-reactive T cells. This form of 'bystander damage' is currently favoured over molecular mimicry as a mechanism of systemic infection-mediated organ-specific autoimmune disease [87].

In addition, during the course of the disease, considerable nonspecific damage can be mediated via release of chemical mediators, such as free radicals, especially NO [88] and soluble enzymes such as matrix metalloproteinases [89, 90]. This will lead to further release of antigen from the tissues and allow continued antigen presentation by APCs to specific T cells.

Effector Cells

The nature of the tissue damage varies depending on the type of effector cell which induces the disease. Experimental PSII is a CD4 + T-cell-mediated dis- ease and recent studies suggest that genetically susceptible individuals covert from a Th2 phenotype to a Th1 phenotype while resistant individuals fail to induce Th1 cells [Caspi, pers. commun.].

Human and experimental studies of IOI indicate that both T cells and macrophages are required for tissue damage and that TNF-α is a major but not essential mediator of tissue damage. The precise role of each cell type in tissue damage is unclear, but it is likely that T cells initiate early cell membrane attack [91] and macrophages are involved in a scavenging role [92]. Various chemokines are actively involved in the recruitment of T cells and macrophages to the tissue including RANTES, MIP-1α and MCP-1–3 [93] (fig. 5). In addition, tissue and inflammatory cell release of angiogenic chemokines may be important in the late phases of the disease in which subretinal neovascularization occurs and may mimic a number of human low-grade inflammatory conditions (see above).

The Cytokine Microenvironment

From the above it is clear that cytokines and chemokines are likely to play a crucial role in the development of IOI. Clinical studies have shown that several cytokines and chemokines are released during the process of IOI including IL-1, IL-2, IL-6, IL-8, RANTES, MIP-1α and MCP-1–3 [39, 81, 94, 95]. In addition, experimental studies with various cytokines such as IL-10, antibodies or similar reagents to other cytokines such as IL-12 and IL-15 or their receptors and TNFα and its receptor [17, 91, 96] have shown how much of the inflammatory response is determined by the levels of pro-inflammatory versus anti-inflammatory cytokines.

At the cellular level, many of these molecules are released by cells in situ such as retinal pigment epithelial cells, endothelial cells and resident tissue macrophage populations, e.g. microglia in the retina. Thus the nature of the final inflammatory reaction is regulated by how the tissues respond. In addition, resident tissue leukocytes, such as macrophages and mast cells, may play a significant part in how the tissues react. For some time it was suspected that experimental animals show a differential susceptibility to IOI depending on the numbers of mast cells which are present in the choroid [97, 98]. However, recent studies have shown that strains of moderate susceptibility have very few mast cells [99].

Other cytokines are also important. For instance, retinal pigment epithelial cells produce large amounts of GM-CSF [see below] when activated by other cytokines such as IL-1. GM-CSF is known to be essential for dendritic cells' survival and maturation and this may regulate how efficiently choroidal dendritic cells present antigen, i.e. either in a tolerogenic form or in an immunogenic form.

Why Do Certain Types of IOI Present the Way They Do?

Since there are so many variables at play during the course of an episode of IOI, including antigens, cell types (both for the induction and effector stages of the disease) and chemical mediators, it is not surprising that there are so many clinical forms of the disease, despite the fact that experimental studies indicate that the differences are likely to be more of degree than nature. Clinically, IOI ranges in severity from advanced retinal vasculitis and necrosis in Behçet's disease or extensive exudative retinal detachment in Vogt-Koyanagi-Harada disease, to much milder but equally sight-threatening forms such as serpiginous choroiditis or ocular histoplasmosis syndrome. Conditions such as pars planitis and peripheral retinal vasculitis occupy a middle position.

Predictions can be made on the basis of experimental work concerning what kind of inflammatory mechanism is taking place in each of these forms of IOI. Thus very severe forms of IOI involving extensive exudative retinal detachment and widespread tissue damage, experimentally at least, are associated with large-scale free radical release [100, 101] and production of large amounts of cytokine such as TNF-α [102]. Low-grade forms of 'healed' inflammatory responses with subretinal neovascularization and fibrosis may be associated with angiogenic chemokine production and B-cell activity. The location of inflammation at the ciliary body and pars plana may be a result of preferential adhesion molecule expression at this site rather than in more posteriorly placed retinal vessels. The questions which clearly arise are related to how such site-selective inflammation occurs and what the local regulatory mechanisms might be.

Regulatory Mechanisms in the Eye and How These Are Disabled in IOI

Many tissues and organs have in place mechanisms which can modulate the immune response. This is particularly true of the eye where 'immune privilege' may exist, in common with other tissues such as the brain, testis, liver and pancreas, see chapter by Streilein [this volume, pp. 11–38]. In the eye, or more particularly in the anterior chamber, this property has been termed anterior chamber-associated immune deviation (ACAID) in which immune responses are curtailed or modified by factors produced in the eye. Initially it was thought that this was due to anatomical factors such as the absence of lymphatics or of tissue resident APCs, but neither of these conditions obtains in the chambers of the eye [103]. It also now seems that a similar situation exists in the CNS where dendritic cells and macrophages are extensively distributed in the meninges and choroid plexus and where they have communication with the nasal lymphatic vessels and cervical lymph nodes [103]. In fact, it has been shown that cytokines (such as TGF-β and IL-10) [104] and peptides (such as MSH-α and VIP) [105] downregulate Th1 cell activity in the eye and 'deviate' the immune response towards a Th2 response in which noninflammatory cytokines are produced [106, 107]. In part this effect correlates with the nature of the antigen [108].

A further recent and important mechanism of local immunoregulation has been shown, namely the constitutive expression of FasL by cells of the anterior and posterior chambers of the eye which are functionally active and induce apoptosis in activated Fas-expressing T cells when they enter the eye [109]. This process also appears to be linked to production of IL-10 by the apoptosing cells [110].

Cells in the posterior chamber, such as retinal pigment epithelial cells, also express FasL [111] and may induce bystander suppression in a similar way. In addition, retinal pigment epithelial cells are known to secrete several immunosuppressive cytokines and mediators such as IL-10, TGF-β, NO and PGE$_2$ [for review, see 112].

A possible mechanism therefore, whereby autoimmune responses may occur, is by release of pro-inflammatory cytokines which override these immunosuppressive mechanisms. Thus it has been shown that exposure of cells of the ciliary epithelium and the retinal pigment epithelium to cytokines such as IL-1 and IFN-γ will induce the release of other pro-inflammatory cytokines and chemokines such as IL-6 and IL-8, GM-CSF and MIP-1α and RANTES which will permit the progression of an autoimmune inflammation [94, 113, 114, and Crane et al., unpubl. data]. Thus a nonspecific viral infection which produces high levels of circulating cytokines such as IFN-γ or TNF-α may alter the tissue microenvironment in such a way that it may promote an autoimmune reaction if the appropriate T cells and APCs are present [112]. Pro-inflammatory cytokines may have a direct effect on APCs by inducing the expression of co-stimulatory factors such as CD40 and B7 on APCs which render them more likely to induce responses in activated T cells. In addition, pro-inflammatory cytokines produced by APCs are necessary for the proper induction of an immune response, in particular IL-12 and IL-15. Recently, it has been shown that live micro-organisms are not necessary for induction of a pathogenic T-cell response since simply incubating antigen-specific T cells in LPS or highly purified bacterial products is sufficient to induce autoimmune disease [72].

An alternative to local tissue regulation of the immune response is the proposal that antigen-specific regulatory T cells are generated in the course of the host's response to antigen and that such cells are essential for the maintenance of central and peripheral tolerance [115]. Induction of tolerance through mechanisms such as mucosal administration of antigen or intravenous injection of antigen have shown that antigen-specific T cells with an immuno-regulatory phenotype can be generated. Such cells appear to be CD4+CD8- and are skewed towards a Th2 phenotype [for review, see 116] although some authorities hold to the view that CD8+ T cells are suppressor in nature [117]. It has also been suggested that regulatory CD8+ T cells expressing the γδ receptor are the relevant population [118] although there may be some redundancy in the system [119]. Regulatory (also termed Th3 by some) T cells appear to mediate their effect through secretion of TGF-β [120].

It has been suggested that regulatory T cells may also be induced through the idiotype network [121]. While the concept of idiotype control over immune responses has been discussed for a considerable time, definite evidence for this mechanism has been difficult to produce. However, in several autoimmune diseases, infusions of polyclonal intravenous immunoglobulins have been shown to be beneficial and it is thought that such immunoglobulins function via the idiotype network [122, 123]. However, evidence from studies of T-cell vaccination procedures in experimental models have suggested that the strong anti-T-cell antibody response which appears to be implicated in the effector mechanism for disease amelioration using T-cell vaccines, was not idiotype-specific although it was IgG in type indicating that it was probably derived from existing antibody networks.

Finally, an important regulatory factor on the development of auto-immune disease is genetic susceptibility. The association between genetic factors and autoimmune diseases such as rheumatoid arthritis, diabetes mellitus and ankylosing spondylitis is well known and does not conflict with the possible association between infective agents and the same disorders since genetic susceptibility (and resistance) to infectious agents is also well-recognized [124]. The MHC genes have particularly been studied in their relationship to auto-immune disease, not only because of their extensive polymorphism, but because of obvious involvement in the immunity and tolerance.

The human DR3 and DR4 genes have been shown to have strong associations with rheumatoid arthritis and diabetes mellitus where the relative risk of developing diabetes mellitus in the DR3/DR4 heterozygotes is 20. Indeed linkage disequilibrium between the DQ3.2 gene and DR4 has been elegantly demonstrated and has been correlated with amino acid substitutions at position 57 of the peptide binding cleft of the DQb chain where possession of the aspartic acid appears to be protective. This protectiveness extends to the diabetes-prone NOD mouse which has serine in the homologous position of the I-Ab chain instead of aspartic acid.

Several ocular disorders also have associations within specific HLA types. In particular, the associations of HLA-B27 with ankylosing spondylitis and acute anterior uveitis is well established, as is the link between HLA-A29 and birdshot retinochoroidopathy in which the peptide-binding motif has been elucidated allowing prediction of potential retinal autoantigenic peptides [125]. More recently, Behçet's disease has been strongly associated with HLA-B5101 [126] while the previously determined association between HLA-DRB1*0405 HLA-DRB*0401 [127] and Vogt-Koyanagi-Harada disease has now been extended to sympathetic ophthalmia [126]. Other ocular conditions with possible genetic associations include ocular pemphigoid and retinal vasculitis, but no clear evidence has yet emerged. Direct implication of specific autoantigens in these conditions has been more difficult to establish (see below).

Precisely how HLA molecules regulate susceptibility to autoimmune disease is not clear but they are most likely to function by influencing the T-cell binding and activation even though many of the polymorphisms do not appear to be embedded in the peptide binding cleft. Most associations between MHC antigens and autoimmune disease are weak (i.e. relative risks in the region 1.5–4) and the significance of such associations is also not clear. They may for instance be important during thymic maturation by permitting some T-cell clones to escape deletion or they may modify the function of regulatory T cells. Finally, the MHC molecule may show sequence homology to certain microbial or autoantigens and in this way lead to inappropriate activation or deletion. Recent studies have in fact shown that homology between retinal S antigen and HLA-B27 exists and this has been proposed as a mechanism for induction of uveitis [67].

Experimental evidence supports the clinical data for genetic susceptibility to autoimmune disease. For instance, several strains of mice are considerably more susceptible to experimental autoimmune encephalomyelitis [128], a model for demyelinating disease, and to EAU [129] than others and the susceptibility is carried by both major and minor histocompatibility antigens as well as non-MHC antigens. Some of this disease susceptibility has been ascribed to mouse T-cell phenotype with some mice responding to antigenic challenge with a more Th1 skewed response than a Th2 response [130]. Similar findings can be applied to other species such as rats and guinea pigs and presumably man. In addition, the T-cell phenotype which predominantly becomes activated or tolerized in response to any one specific antigen or in any type of autoimmune disease, may also be significantly restricted. For instance, the Vβ8.2 TCR [131] cell phenotype may be involved in both the immune response or be expressed on regulatory T cells involved in tolerance.

Conclusion

In conclusion, this overview attempts to synthesize much of what is known about uveitis. Specifically, the aim has been to highlight the clinical problem and to place it in the context of autoimmune disease generally by discussing the evidence for uveitis as an autoimmune disease. In particular, mechanisms of both immunity and tolerance within the eye appear to be organ-specific and unique immunoregulatory mechanisms may be involved in the control of the immune response within the eye and the CNS [103].

References

1 Forrester JV, Okada AA, Ben Ezra D, Ohno S: Posterior Segment Intraocular Inflammation: Guidelines. The Hague, Kugler Publications, 1998.
2 Wacker WB, Kalsow CM, Yankeelov JA, Organisciack DT: Experimental allergic uveitis. Isolation, characterisation and localisation of a soluble uveitopathogenic antigen from bovine retina. J Immunol 1977;119:1949–1958.
3 Wacker WB: Experimental allergic uveitis: Investigations of retinal autoimmunity and the immunopathologic responses evoked: Proctor Lecture. Invest Ophthalmol Vis Sci 1991;32:3119–3129.
4 Broekhuyse RM, Kuhlmann ED,Winkens HJ: Experimental autoimmune posterior uveitis accompanied by epithelioid cell accumulation. A new type of experimental ocular disease inducd by immunisation with PEP-65, a pigment epithelial polypeptide preparation. Exp Eye Res 1992;55:819–829.
5 Broekhuyse RM, Kuhlmann ED,Winkens HJ: Experimental autoimmune anterior uveitis. III. Induction by immunisation with purified uveal and skin melanins. Exp Eye Res 1993;56:401–411.
6 Dua HS, Lee RH, Lolley RN, Barrett JA, Abrahams M, Forrester JV, Donoso LA: Induction of experimental autoimmune uveitis by the retinal photoreceptor cell protein, phosducin. Curr Eye Res 1992;11(suppl):107–112.
7 Gery I: Retinal antigens and the immunopathologic process they provoke. Prog Retinal Eye Res 1986;5:75–109.
8 Gery I, Chanaud NP, Anglade E: Recoverin is highly uveitogenic in Lewis rats. Invest Ophthalmol Vis Sci 1994;35:3342–3345.
9 Forrester JV, Liversidge JM, Dua HS, Towler HM, McMenamin PG: Comparison of clinical and experimental uveitis. Curr Eye Res 1990;9(suppl):75–84.
10 Forrester JV, Borthwick GM, McMenamin PG: Ultrastructural pathology of S-antigen uveoretinitis. Invest Ophthal Vis Sci 1985;26:1281–1292.
11 Forrester JV: Uveitis. Br J Ophthalmol 1990;74:620–622.
12 Forrester JV: Uveitis: Pathogenesis. Lancet 1991;338:1498–1501.
13 Inomata H: Necrotic changes of choroidal melanocytes in sympathetic ophthalmia. Arch Ophthalmol 1988;106:239–242.
14 Inomata H, Sakamoto T: Immunohistochemical studies of Vogt-Koyanagi-Harada disease with sunset sky fundus. Curr Eye Res 1990;95:35–40.
15 Nowack R, Flores-Suarez LF, van der Woude FJ: New developments in pathogenesis of systemic vasculitis. Curr Opin Rheumatol 1998;10:3–11.
16 Baggia S, Lyons JL, Angell E, Barkhuizen A, Han YB, Planck SR, Taurog JD, Rosenbaum JT: A novel model of bacterially-induced acute anterior uveitis in rats and the lack of effect from HLA-B27 expression. J Invest Med 1997;45:295–301.

17   Hayashi S, Chan CC, Gazzinelli RT, Pham NT, Cheung MK, Roberge FG: Protective role of nitric oxide in ocular toxoplasmosis. Br J Ophthalmol 1996;80:644–648.

18   Rao NA: Mechanisms of inflammatory response in sympathetic ophthalmia and VKH syndrome. Eye 1997;11:213–216.

19   de Smet MD, Mochizuki M, Gery I, Singh VJ, Shinohara T, Wiggert B, Chader GJ, Nussenblatt RB: Cellular immune responses of patients with uveitis to retinal antigens and their fragments. Am J Ophthalmol 1991;110:135–142.

20   de Smet MD, Dayan M, Nussenblatt RB: A novel method for the determination of T-cell proliferative responses in patients with uveitis. Ocul Immunol Inflamm 1998;6:139–207.

21   Doekes G, van der Gaag R, Rothova A, van Koojk Y, Broersma L, Zaal MJM, Dijkman G, Fortuin ME, Baarsma GS, Kijlstra A: Humoral and cellular immune responsiveness to human S-antigen in uveitis. Curr Eye Res 1987;6:909–919.

22   Forrester JV, Stott D, Hercus K: Naturally occurring antibodies to bovine and human retinal S antigen: A comparison between uveitis patients and healthy volunteers. Br J Ophthalmol 1989;73:155–159.

23   Froebel KS, Armstrong SS, Urbaniak SJ, Forrester JV: An investigation of the general immune status and specific immune responsiveness to retinal S-antigen in patients with chronic posterior uveitis. Eye 1989; 3:263–270.

24   Nussenblatt RB, Mittal KK, Ryan S, Green WR, Maumenee AE: Birdshot retinochoroidopathy associated with HLA-A29 antigen and immune responsiveness to retinal S antigen. Am J Ophthalmol 1982;94:147–158.

25   Opremcak EM, Cowans AB, Orosz CG, Adams PW, Whisler RL: Enumeration of autoreactive helper T lymphocytes in uveitis. Invest Ophthalmol Vis Sci 1991;32:2561–2567.

26   Nussenblatt RB, Gery I, Weiner HL, Ferris FL, Shiloach J, Remaley N, Perry C, Caspi RR, Hafler DA, Foster C, Whitcup SM: Treatment of uveitis by oral administration of retinal antigens: Results of a phase I/II randomized masked trial. Am J Ophthalmol 1997;123:583–592.

27   Dubey JP: Bradyzoite-induced murine toxoplasmosis: Stage conversion, pathogenesis, and tissue cyst formation in mice fed bradyzoites of different strains of *Toxoplasma gondii*. J Eukaryot Microbiol 1996;44:592–602.

28   Araujo F, Slifer T, Kim S: Chronic infection with *Toxoplasma gondii* does not prevent acute disease or colonization of the brain with tissue cysts following reinfection with different strains of the parasite. J Parasitol 1997;83:521–522.

29   Dutton GN, McMenamin PG, Hay J, Cameron S: The ultrastructural pathology of congenital murine toxoplasmic retinochoroiditis. I. The localisation of the toxoplasma cysts in the retina. Exp Eye Res 1986;43:529–543.

30   McMenamin PG, Dutton GN, Hay J, Cameron S: The ultrastructural pathology of congenital murine toxoplasmic retinochoroiditis. II. The morphology of the inflammatory changes. Exp Eye Res 1986;43:545–560.

31   Bruggeman CA, Li F, Stals FS: Pathogenicity: Animal models. Scand J Infect Dis 1995;99 (suppl): 43–50.

32   Persoons MC, Stals FS, van dam Mieras MC, Bruggeman CA: Multiple organ involvement during experimental cytomegalovirus infection is associated with disseminated vascular pathology. J Pathol 1998;184:103–109.

33   Sutherland MR, Raynor CM, Leenknegt H, Wright JF, Pryzdial EL: Coagulation initiated on herpes viruses. Proc Natl Acad Sci USA 1997;94:13510–13514.

34   Craigen JL, Yong KL, Jordan NJ, MacCormac LP, Westwick J, Akbar AN, Grundy JE: Human cytomegalovirus infection up-regulates interleukin-8 gene expression and stimulates neutrophil trans-endothelial migration. Immunology 1997;92:138–145.

35   Rothova A, Suttorp-van Schulten MS, Frits Treffers W, Kijlstra A: Causes and frequency of blindness in patients with intraocular inflammatory disease. Br J Ophthalmol 1996;80:332–336.

36   Careless DJ, Chiu B, Rabinovitch T, Wade J, Inman RD: Immunogenetic and microbial factors in acute anterior uveitis. J Rheumatol 1997;24:102–108.

37   Sprenkels SH, Van Kregten E, Feltkamp TE: IgA antibodies against *Klebsiella* and other Gram-negative bacteria in ankylosing spondylitis and acute anterior uveitis. Clin Rheumatol 1996; 15(suppl 1):48–51.

38   de Boer JH, Verhagen C, Bruinenberg M, Rothova A, de Jong PT, Baarsma GS, Van der Lelij A, Ooyman FM, Bollemeijer JG, Derhaag PJ, Kijlstra A: Serologic and polymerase chain reaction of intraocular fluids in the diagnosis of infectious uveitis. Am J Ophthalmol 1996;121:650–658.

39   Muhaya M, Calder V, Towler HM, Shaer B, McLauchlan M, Lightman S: Characterization of T cells and cytokines in the aqueous humour in patients with Fuchs' heterochromic cyclitis and idiopathic anterior uveitis. Clin Exp Immunol 1998;111:123–128.

40   Dua HS, Dick AD, Watson NJ, Forrester JV: A spectrum of clinical signs in anterior uveitis. Eye 1993;7:68–73.

41   La Heij E, Kuijpers RW, Baarsma SG, Kijlstra A, van der Weiden M, Mooy CM: Adhesion molecules in iris biopsy specimens from patients with uveitis. Br J Ophthalmol 1998;82:432–437.

42   Liversidge J, Dick A, Cheng YF, Scott GB, Forrester JV: Retinal antigen specific lymphocytes, TCR-$\gamma\delta$ T cells and CD5+ B cells cultured from the vitreous in acute sympathetic ophthalmitis. Autoimmunity 1993;15:1–10.

43   Verbraeken HS: Diagnostic vitrectomy and chronic uveitis. Graefes Arch Clin Exp Ophthalmol 1996;234(suppl 1):2–7.

44   George RK, Chan CC, Whitcup SM, Nussenblatt RB: Ocular immunopathology of Behçet's disease. Surv Ophthalmol 1997;42:157–162.

45   Chan CC, Matteson DM, Li Q, Whitcup SM, Nussenblatt RB: Apoptosis in patients with posterior uveitis. Arch Ophthalmol 1997;115:1559–1567.

46   Cohen SY, Laroche A, Leguen Y, Soubrane G, Coscas GJ: Etiology of choroidal neovascularization in young patients. Ophthalmology 1996;103:1241–1244.

47   Dees C, Arnold JJ, Forrester JV, Dick AD: Immunosuppressive treatment of choroidal neovascularization associated with endogenous posterior uveitis. Arch Ophthalmol 1998;116:1456–1464.

48   Forrester JV, Worgul BV, Merriam GR: Endotoxin-induced uveitis in the rat. Graefes Arch Clin Exp Ophthalmol 1980;213:221–233.

49   Rosenbaum JT, McDevitt HO, Guss RB, Egbert PR: Endotoxin-induced uveitis in rats as a model for human disease. Nature 1980;286:611–613.

50   Pouvreau I, Zech JC, Thillaye-Goldenberg B, Naud MC, Van Rooijen N, de Kozak Y: Effect of macrophage depletion by liposomes containing dichloromethylene-diphosphonate on endotoxin-induced uveitis. J Neuroimmunol 1998;86:171–181.

51   Bora NS, Kim MC, Kabeer NH, Simpson SC, Tandhasetti MT, Cirrito TP, Kaplan AD, Kaplan HJ: Experimental autoimmune anterior uveitis. Induction with melanin-associated antigen from the iris and ciliary body. Invest Ophthalmol Vis Sci 1995;36:1056–1066.

52   Bora NS, Woon MD, Tandhasetti MT, Cirrito TP, Kaplan HJ: Induction of experimental autoimmune anterior uveitis by a self antigen: Melanin complex without adjuvant. Invest Ophthalmol Vis Sci 1997;38:2171–2175.

53   McKechnie NM, Gurr W, Braun G: Immunization with the cross-reactive antigens Ov39 from *Onchocerca volvulus* and hr44 from human retinal tissue induces ocular pathology and activates retinal microglia. J Infect Dis 1997;176:1334–1343.

54   Gazzinelli RT, Brezin A, Li Q, Nussenblatt RB, Chan CC: *Toxoplasma gondii*: Acquired ocular toxoplasmosis in the murine model, protective role of TNF-alpha and IFN-gamma. Exp Parasitol 1994;78:217–229.

55   von Herrath MG, Oldstone MB: Virus-induced autoimmune disease. Curr Opin Immunol 1996;8:878–885.

56   Gery I, Streilein JW: Autoimmunity in the eye and its regulation. Curr Opin Immunol 1994;6:938–945.

57   Constantinescu CS, Hilliard B, Fujioka T, Bhopale MK, Calida D, Rostami AM: Pathogenesis of neuroimmunologic diseases. Experimental models. Immunol Res 1998;17:217–227.

58   Smith RE, Ganley JP: An epidemiologic study of presumed ocular histoplasmosis. Trans Am Acad Ophthalmol Otolaryngol 1971;75:994–1005.

59   Suttorp-Schulten MS, Bollemeijer JG, Bos PJ, Rothova A: Presumed ocular histoplasmosis in The Netherlands – An area without histoplasmosis. Br J Ophthalmol 1997;81:7–11.

60 Wucherpfennig KW, Strominger JL: Molecular mimicry in T cell-mediated autoimmunity: Viral peptides activate human T cell clones specific for myelin basic protein. Cell 1995;80:695–705.

61 Matzinger P: Tolerance, danger, and the extended family. Annu Rev Immunol 1994;12:991–1045.

62 Kurts C, Carbone FR, Barnden M, Blanas E, Allison J, Heath WR, Miller JF: CD4+ T cell help impairs CD8+ T cell deletion induced by cross-presentation of self antigens and favors autoimmunity. J Exp Med 1997;186:2057–2062.

63 Mason D: A very high level of cross-reactivity is an essential feature of the T-cell receptor. Immunol Today 1998;19:395–404.

64 Hausmann S, Wucherpfennig KW: Activation of autoreactive T cells by peptides from human pathogens. Curr Opin Immunol 1997;9:831–838.

65 Vreugdenhil GR, Geluk A, Ottenhoff TH, Melchers WJ, Roep BO, Galama JM: Molecular mimicry in diabetes mellitus: The homologous domain in coxsackie B virus protein 2C and islet autoantigen GAD65 is highly conserved in the coxsackie B-like enteroviruses and binds to the diabetes-associated HLA-DR3 molecule. Diabetalogia 1998; 41:40–46.

66 Brezin AP, Massin-Korobelnik P, Boudin M, Gaudric A, LeHoang P: Acute posterior multifocal placoid pigment epitheliopathy after hepatitis B vaccine. Arch Ophthalmol 1995;113:297–300.

67 Wildner G, Thurau SR: Cross-reactivity between an HLA-B27-derived peptide and a retinal autoantigen peptide: A clue to major histocompatibility complex association with autoimmune disease. Eur J Immunol 1994;24:2597–2685.

68 Bora NS, Bora PS, Tandhasetti MT, Cirrito TP, Kaplan HJ: Molecular cloning, sequencing, and expression of the 36 kDa protein present in pars planitis. Sequence homology with yeast nucleopore complex protein. Invest Ophthalmol Vis Sci 1996;37:1877–1883.

69 Bora NS, Bora PS, Kaplan HJ: Identification, quantitation, and purification of a 36 kDa circulating protein associated with active pars planitis. Invest. Ophthalmol Vis Sci 1996;37:1870–1896.

70 Lehner T: The role of heat shock protein, microbial and autoimmune agents in the aetiology of Behçet's disease. Int Rev Immunol 1997;14:21–31.

71 Schattner A: Virus-induced autoimmunity. Rev Infect Dis 1990;12:204–222.

72 Schiffenbauer J, Soos J, Johnson H: The possible role of bacterial superantigens in the pathogenesis of autoimmune disorders. Immunol Today 1998;19:117–120.

73 Friedman SM, Tumang JR, Crow MK: Microbial superantigens as etiopathogenic agents in autoimmunity. Rheum Dis Clin North Am 1993;19:207–222.

74 Lerner MP, Donoso LA, Nordquist RE, Cunningham MW: Immunological mimicry between retinal S-antigen and group A streptococcal M proteins. Autoimmunity 1995;22:95–106.

75 Shinohara T, Singh VK, Tsuda M, Yamaki K, Abe T, Suzuki S: S-antigen: From gene to autoimmune uveitis. Exp Eye Res 1990;50:751–757.

76 Zhao ZS, Granucci F, Yeh L, Schaffer PA, Cantor H: Molecular mimicry by herpes simplex virustype 1: Autoimmune disease after viral infection. Science 1998;279:1344–1347.

77 Esin S, Gul A, Hodara V, Jeddi-Tehrani M, Dilsen N, Konice M, Andersson R, Wigzell H: Peripheral blood T cell expansions in patients with Behçet's disease. Clin Exp Immunol 1997;107:520–527.

78 Tighe PJ, Liversidge J, Forrester JV, Sewell HF: Analysis of the T-cell receptor beta chain repertoire expressed in endogenous posterior uveitis. Ann NY Acad Sci 1995;756:421–423.

79 Feron EJ, Calder VL, Lightman SL: Oligoclonal activation of CD4+ T lymphocytes in posterior uveitis. Clin Exp Immunol 1995;99:412–418.

80 Dick AD, Cheng YF, Purdie AT, Liversidge J, Forrester JV: Immunocytochemical analysis of blood lymphocytes in uveitis. Eye 1992;6:643–647.

81 Xu H, Rizzo LV, Silver PB, Caspi RR: Uveitogenicity is associated with a Th1-like lymphokine profile: Cytokine-dependent modulation of early and committed effector T cells in experimental autoimmune uveitis. Cell Immunol 1997;178:69–78.

82 McMenamin PG, Holthouse I, Holt PG: Class II MHC (Ia) antigen-bearing dendritic cells within the iris and ciliary body of the rat eye: Distribution, phenotype, ontogeny, and relation to retinal microglia. Immunology 1992;77:385–393.

83 McMenamin PG, Crewe J, Morrison S, Holt PG: Immunomorphological studies of macrophages and MHC class II-positive dendritic cells in the iris and ciliary body of the rat, mouse and human eye. Invest Ophthalmol Vis Sci 1994;35:3234–3250.

84   Forrester JV, McMenamin PG, Holthouse I, Lumsden L, Liversidge J: Localisation and characteri-
      sation of major histocompatibility complex class II-positive cells in the posterior segment of the
      eye: Implications for the induction of autoimmune uveoretinitis. Invest Ophthalmol Vis Sci 1994;
      35:64–77.

85   Egan RM, Yorkey C, Black R, Loh WK, Stevens JL, Woodward JG: Peptide-specific T cell clonal
      expansion in vivo following immunization in the eye, an immune-privileged site. J Immunol 1996;
      157:2262–2271.

86   Forrester JV: Duke Elder Lecture: New concepts on the role of autoimmunity in the pathogenesis
      of uveitis. Eye 1992;6:433.

87   Benoist A, Mathis D: The pathogen connection. Nature 1998;394:227–228.

88   Kolb H, Kolb-Bachofen V: Nitric oxide in autoimmune disease: Cytotoxic or regulatory mediator?
      Immunol Today 1998;19:556–561.

89   Kieseier BC, Kiefer R, Clements JM, Miller K, Wells GM, Schweitzer T, Gearing AJ, Hartung
      HP: Matrix metalloproteinase-9 and -7 are regulated in experimental autoimmune encephalomyelitis.
      Brain 1998;121:159–166.

90   Liedtke W, Cannella B, Mazzaccaro RJ, Clements JM, Miller KM, Wucherpfennig KW, Gearing
      AJ, Raine CS: Effective treatment of models of multiple sclerosis by matrix metalloproteinase
      inhibitors. Ann Neurol 1998;44:35–46.

91   Dick AD, McMenamin PG, Korner H, Scallon BJ, Ghrayeb J, Forrester JV, Sedgwick JD: Inhibition
      of tumor necrosis factor activity minimizes target organ damage in experimental autoimmune
      uveoretinitis despite quantitatively normal activated T cell traffic to the retina. Eur J Immunol
      1996;26:1018–1025.

92   Forrester JV, Huitinga I, Lumsden L, Dijkstra CD: Marrow-derived activated macrophages are
      required during the effector phase of experimental autoimmune uveoretinitis in rats. Curr Eye Res
      1998;17:426–437.

93   Sacca R, Cuff CA, Ruddle NH: Mediators of inflammation. Curr Opin Immunol 1997;9:851–
      857.

94   Crane IJ, Kuppner MC, McKillop-Smith S, Knott RM, Forrester JV: Cytokine regulation of
      RANTES production by human retinal pigment epithelial cells. Cell Immunol 1998;184:37–44.

95   Verma MJ, Lloyd A, Rager H, Strieter R, Kunkel S, Taub D, Wakefield D: Chemokines in acute
      anterior uveitis. Curr Eye Res 1997;16:1202–1208.

96   Guex-Crosier Y, Raber J, Chan CC, Kriete MS, Benichou J, Pilson RS, Kerwin JA, Waldmann TA,
      Hakimi J, Roberge FG: Humanized antibodies against the alpha-chain of the IL-2 receptor and
      against the beta-chain shared by the IL-2 and IL-15 receptors in a monkey uveitis model of
      autoimmune diseases. J Immunol 1997;158:452–458.

97   Li Q, Fujino Y, Caspi RR, Najafian F, Nussenblatt RB, Chan CC: Association between mast cells
      and the development of experimental autoimmune uveitis in different rat strains. Clin Immunol
      Immunopathol 1992;65:294–299.

98   Li Q, Peng B, Whitcup SM, Jang SU: Endotoxin-induced uveitis in the mouse: Susceptibility and
      genetic control. Exp Eye Res 1995;61:629–632.

99   Steptoe RJ, McMenamin PG, McMenamin CC: Choroidal mast cell dynamics during experimental
      autoimmune uveoretinitis in rat strains of differing susceptibility. Ocul Immunol Inflamm 1994;2:
      7–22.

100   Rao NA, Romero JL, Fernandez MA, Sevanian A, Marak GE Jr: Role of free radicals in uveitis.
      Surv Ophthalmol 1987;32:209–213.

101   Ishimoto S, Wu GS, Hayashi S, Zhang J: Free radical tissue damages in the anterior segment of
      the eye in experimental autoimmune uveitis. Invest Ophthalmol Vis Sci 1996;37:630–636.

102   Nakamura S, Yamakawa T, Sugita M, Kijima M, Ishioka M, Tanaka S: The role of tumor necrosis
      factor-alpha in the induction of experimental autoimmune uveoretinitis in mice. Invest Ophthalmol
      Vis Sci 1994;35:3884–3889.

103   McMenamin PG, Forrester JV: Dendritic Cells in the Central Nervous System and the Eye and
      Their Associated Supporting Tissues. San Diego, Academic Press, 1998.

104   D'Orazio TJ, Niederkorn JY: A novel role for TGF-beta and IL-10 in the induction of immune
      privilege. J Immunol 1998;160:2089–2098.

Immunopathogenic Mechanisms in Intraocular Inflammation   183

105 Ferguson TA, Fletcher S, Herndon J, Griffith TS: Neuropeptides modulate immune deviation induced via the anterior chamber of the eye. J Immunol 1995;155:1746–1756.

106 Li XY, D'Orazio LT, Niederkorn JY: Role of Th1 and Th2 cells in anterior chamber-associated immune deviation. Immunology 1996;89:34–40.

107 Wang Y, Goldschneider I, Foss D, Wu DY, O'Rourke J: Direct thymic involvement in anterior chamber-associated immune deviation: Evidence for a nondeletional mechanism of centrally induced tolerance to extrathymic antigens in adult mice. J Immunol 1997;158:2150–2155.

108 D'Orazio TJ, Niederkorn JY: The nature of antigen in the eye has a profound effect on the cytokine milieu and resultant immune response. Eur J Immunol 1998;28:1544–1553.

109 Griffith TS, Yu X, Herndon JM, Green DR, Ferguson TA: CD95-induced apoptosis of lymphocytes in an immune privileged site induces immunological tolerance. Immunity 1996;5:7–16.

110 Gao Y, Hendon JM, Zhang H, Griffiths TS, Ferguson TA: Anti-inflammatory effects of CD95 ligand (FasL)-induced apoptosis. J Exp Med 1998;188:887–896.

111 Jorgensen A, Wiencke AK, la Cour M, Kaestel CG, Madsen HO, Hamann S, Lui GM, Scherfig E, Prause JU, Svejgaard A, Odum N, Nissen MH, Ropke C: Human retinal pigment epithelial cell-induced apoptosis in activated T cells. Invest Ophthalmol Vis Sci 1998;39:1590–1599.

112 Forrester JV, Lumsden L, Liversidge J, Kuppner MM: Immunoregulation of uveoretinal inflammation. Prog Retinal Eye Res 1995;14:393–412.

113 Kuppner MC, McKillop-Smith S, Forrester JV: Transforming growth factor-β and IL-1 act in synergy to enhance IL-6 and IL-8 mRNA levels and IL-6 production by human retinal pigment epithelial cells. Immunology 1995;84:265–271.

114 Crane IJ, Kuppner MC, McKillop-Smith S, Wallace CA, Forrester JV: Production of granulocyte-macrophage colony-stimulating factor by human retinal pigment epithelial cells. Clin Exp Immunol 1998;115:288–293.

115 Mason D, Powrie F: Control of immune pathology by regulatory T cells. Curr Opin Immunol 1998;10:649–655.

116 Weiner HL: Oral tolerance: Immune mechanisms and treatment of autoimmune diseases. Immunol Today 1997;18:335–343.

117 Nussenblatt RB, Caspi RR, Mahdi R, Chan CC, Roberge F, Lider O, Weiner HL: Inhibition of S-antigen induced experimental autoimmune uveoretinitis by oral induction of tolerance with S-antigen. J Immunol 1990;144:1689–1695.

118 McMenamin C, Pimm C, McKersey M, Holt PG: Regulation of IgE responses to inhaled antigen in mice by antigen-specific gamma delta T cells. Science 1994;265:1869–1871.

119 Seymour BW, Gershwin LJ, Coffman RL: Aerosol-induced immunoglobulin E unresponsiveness to ovalbumin does not require CD8 + or T cell receptor-gamma/delta + T cells or interferon-gamma in a murine model of allergen. J Exp Med 1998;187:721–723.

120 Chen Y, Inobe J, Marks R, Gonnella P, Kuchroo VK, Weiner H: Peripheral deletion of antigen-reactive T cells in oral tolerance. Nature 1995;376:177–180.

121 Thierfelder S, Mocikat R, Mysliwietz J, Lindhofer H, Kremmer E: Immunosuppression by Fc region-mismatched anti-T cell antibody treatment. Eur J Immunol 1995;25:2242–2246.

122 Ballow M: Mechanisms of action of intravenous immune serum globulin in autoimmune and inflammatory diseases. J Allergy Clin Immunol 1997;100:151–157.

123 Stangel M, Hartung HP, Marx P, Gold R: Intravenous immunoglobulin treatment of neurological autoimmune diseases. J Neurol Sci 1998;153:203–214.

124 Van Noort JM, Amor S: Cell biology of autoimmune diseases. Int Rev Cytol 1998;178:127–206.

125 Boisgerault F, Khalil I, Tieng V, Connan F, Tabary T, Cohen JH, Choppin J, Charron D: Definition of the HLA-A29 peptide ligand motif allows prediction of potential T-cell epitopes from the retinal soluble antigen, a candidate autoantigen in birdshot retinopathy. Proc Natl Acad Sci USA 1996;93:3466–3470.

126 Shindo Y, Ohno S, Usui M, Ideta H, Harada K, Masuda H, Inoko H: Immunogenetic study of sympathetic ophthalmia. Tissue Antigens 1997;49:111–115.

127 Shindo Y, Inoko H, Yamamoto T, Ohno S: HLA-DRB1 typing of Vogt-Koyanagi-Harada's disease by PCR-RFLP and the strong association with DRB1*0405 and DRB1*0410. Br J Ophthalmol 1994;78:223–226.

128 Butterfield RJ, Sudweeks JD, Blankenhorn EP, Korngold R, Marini JC, Todd JA, Roper RJ, Teuscher C: New genetic loci that control susceptibility and symptoms of experimental allergic encephalomyelitis in inbred mice. J Immunol 1998;161:1860–1867.

129 Caspi RR, Chan CC, Fujino Y, Oddo S, Najafian F, Bahmanyar S, Heremans H, Wilder RL, Wiggert B: Genetic factors in susceptibility and resistance to experimental autoimmune uveoretinitis. Curr Eye Res 1992;11(suppl):81–86.

130 Sun B, Rizzo LV, Sun SH, Chan CC, Wiggert B, Wilder RL, Caspi RR: Genetic susceptibility to experimental autoimmune uveitis involves more than a predisposition to generate a T helper-1-like or a T helper-2-like response. J Immunol 1997;159:1004–1011.

131 Vainiene M, Burrows GG, Ariail K, Robey I, Vandenbark AA, Offner H: Neonatal injection of Lewis rats with recombinant V beta 8.2 induces T cell but not B cell tolerance and increased severity of experimental autoimmune encephalomyelitis. J Neurosci Res 1996;45:475–486.

John V. Forrester, MD, Department of Ophthalmology, University of Aberdeen,
Medical School, Foresterhill, Aberdeen AB25 2ZD (UK)
Tel. +44 1224 681818, Fax +44 1224 685158, E-Mail j.forrester@abdn.ac.uk

Streilein JW (ed): Immune Response and the Eye.
Chem Immunol. Basel, Karger, 1999, vol 73, pp 186–206

....

Immunobiology and Immunopathology of Corneal Transplantation

J. Wayne Streilein

Schepens Eye Research Institute, Harvard Medical School, Boston, Mass., USA

History and Clinical Experience

Since the first orthotopic corneal allotransplantation was performed successfully in human beings at the turn of this century [1], this procedure has emerged as the most common form of solid tissue transplantation. At present, more than 50,000 corneal transplants are performed each year in the United States alone. Moreover, the success rate of corneal transplantation performed in human beings is very high [2, 3]. In uncomplicated cases, the 2-year survival rate for initial corneal allografts placed in avascular corneal beds is estimated to be more than 90%. There is good reason to believe that the unique molecular and cellular features of the cornea and anterior chamber of the eye – which in aggregate give rise to the phenomenon of immune privilege – are responsible for this success rate. However, the extraordinary success of primary corneal transplants tends to overshadow the considerably less satisfactory clinical experience when corneal transplants are placed in so-called 'high-risk' eyes [4–7]. In patients with vascularized corneas, with previously failed corneal grafts, or with glaucoma, corneal allografts experience a much lower rate of success. To place this information in perspective, the results of corneal transplantation in high-risk recipient eyes are actually worse than first allografts of kidney, heart, or liver. In the overwhelming number of cases, immune rejection is thought to be the proximate cause of corneal graft failure.

Experimental analysis of corneal allograft rejection in animal model systems dates to the pioneering efforts of Maumanee [8]. On the one hand, these investigators recognized that orthotopic corneal allografts were subject to the same rules of transplantation immunology as other solid tissue grafts, while on the other hand, they correctly perceived that corneal allografts suffered rejection less often, and less acutely than did orthotopic skin grafts. Following on Medawar's formulation of the phenomenon of immune privilege [9], Maumanee and his collaborators ascribed the high success rate of orthotopic corneal allografts in rabbits to immune privilege. But the role of immune privilege remained of questionable importance, since in succeeding years, various investigators, especially Silverstein and Khoudadoust [10, 11], demonstrated that corneal tissues express transplantation antigens, that recipients of both heterotopic and orthotopic corneal grafts make identifiable immune responses to these antigens, and that immunity directed at corneal antigens can lead to graft rejection. As this field entered the 1970s, the cornea as a transplant offered a paradox. On the one hand, the cornea as a graft appeared to experience immune privilege when placed orthotopically, while, on the other hand, graft failure typically resulted from immune-mediated rejection. Since immune privilege was considered to be a static state, the field of investigators segregated into two camps: one camp focused on corneal graft failure and declaimed the existence and importance of immune privilege, considering cornea grafts to be similar to any other type of solid tissue graft; the other camp focused on graft success and championed the importance of immune privilege. Now that it is generally accepted that immune privilege is a dynamic, rather than a static, state [12–18], it is possible to explain – in the context of a single paradigm – a high rate of graft acceptance of orthotopic corneal allografts in so-called low-risk eyes, and the high rate of graft rejection in high-risk eyes.

Two important facts have been learned which have transformed our understanding of why penetrating keratoplasties fail and why they succeed. *First*, we now know that the quality of the recipient bed plays an important role in dictating graft outcome. The concept of 'high-risk' eyes – in which penetrating keratoplasties have a high risk of succumbing to immune rejection – has been embraced by both clinicians and laboratory scientists [19–22]. This concept relates directly to the phenomenon of immune privileged sites, since certain types of 'high-risk' eyes (those with neovascularized and inflamed corneas, or those that have previously experienced a rejection) no longer function as immune privileged sites [23, 24]. Only within the past few years have animal models with 'high-risk' ocular graft beds been used extensively. As a consequence, information is now being gathered that is particularly relevant to the clinical situation, since corneal graft rejection in humans is highly correlated with 'high-risk' eyes. *Second*, unique features of corneal tissues confer upon the corneal graft the properties responsible for 'immune privilege'. Numerous studies have demonstrated that the deficit of antigen presenting cells (APC) in the normal cornea is a critical component of corneal immune privilege [25–28]. Experimental manipulations that cause Langerhans' cells to migrate into corneal epithelium render cornea grafts highly vulnerable to rejection. Moreover, the recent discovery of constitutive expression of Fas ligand (CD95L) on corneal cells [29–31] has led to the conclusion that corneal grafts can protect themselves from immune rejection by expressing a molecule that triggers apoptosis among attacking CD95 + effector cells. These two examples emphasize that the cornea graft itself is immune privileged.

Since 1-year survival rates of keratoplasties in human beings approaches 90% in the virtual absence of systemic immunosuppression, it is small wonder that HLA matching has been found to influence graft outcome very little [32–36]. However, even in high-risk eyes, where local immune privilege is compromised, and where the rate of graft rejection is much higher (35–65%), it has been difficult (some studies) or impossible (other studies) to demonstrate a significant effect of matching donor and recipient for either HLA class I or class II antigens on graft outcome [37]. In fact, two studies have even suggested that grafts that share one HLA class II antigen in common suffer a higher rate of rejection in high-risk eyes [38, 39]. Recent studies in laboratory animals have given insight into this curious aspect of human cornea grafting, and the insight relates, on the one hand, to reduced expression of MHC-encoded molecules on corneal parenchymal cells [40, 41], and, on the other hand, to the absence of APC (passenger leukocytes) [25] in the normal cornea as a graft (see below).

Another remarkable difference between orthotopic corneal grafts in human beings and other solid tissue allografts is the lack of need for systemic immunosuppressive therapy. In low-risk eyes, systemic immunosuppressive therapy is almost never necessary to reverse a rejection reaction within a cornea graft. By contrast, systemic immunosuppression is de riguer for allografts of heart, liver, skin, kidney, etc. Even in high-risk eyes, intensive local immuno-suppressive therapy, sometimes involving subconjunctival injection of drugs, usually succeeds in reigning in a progressive rejection reaction. Another way of considering these same sets of results is that when a corneal graft suffers a severe rejection reaction that cannot be controlled locally, systemic therapy is often of no avail – in part because of the hesitancy of the ophthalmologist to recommend a therapy that may threaten life for a condition that (merely) threatens sight.

Orthotopic Corneal Allografts in Laboratory Animals

As mentioned previously, the first important studies of the pathogenesis of corneal graft rejection were conducted in rabbits. While much was gained from these studies, lack of genetically defined strains combined with a very limited repertoire of immune reagents made it difficult to study the mechanisms of graft rejection in a contemporary manner. A significant advance came when Williams and Coster [42] developed a model for orthotopic corneal transplantation in laboratory rats in the mid-1980s, and the situation further improved within a decade when She et al. [43] described a method of cornea transplantation in mice.

Fate of Orthotopic Corneal Allografts in Normal and High-Risk Situations

From the many studies that have been performed in the last decade and a half on the fate of orthotopic corneal allografts in rats and mice, a short summary of generally accepted results can be devised [44, 45]: (a) In uncomplicated, normal recipient eyes, a significant proportion of allogeneic cornea grafts are accepted without evidence of the acute rejection (within 7–14 days) that is observed with other orthotopic solid organ grafts; a high proportion of allogeneic cornea grafts survive indefinitely without evidence of rejection reactions and without the aid of local or systemic immunosuppressive therapy; and grafts that confront their recipients with only MHC-encoded alloantigens succeed more often than grafts that confront their recipients with minor histocompatibility antigens alone [46–49]. (b) In experimentally induced high-risk eyes, acute, irreversible graft rejection is common (within 7–14 days); a much lower proportion of allogeneic cornea grafts survive beyond the acute postgraft interval, and very few of these grafts survive indefinitely; grafts that express minor histocompatibility antigens alone fare more poorly than grafts that only express MHC-encoded disparate antigens.

The general conclusions drawn from these studies are that: (a) the normal eye is an immune privileged site for orthotopic corneal allografts, and that privilege is compromised when the eye is high-risk; (b) long-term graft acceptance is limited to eyes that display immune privilege, and (c) minor histocompatibility antigens, rather than MHC-encoded antigens, are the more important barriers to corneal allograft acceptance.

In human beings, keratoplasties are frequently performed in patients that may have been sensitized previously to transplantation antigens on the graft. In fact, such patients are regarded as 'high-risk'. When rats and mice are preimmunized to transplantation antigens that are expressed on subsequent orthotopic corneal allografts, the incidence and rate of rejection is considerably enhanced [47, 50]. These findings were derived from experiments in which the recipient eyes were normal, i.e. not high-risk. As such, the results confirm that rejection caused by specific immune factors can occur within the eye, and that this vulnerability exists even when the eye is ostensibly 'immune privileged'.

Experimental Manipulations Designed to Alter the Fate of Orthotopic Corneal Allografts

While the precise immune effectors responsible for rejection of orthotopic corneal allografts remain unclear (see below), T lymphocytes are thought to play a dominant role. Corneal allografts placed in eyes of severe combined immune-deficient mice survive indefinitely, irrespective of the degree of immunogenetic disparity. This indicates that cells of the adaptive immune system are essential to the rejection process. Several studies have explored the possible role of donor-specific antibodies, and the current view is that antibodies play no role in rejection of cornea grafts [51–53]. To gain more insight into the T cells responsible for cornea rejection, recipients of orthotopic corneal allografts have been treated systemically, and even locally, with monoclonal antibodies directed at molecules expressed on T cells and/or APC [54–56]. The results indicate that rejection is impaired with antibodies directed at CD4, but not CD8, and that anti-ICAM-1 antibodies interfere with graft rejection, but anti-LFA-1 has little effect. These results have pointed to the CD4+ T cell as the key player in instigating acute rejection of cornea grafts. In a similar vein, transgenic mice with genes disrupted by homologous recombination have helped refine our understanding of the mediators of cornea graft rejection. Graft rejection occurs without impediment in mice lacking the Ig μ chain gene (these mice are deficient in both B cells and antibodies) [53]. Similarly, mice lacking the third component of complement reject grafts in a conventional fashion [53]. Finally, Van der Veen et al. [57] have inhibited corneal graft rejection by injection of toxic liposomes into the subconjunctival space. These liposomes selectively kill activated, phagocytic macrophages, implying that these cells participate in graft rejection. Since macrophages are typically recruited and activated by CD4+ T cells of the Th1 type, the current view is that T cells – especially the cells that are CD4+ and secrete proinflammatory cytokines such as IFN-γ and TNF-α – govern the cornea graft rejection process.

Features of the Cornea Important to Its Success as an Allograft

Billingham and Boswell [58] first reported almost 40 years ago that the cornea is an immune privileged tissue. By calling the cornea an immune privileged tissue, they called attention to the fact that certain tissues of the body inherently resist immune rejection, the cornea being one of them. By now, investigators have accumulated a large body of experimental data attesting to this fact. First, as mentioned above, expression of MHC class I and class II molecules is reduced and impaired on the parenchymal cells of the cornea, especially on the corneal endothelium [59–61]. The net antigenic load of corneal tissue is thus reduced compared to other tissues, which has a mitigating effect on both induction and expression of alloimmunity. Second, the cornea lacks blood and lymph vessels. The absence of these vascular structures isolates the cornea graft from the immune system in a manner that inhibits antigenic information from escaping from the tissue while at the same time inhibiting blood-borne immune effectors from gaining access to the tissue. Third, the cornea is deficient in bone marrow-derived cells, especially Langerhans' cells [25]. Mobile cells of this type are present in all other solid tissues where, in grafts, they are referred to as 'passenger leukocytes' [62–64]. Passenger leukocytes are one important way in which antigenic information from a solid tissue graft alerts cells of the immune system in regional lymph nodes to its presence. The absence of APC from the cornea dramatically lengthens the time it takes for the recipient immune system to become aware of the graft's existence. Fourth, cells of the cornea constitutively secrete molecules with immunosuppressive properties [65–69]. Cells of all three corneal layers secrete TGF-β, as well as yet-to-be-defined inhibitory molecules. In addition, corneal epithelial cells and keratocytes constitutively produce an excess of IL-1 receptor antagonist, compared to the endogenous production of IL-1α [70]. These immunosuppressive molecules have powerful modulatory effects on APC, T cells, B cells, NK cells and macrophages, and can act during induction and expression of alloimmunity to prevent or inhibit graft rejection. Fifth, cells of the cornea constitutively express surface molecules that inhibit immune effectors. Corneal endothelial cells display on their surface DAF, CD59 and CD46 – molecules that inhibit complement effector functions [71]. These inhibitors protect corneal endothelial cells from injury by complement molecules generated during an alloimmune response. Recently, corneal cells have been found to express CD95L (Fas ligand), and expression of this molecule on mouse cornea grafts has been formally implicated in protecting the grafts from attack by CD95 + T cells and other leukocytes [29, 30]. Finally, the cornea graft forms the anterior surface of the anterior chamber; antigens released from the graft endothelium escape into aqueous humor. Antigen presented to the systemic immune system in this manner induces a stereotypic, deviant immune response that is selectively deficient in delayed hypersensitivity and complement fixing antibodies [72, 73]. Experimental evidence indicates that allogeneic cornea grafts induce donor-specific ACAID in recipients [74, 75], and the inability of these recipients to acquire donor-specific delayed hypersensitivity plays a key role in maintaining the integrity of accepted grafts.

The unusual expression of MHC-encoded molecules on corneal cells is worthy of special comment. Class I MHC antigens are expressed strongly on the epithelial cells of the cornea, comparable in intensity to their expression on epidermal cells of skin. Keratocytes express less class I than conventional fibroblasts, and corneal endothelial cells express only small amounts of class I antigens under normal circumstances. Except at the periphery near the limbus, the cornea contains no 'adventitial cells', i.e. cells of bone marrow origin [25]. Therefore, under normal conditions, the burden of class II MHC antigens expressed by corneal grafts is minimal. Corneal epithelial and endothelial cells resemble other cells of the body in responding to IFN-γ by upregulation of class I antigen expression. Among IFN-γ-treated epithelial cells, class II antigens are also expressed. However, corneal endothelial cells resist expression of class II antigens [76–78]. Since class II antigens, especially those expressed on bone marrow-derived cells, are extremely important in providing solid tissue grafts with their ability to evoke transplantation immunity, the deficit of these antigens on corneal cells offers a significant barrier to sensitization.

The unusual tissue expression of MHC-encoded molecules may help to explain the confusion surrounding the effects (or lack thereof) of HLA matching on corneal allograft success. As mentioned above, minor transplantation antigens offer the more significant barrier to graft success in rodents [46–49, 79]. Two factors seem to be important in this outcome. First, the reduced expression of MHC antigens on corneal grafts renders these grafts less immunogenic than other solid tissue grafts. Second, corneal antigens are only detected by the recipient immune system when the recipient's own APC infiltrate the graft and capture donor antigens. Graft cells are, of course, the source of donor antigens that lead to alloimmune sensitization. Apparently in the cornea, minor transplantation antigens are quantitatively more numerous than MHC antigens. Therefore, the recipient mounts an immune response directed primarily at minor transplantation antigens. Since tissue typing is unable at present to match organs and donors for minor histocompatibility antigens, it is no surprise that current tissue typing has proven ineffectual at improving corneal allograft success.

Unusual expression of MHC-encoded antigens by corneal cells, combined with the absence of indigenous passemger leukocytes, also helps to explain the transcendent importance of minor, as opposed to MHC, alloantigens in corneal allograft immunity. These two features of the cornea relate to the relative roles that two different sets of alloreactive T cells play in rejection of solid tissue grafts [80–82]. One set, called *indirect alloreactive T cells*, recognizes peptides derived from alloantigenic proteins expressed on graft parenchymal cells. These proteins are taken up by infiltrating APC, cleaved into peptides, loaded onto class I and II molecules, and expressed on the cell surface. If the APC are of recipient origin, responding T cells recognize donor-derived peptides in association with self-MHC molecules. Other T cells, called *direct alloreactive T cells*, recognize allogeneic MHC class I and II molecules directly. T cells of the direct type are the cells that proliferate in the conventional mixed lymphocyte reaction.

For most solid tissue grafts (e.g. kidney, heart, skin), acute rejection is triggered by T cells that recognize donor class I and II MHC molecules directly. As mentioned above, most solid tissue grafts contain a population of bone marrow-derived cells (dendritic cells, macrophages) that constitutively express high levels of both class I and II MHC molecules. These passenger leukocytes are primarily responsible for sensitization of direct alloreactive T cells. Sensitization occurs when passenger leukocytes migrate out of the graft, through lymphatics, to the draining lymph node. At this site, naive direct alloreactive T cells are activated, differentiate into effectors, and then return to the graft and destroy it. Grafts rendered deficient experimentally of passenger leukocytes fail to activate 'direct' alloreactive T cells, and acute rejection is not observed. The normal cornea is, in a sense, an 'experiment of nature' in which passenger leukocytes are excluded. The findings described above, in which minor H-incompatible cornea grafts suffer more rejection that MHC-incompatible grafts, are explained by the paucity of MHC expression on corneal cells, combined with the absence of passenger leukocytes from the normal cornea. These findings help us further to understand why in humans HLA matching of donor and host in corneal transplantation has not been found to be particularly useful.

Very recently, our laboratory has explored directly the issue of immune privilege of corneal tissue by implanting allogeneic cornea beneath the kidney capsule. This site has been used traditionally by transplantation immunologists as a suitable nonprivileged, heterotopic site for the study of solid tissue allografts. Hori and Streilein [83, and under review] have found that allogeneic cornea tissue, from which the epithelium had been removed, survived beneath the kidney capsule indefinitely, without evidence of rejection. The grafts appeared clear when inspected grossly, were devoid of inflammation and neovascularization, and when examined immunohistochemically donor-derived endothelial cells were detected as late as 8 weeks after implantation. However, similar allografts prepared from mice lacking the ability to express CD95 ligand suffered acute rejection beneath the kidney capsule. These findings strengthen the idea that corneal tissues possesses inherent immune privilege, and they confirm that CD95L expression on corneal cells makes an important contribution to the privileged status.

Mechanisms of Rejection of Orthotopic Corneal Allografts

The simple fact that in experimental animals some orthotopic corneal allografts fail, whereas virtually no syngeneic grafts fail, reflects the powerful role of immunity against antigens expressed on the graft in causing rejection. However, the precise cellular and molecular mechanisms that mediate rejection are only incompletely understood. Part of the confusion regarding rejection mechanisms derives from the fact that orthotopic corneal allografts can suffer different forms of rejection in rodents. In a manner similar to other solid tissue grafts, cornea allografts can experience acute rejection (arbitrarily defined as between 7 and 14 days postgrafting), subacute rejection (arbitrarily defined as between 14 and 56 days), and chronic rejection (arbitrarily defined as rejection beyond 56 days). However, cornea grafts differ from other types of solid tissue grafts in that they do not appear to suffer from hyperacute rejection (arbitrarily defined as rejection within hours to a few days of engraftment). Different immunopathogenic mechanisms are known to participate in acute, subacute, and chronic rejection of solid tissue allografts, but in these circumstances complete understanding and agreement about effector mechanisms has not been reached. In general, so-called acute rejection of cornea grafts occurs primarily in the setting of high-risk eyes, whereas subacute rejection is typical of rejection in normal eyes.

Several laboratories, including ours, have examined recipients of orthotopic corneal allografts for evidence of donor antigen-specific delayed hypersensitivity, cytotoxic T cells, and antibodies. Whereas antibodies have often not been found when allogeneic cornea is grafted into normal eyes, delayed hypersensitivity is routinely found [84]. In our experience, cornea allografts placed in normal eyes generate donor-specific delayed hypersensitivity within 4 weeks, and this reactivity is directed almost exclusively at minor histocompatibility antigens. When grafts are placed in high-risk eyes, then delayed hypersensitivity to both major and minor H antigens is detected. These findings, in consort with the effectiveness of anti-CD4 antibodies in suppressing graft rejection, argue strongly for a central role in graft rejection of CD4+ T cells that mediate delayed hypersensitivity (i.e. Th1). Confirmatory evidence comes from experiments in which cornea graft rejection proceeds normally in mice that are deficient in (a) MHC class I expression (β_2-microglobulin knockout), or (b) CD4 expression (CD4 KO) [Yamada and Streilein, under review]. Supportive data also comes from experiments in which mice with immune systems heavily biased toward Th2 responses received orthotopic corneal allografts. In Th2-biased mice, minor H-incompatible corneal grafts placed in high-risk eyes experienced significantly enhanced survival [85].

With all of this evidence in favor of a central role for CD4+ Th1 cells in rejection of corneal allografts, sight cannot be lost of the potential importance of CD8 + cytotoxic T cells (Tc). The findings that graft rejection proceeds conventionally in mice genetically incapable of generating cytotoxic Tc, and that anti-CD8 antibodies have little influence on graft outcome cannot force the conclusion that CD8 + Tc are irrelevant to graft outcome. We, and others, have reported that donor-specific Tc are generated when mice receive ortho-topic corneal allografts [86, 87]. In our experience, virtually all of the donor-specific Tc are self-restricted, meaning that they have detected donor-derived antigens processed by recipient APC – the indirect pathway of allorecognition. Based on relative expression of MHC and minor H antigens on corneal tissue, it comes as no surprise that the vast majority of the Tc are directed at donor minor H antigens. However, *direct* alloreactive Tc are generated in certain circumstances. Recipients of allografts in high-risk eyes regularly develop direct Tc, and C57BL/6 recipients of BALB/c corneas (MHC disparate) also display activated direct Tc [Yamada et al., in prep.]. Detection of these types of cells may help us understand the pathogenesis of cornea graft rejection. Only direct alloreactive Tc can recognize the parenchymal cells of the cornea graft. Indirect alloreactive Tc, by definition, cannot recognize donor antigens on corneal parenchymal cells because the wrong MHC class I molecules are expressed. In the instance where donor and recipient share one class I MHC antigen, indirect alloreactive Tc are able to bind to corneal cells directly. This would argue, then, that cornea grafts which share an HLA, A, B or C specificity with their recipient should be more, not less, vulnerable to immune rejection.

What is particularly difficult to understand is how corneal allografts are rejected in the setting where donor and recipient are completely mismatched at the MHC, and where only indirect alloreactive Tc are generated. The only 'targets' that could be present within the graft are recipient-derived cells that migrate in, and then process and present donor antigens. It is hard to imagine how recipient APC – which are relatively low in number – presenting donor antigen within a cornea allograft can serve as sufficient targets of Tc to cause graft rejection. It is for this reason that most investigators currently believe that CD4 + Tc mediate graft rejection, since these cells – also indirectly allore-active – can respond to donor antigens presented on recipient APC within the graft and secrete proinflammatory cytokines that cause destructive delayed hypersensitivity, and 'innocent bystander injury' to corneal parenchymal cells.

The previous discussion concerns the immunopathogenesis of graft failure of the acute and subacute types. Almost nothing is known about mechanisms responsible for chronic rejection, or perhaps more particularly, graft rejection that is extremely delayed. Such rejections are very uncommon in laboratory animals, but more common in human beings. We have recently observed [Yamada et al., under review] that CD4 knockout mice, which do not reject corneal allografts within 8 weeks, eventually destroy their orthotopic grafts –

sometimes as late as 10–16 weeks postgrafting. Since these mice contain neither CD4+ Tc, nor activated donor-specific Tc, the mechanism of graft failure is obscure.

Mechanisms of Sensitization of Recipients of Orthotopic Corneal Allografts

Although much remains to be learned about the effector mechanisms responsible for acute and subacute graft rejection, considerably more has been learned about the means by which orthotopic corneal allografts sensitize their recipients. It is generally believed that solid tissue grafts sensitize their recipients when antigens of graft origin are delivered via lymphatic to draining lymph nodes. Moreover, passenger leukocytes [62–64] within the grafts are thought to be the primary immunogens for three reasons: (a) these cells express the full range of MHC class I and II molecules, plus minor H antigens, of the donor; (b) passenger cells are mobile, which enables them to carry their burden of antigens to the draining lymph node, and (c) passenger cells express costimulation molecules that are necessary for initial activation of naive T cells. However, the normal cornea lacks such cells, and recent evidence indicates that sensitization to donor antigens awaits the migration of recipient Langerhans' cells into the graft from the limbus [88]. Several lines of evidence point to this conclusion. First, the rate of Langerhans' cell migration into corneal allografts in low- and high-risk graft beds has been assessed [Sano et al., in prep.]. Langerhans' cells move into grafts in high-risk beds much faster than into grafts in low-risk beds. Onset of donor-specific delayed hypersensitivity correlates temporally with Langerhans' cells migration, i.e. systemic donor-specific delayed hypersensitivity is detected much earlier when grafts are placed in high-risk beds. In addition, Langerhans' cell migration into cornea grafts is inhibited by topical application of soluble IL-1 receptor antagonist (IL-1ra), and topical treatment with this agent not only inhibits the onset of donor-specific delayed hypersensitivity, but reduces the incidence and frequency of graft failure [89–91]. Finally, the strongest evidence for a role for Langerhans' cells comes from experiments where donor grafts have been manipulated to contain Langerhans' cells in the corneal epithelium at the time of grafting [Sano et al., in prep.]. In this instance, recipient sensitization to donor antigen is very swift, and graft rejection occurs acutely. Thus, orthotopic corneal allografts sensitize their recipients when the grafts become infiltrated with recipient APC. The donor-reactive T cells that are activated by this process are exclusively of the 'indirect' alloreactive type. Not surprisingly, when the cornea graft already contains Langerhans' cells at the time of grafting, 'direct' alloreactive T cells are also activated. Williams et al. [28] first called attention to this potential role of bone marrow-derived cells by demonstrating that human cornea grafts were more likely to be rejected if the donor rim contained Langerhans' cells at the time the graft was removed.

What has not been formally demonstrated is the pathway by which Langerhans' cells within cornea grafts induce systemic sensitization within recipients. While it would be simple to suggest that the cells merely migrate centrifugally to the limbus, then enter lymphatic channels and are carried to the cervical lymph nodes, no such path has been documented experimentally. Rather, the flow of epithelium of the corneal surface is centripetal, rather than centrifugal. Since Langerhans' cells in the corneal epithelium rob the eye of immune privilege and the capacity to support ACAID induction, the possibility exists that Langerhans' cells may escape from the donor cornea by an unconventional route, e.g. into the anterior chamber and out the trabecular meshwork.

It is important to point out that the constitutive expression of CD95L on corneal cells, which has been presumed to promote allograft acceptance by deleting T cells that encounter the cells of the graft, has no discernible impact on the T-cell repertoire of the recipient immune apparatus. That is to say, the peripheral T cells of mice bearing healthy orthotopic corneal allografts retain their capacity to respond to donor antigens in mixed lymphocytes reactions and in cell-mediated cytotoxicity reactions. Thus, widespread deletion of clones of T cells reactive with donor antigens does not take place systemically. Eventually, however, mice with long-standing, healthy corneal allografts acquire donor-specific ACAID [74, 75, 91]. Attempts to immunize these recipients with donor antigens fails to result in the development of delayed hypersensitivity. Since ACAID does not emerge in animals that reject their orthotopic corneal allografts, this evidence suggests that ACAID may have a role to play in the long-term mainenance of successful allografts.

Before leaving this discussion of the capacity of orthotopic corneal allografts to sensitize their recipients, two related lines of experimental evidence need to be mentioned. First, allogeneic corneas have been grafted heterotopically to the body wall, subcutaneously, and (most recently) beneath the kidney capsule. Corneas grafted to the skin and subcutaneous tissue are profoundly immunogenic to their recipients, leading not only to prompt rejection, but to the induction of cytotoxic T cells. However, only when the grafts contain Langerhans' cells do the recipients respond by generating donor-specific delayed hypersensitivity. Thus, Langerhans' cells appear to be crucial to the multicellular process by which the T cells that mediate delayed hypersensitivity are activated following implantation of cornea grafts in the skin [92]. A different situation appears to unfold when cornea grafts are placed beneath the kidney capsule. As mentioned above, corneal allografts placed beneath the kidney capsule survived indefinitely, and failed to induce donor-specific delayed hyper-sensitivity. This is true, however, only when the cornea used for grafting has been stripped of its epithelial layer. Cornea allografts that include the epithelium which are placed beneath the kidney capsule induce donor-specific delayed hypersensitivity [83]. The evidence suggests that corneal epithelium may have a selective property of promoting reactivity of the delayed hypersensitivity type. But the corneal epithelium is not the only component of the cornea relevant to induction of delayed hypersensitivity when the tissue is placed beneath the kidney capsule. Hori and Streilein [83] have discovered that epithelium-deprived corneal allografts that lack expression of CD95L (from *gld* mice) are rejected within 2 weeks when placed beneath the kidney capsule, and such grafts induce readily detectable, donor-specific delayed hypersensitivity. Thus, constitutive expression of CD95L by corneal endothelium and keratocytes serves to prevent the recipient from acquiring this form of cell-mediated immunity, presumably by deleting alloreactive T cells that express CD95.

Second, fragments of allogeneic cornea have been implanted into the anterior chamber of the eye [75, Sonoda et al., under review]. Such fragments – with or without an epithelial layer – survive indefinitely without any evidence of inflammation or rejection. However, fragments with epithelium intact induce systemic delayed hypersensitivity, albeit transiently, whereas epithelium-deprived fragments never induce delayed hypersensitivity. Once again, there is a linkage between the presence of an allogeneic epithelium, and the induction of delayed hypersensitivity. But we are unable to explain the basis for that link.

Opportunities for Enhancing Corneal Allograft Survival

It is a truism that a large majority of corneal allografts placed orthotopically in low-risk human eyes survive and provide sight for those with corneal blindness. It is also true that virtually all of these eyes are treated with local instillation of corticosteroids, and that episodes of rejection reaction are often reversed with increased doses of topical steroids. For grafts in high-risk eyes, more intensive topical steroid therapy is used, and for intractable graft rejection local injection of cyclosporin A is used. In the most severe cases of rejection, systemic treatment with large-dose steroids supplemented with cyclosporin are attempted. Throughout this ever-escalating therapeutic strategy, an ever-escalating set of complications accrue, ranging from ocular herpes infection to exacerbation of glaucoma. It is sobering to remember that the rate of rejection of corneas grafted into high-risk eyes exceeds the rate of rejection of kidney, heart and liver grafts. The need for more physiologic and less pharmacologic (and therefore less toxic) approaches to the prevention and treatment of immune rejection is readily apparent, and, in part, this need motivates many of the studies of orthotopic corneal grafting in animal models.

Because the last two decades have witnessed a resurgence of experimental interest in corneal transplantation, and because major advances in understanding of the pathogenesis of graft failure have been made, a relatively wide range of possible new treatment strategies has been advanced. Some of these strategies are not novel to the eye, and their logic derives from studies of transplantation immunology of other solid organ transplants. This large field of work is beyond the scope of this paper, and suitable reviews are available. Instead, this portion of the discussion will be directed to novel therapies that are predicated on unique features of the eye and the cornea as a transplantation site and graft.

Strategies Designed to Prevent the Induction of Alloimmunity by Orthotopic Corneal Allografts

An overwhelming amount of evidence points to the alloreactive CD4+ Th1 cell as the main mediator of acute and subacute rejection of corneal allografts. This cell, which preferentially secretes IL-2, IFN-γ and TNF-α, and mediates destructive delayed hypersensitivity reactions, is activated initially by professional APC that express high levels of class II MHC molecules. Based on the information presented above, the APC primarily responsible for activation of alloreactive Th1 cells in corneal allografts are recipient Langerhans' cells that have migrated into the cornea and captured and presented alloantigens from the parenchymal cells of the grafts in the context of recipient (self) class II molecules. The costimulatory molecules expressed by these APC force naive T cells to differentiate down the Th1 pathway. Three novel therapies have been tried experimentally to prevent the generation of these graft-destructive Th1 cells.

Strategy 1

The afferent limb of the reflex arc that leads to Th1 activation begins when recipient Langerhans' cells migrate from the limbus into the cornea graft. While the precise molecular details of this migratory process remain to be elucidated, there is considerable evidence that an important, initial player is IL-1 – presumably secreted by cells of the graft. Injection of IL-1 into the corneal stroma causes Langerhans' cells to stream into the central epithelium. Dana et al. [89, 91] and Yamada et al. [90] have completed an important series of studies examining the possibility that Langerhans' cell migration, and therefore activation of donor-specific alloreactive Th1 cells, can be suppressed by topical application of IL-1 receptor antagonist. The results of these experiments indicate that topical IL-1ra inhibits Langerhans' cell migration into allografts placed in both low- and high-risk mouse eyes. Moreover, this local therapy delays and even prevents the emergence of donor-specific, systemic delayed hypersensitivity. Finally, topical IL-1ra significantly delays the onset of rejection reactions in orthotopic corneal allografts, and enhances the rate of corneal allograft acceptance in low- and high-risk eyes.

Strategy 2

Activation of Th1 cells under normal circumstances reflects the costimulatory environment provided by APC. Chiefly, APC that secrete IL-12 and IL-1β, and express CD40 encourage responding T cells to become Th1, rather than Th2 cells. If the microenvironment surrounding initial activation of alloreactive T cells is altered to contain IL-4, IL-10 and other cytokines secreted by Th2 cells, responding alloreactive T cells are deflected down the Th2 pathway. Yamada et al. [85] have recently demonstrated that mice with systemic immune systems preemptively biased toward Th2 responses are more likely to accept orthotopic corneal allografts. Specifically, these investigators have found that immunizing normal mice with keyhole limpet hemocyanin (KLH) plus incomplete Freund's adjuvant generates a potent, systemic KLH-specific Th2 response. When corneal allografts are placed in high-risk eyes of mice pretreated with KLH in this manner, the incidence of rejection reactions is significantly delayed with many grafts suffering no evidence of immune injury. T cells removed from these mice respond in vitro to graft alloantigens by secreting typical Th2-like cytokines (IL-4, IL-10). More important, the same T cells, when adoptively transferred into naive syngeneic recipients, enable the recipients to accept corneal allografts genetically identical to the original corneal allograft.

Strategy 3

The orthotopic corneal allograft forms the anterior surface of the anterior chamber – an immune-privileged site. Antigens placed in the anterior chamber induce a deviant systemic immune response called ACAID. In ACAID, there is a selective suppression of T cells that mediate delayed hypersensitivity. Several years ago, Sonoda and Streilein [74] reported that long-standing, healthy corneal allografts induce donor-specific ACAID. However, in the setting of the orthotopic corneal graft, considerable time passes before ACAID emerges – at least 8 weeks. Therefore, while ACAID may promote long-term graft acceptance, the graft is unable to generate ACAID quickly enough to reduce its vulnerability to acute rejection. Altenatively, several laboratories have now demonstrated that preemptive induction of ACAID to graft antigens has a positive effect on graft survival. She et al. [93] first reported that injection of allogeneic lymphocytes into the anterior chamber of the eye induced ACAID. Okamoto et al. [94] then found that allogeneic APC, incubated in vitro with TGF-β-containing fluid, induced ACAID when injected intravenously into naive mice. More recently, several laboratories [95–97] have used this method to induce donor-specific ACAID in normal mice with high-risk eyes. When corneal allografts, genetically identical to the ACAID-inducing cells, were grafted into high-risk eyes, there was a significant increase in graft acceptance and longevity.

Niederkorn and coworkers [98] have taken a different approach to altering the ability of graft recipients to mount destructive alloimmune responses. These investigators have induced tolerance in mice by feeding the animals cells bearing alloantigens. Oral tolerance of this type is deficient in T cells that mediate delayed hypersensitivity. Grafts placed in eyes of mice rendered orally tolerant to donor antigens enjoyed an extremely high level of success. Holan et al. [99] have also demonstrated recently that induction of neonatal transplantation tolerance permits the long-term acceptance of corneal allografts in mice.

Strategies Designed to Prevent the Expression of Alloimmunity That Destroys Orthotopic Corneal Allografts

Of the therapeutic strategies described above, all except topical IL-1ra result in a deviant systemic immune response in which there is suppression of expression of donor-specific delayed hypersensitivity, as well as inhibition of induction of Th1-type cells. However, there are other novel strategies that selectively target the rejection reaction within the cornea graft itself. Niekerkorn and coworkers [54, 55] as well as Hori et al. [56] have demonstrated that systemic treatment of mice with anti-ICAM-1 antibodies and anti-CD4 antibodies suppress cornea graft rejection. In the case of Niederkorn group's experiments [54, 55], evidence was presented to indicate that the effect of the anti-ICAM-1 antibodies was exerted on the induction, rather than expression, of graft-specific alloimmunity. More recently, Pleyer et al. [100] have used topical anti-ICAM-1 and found that they could reduce the incidence and intensity of graft rejection. We might anticipate that topical treatment with other antibodies of interest will be advanced in the near future.

Many features of the cornea (thin, simple tissue with only three different cell types, no blood or lymph vessels) render it a highly suitable candidate as a graft for a gene therapeutic approach to preventing rejection [101]. Corneal cells normally express CD95L and secrete immunosuppressive factors – both of which have been implicated in the success of orthotopic allografts. It is possible to envision gene therapies that would cause overexpression of these molecules in cells of the grafts. In addition, transfection of corneal cells with genes encoding other proteins that promote graft success has also been envisioned – for example, by inserting a gene that prevents neovascularization or immigration of inflammatory cells. It is even possible that corneas can be genetically manipulated in a manner that limits or even prevents their ability to express strong transplantation antigens. Experiments of this type are currently underway, and it is too early to report results, except to say that corneas have been genetically manipulated, and the manipulated tissue expresses properties likely to promote graft acceptance.

Acknowledgments

Supported by USPHS grant EY.

References

1   Zirm E: Albrecht von Graefes Arch Ophthalmol 1906;64:580–593.
2   Brady SE, Rapuano CJ, Arentsen JJ, Cohen EJ, Laibson PR: Clinical indications for and procedures associated with penetrating keratoplasty. Am J Ophthalmol 1989;108:983–988.
3   Price FW, Whitson WE, Marks RG: Progression of visual acuity after penetrating keratoplasty. Ophthalmology 1991;98:1177–1185.
4   Smith RE, McDonald HR, Nesburn AB, Minckler DS: Penetrating keratoplasty: Changing indications. Arch Ophthalmol 1980;98:1947–1978.
5   Volker-Dieben HJM, Kok-van Alphen CC, Lansbergen Q, Persijn GG: Different influences on corneal graft survival in 539 transplants. Acta Ophthalmol 1982;60:190–202.
6   Wilson SE, Kaufman HE: Graft failure after penetrating keratoplasty. Surv Ophthal 1990;34: 325–356.
7   Mader TH, Stulting RD: The high-risk penetrating keratoplasty. Ophthalmol Clin North Am 1991; 4:411–426.
8   Maumanee AE: The influence of donor-recipient sensitization on corneal grafts. Am J Ophthalmol 1951;34:142–152.
9   Medawar P: Immunity to homologous grafted skin. III. The fate of skin homografts transplanted to the brain, to subcutaneous tissue, and to the anterior chamber of the eye. Br J Exp Pathol 1948; 29:58–69.
10   Khodadoust AA, Silverstein AM: Studies on the nature of the privilege enjoyed by corneal allografts. Invest Ophthalmol Vis Sci 1972;11:137–148.
11   Khoudadoust AA, Silverstein AM: Transplantation and rejection of the individual cell layers of the cornea. Invest Ophthal 1969;8:180–190.
12   Barker CF, Billingham RE: Immunologically privileged sites. Adv Immunol 1977;25:1–54.
13   Niederkorn JY, Peeler JS, Ross J, Callanan D: The immunogenic privilege of corneal allografts. Reg Immunol 1989;2:117–124.
14   Niederkorn JY: Immune privilege and immune regulation in the eye. Adv Immunol 1990;48:191–226.

15 Streilein JW: Immune privilege and the cornea; in Pleyer U, Hartmann C, Sterry W (eds): Proceedings of Symposium: Bullous Oculo-Muco-Cutaneous Disorders. Buren, Aeolus Press, 1997, pp 43–52.

16 Ksander BR, Streilein JW: Regulation of the immune response within privileged sites. Chem Immunol 1994;58:117–145.

17 Streilein JW: Unraveling immune privilege. Science 1995;270:1158–1159.

18 Streilein JW, Ksander BR, Taylor AW: Immune deviation in relation to ocular immune privilege. J Immunol 1997;158:3557–3560.

19 Volker-Dieben HJM: The effect of immunological and non-immunological factors on corneal graft survival. A single center study. Doc Ophthalmol 1982;57:1–153.

20 Volker-Dieben HJM, Kok-van Alphen CC, Lansbergen Q, Persijn GG: Different influences on corneal graft survival in 539 transplants. Acta Ophthalmol 1982;60:190–202.

21 Stark W, Stulting D, Maguire M, Streilein JW: The Collaborative Corneal Transplantation Studies (CCTS): Effectiveness of histocompatibility matching of donors and recipients in high risk corneal transplantation. Arch Ophthalmol 1992;110:1392–1403.

22 Maguire MG, Stark WJ, Gottsch JD, Stulting RD, Sugar A, Fink NE, Schwartz A: Risk factors for corneal graft failure and rejection in the Collaborative Corneal Transplantation Studies (CCTS). Ophthalmology 1994;101:1536–1547.

23 Streilein JW, Bradley D, Sano Y, Sonoda Y: Immunosuppressive properties of tissues obtained from eyes with experimentally manipulated corneas. Invest Ophthalmol Vis Sci 1996;37:413.

24 Sano Y, Ksander BR, Streilein JW: Fate of orthotopic corneal allografts in eyes that cannot support anterior chamber-associated immune deviation induction. Invest Ophthalmol Vis Sci 1995;36:2176–2185.

25 Streilein JW, Toews GB, Bergstresser PR: Corneal allografts fail to express Ia antigens. Nature 1979;282:325–327.

26 Gillette TE, Chandler JW, Greiner JW: Langerhans' cells of the coular surface. Ophthalmology 1982;89:700.

27 Rubsamen PE, McCulley J, Bergstresser PR: Streilein JW: On the Ia immunogenicity of mouse corneal allografts infiltrated with Langerhans' cells. Invest Ophthalmol Vis Sci 1984;25:513–518.

28 Williams K, Ash JK, Coster DJ: Histocompatibility antigen and passenger cell content of normal and diseased human cornea. Transplantation 1985;39:265–269.

29 Griffith TS, Brunner T, Fletcher SM, Green DR, Ferguson TA: Fas ligand-induced apoptosis as a mechanism of immune privilege. Science (Wash) 1995;270:1189–1192.

30 Stuart PM, Griffith TS, Usui N, Pepose J, Yu X, Ferguson TA: CD95 ligand (FasL)-induced apoptosis is necessary for corneal allograft survival. J Clin Invest 1997;99:396–402.

31 Yamagami S, Kawashima H, Tsuru T, Yamagami H, Kayagaki N, Yagita H, Gregerson DS: Role of Fas-Fas ligand interactions in the immunorejection of allogeneic mouse corneal transplants. Transplantation 1997;64:1107–1111.

32 Ehlers N, Ahrons S: Corneal transplantation and histocompatibility. Acta Ophthalmol 1971;49:513–527.

33 Allansmith MR, Fine M, Payne R: Histocompatibility typing and corneal transplantation. Trans Am Acad Ophthalmol Otolaryngol 1974;78:445–460.

34 Batchelor JR, Casey TA, Gibbs DC, Prasad SS, Lloyd DF, James A: HLA matching and corneal grafting. Lancet 1976;i:551–554.

35 Stark WJ, Taylor HR, Bias WB, Maumenee AE: Histocompatibility (HLA) antigens and keratoplasty. Am J Ophthalmol 1978;86:595–604.

36 Boisjoly HM, Roy R, Dube I, Laughrea PA, Michaud R, Douville P, Hebert J: HLA-A,B and DR matching in corneal transplantation. Ophthalmology 1982;93:1290–1297.

37 Vail A, Gore SM, Bradley BA, Easty DL, Rogers CA, Armitage WJ: Influence of donor and histocompatibility factors on corneal graft outcome. Transplantation 1994;58:1210–1216.

38 The Collaborative Corneal Transplantation Studies Research Group: The collaborative corneal transplantation studies (CCTS). Effectiveness of histocompatibility matching in high-risk corneal transplantation. Arch Ophthalmol 1992;110:1392.

39 Gore SM, Vail A, Bradley BA, Rogers CA, Easty DL, Armitage WJ: HLA-DR matching in corneal transplantation. Systemic review of published evidence. Transplantation 1995;60:1033–1039.

40   Wang HM, Kaplan HJ, Chan WC, Johnson M: The distribution and ontogeny of MHC antigens in murine ocular tissues. Invest Ophthalmol Vis Sci 1987;28:1383–1389.

41   Abi-Hanna D, Wakefield D, Watkins S: HLA antigens in ocular tissues. Transplantation 1998;45: 610–613.

42   Williams KA, Coster DJ: Penetrating corneal transplantation in the inbred rat: A new model. Invest Ophthalmol Vis Sci 1985;26:23–30.

43   She SH, Steahly LP, Moticka EJ: A method for performing full-thickness, orthotopic, penetrating keratoplasty in the mouse. Ophthalmic Surg 1990;21:7810–7817.

44   Katami M, Madden PW, White DJG, Watson PG, Kamada N: The extent of immunological privilege of orthotopic corneal grafts in the inbred rat. Transplantation 1989;48:371–376.

45   Callanan D, Peeler J, Niederkorn JY: Characteristics of rejection of orthotopic corneal allografts in the rat. Transplantation 1988;45:437–443.

46   Nicholls SM, Bradley BB, Easty DL: Effect of mismatches of major histocompatibility complex and minor antigens on corneal graft rejection. Invest Ophthalmol Vis Sci 1991;32:2729–2734.

47   Sonoda Y, Streilein JW: Orthotopic corneal transplantation in mice. Evidence that the immuno-genetic rules of rejection do not apply. Transplantation 1992;54:694–703.

48   Joo C, Pepose JC, Stuart PM: T cell mediated responses in a murine model of orthotopic corneal transplantation. Invest Ophthalmol Vis Sci 1995;36:1530–1540.

49   Sano Y, Ksander BR, Streilein JW: Murine orthotopic corneal transplantation in 'high-risk' eyes. Rejection is dictated primarily by weak rather than strong alloantigens. Invest Ophthalmol Vis Sci 1997;38:1130–1138.

50   Ross J, He YG, Niederkorn JY: Class I disparate corneal grafts enjoy afferent but not efferent blockade of the immune response. Curr Eye Res 1991;19:889–892.

51   Hutchinson IV, Alam Y, Ayliffe WR: The humoral response to an allograft. Eye 1995;9:155.

52   Hegde S, Hargrave S, Mellon J, Niederkorn JY: Antibody and cell mediated immune responses during rejection of a murine orthotopic corneal graft. Invest Ophthalmol Vis Sci 1998;39:S455.

53   Goslings WRO, Yamada J, Dana MR, Streilein JW, Prodeus AP, Carroll MC, Jager MJ: Corneal transplant survival in antibody – and complement-deficient mice. Invest Ophthalmol Vis Sci 1998; 40:250–256.

54   He YG, Ross J, Niederkorn JY: Promotion of murine orthotopic corneal allograft survival by systemic administration of anti-CD4 monoclonal antibody. Invest Ophthalmol Vis Sci 1991;32: 2723–2728.

55   He Y, Mellon J, Apte R, Niederkorn JY: Effect of LFA-1 and ICAM-2 antibody treatment on murine corneal allograft survival. Invest Ophthalmol Vis Sci 1994;35:3218–3225.

56   Hori J, Isobe M, Yamagami S, Mizuochi T, Truru T: Specific immunosuppression of corneal allograft rejection by combination of anti-VLA-4 and anti-LFA-1 monoclonal antibodies in mice. Exp Eye Res 1997;65:89–98.

57   Van der Veen G, Broersma L, Dijkstra CD, Van Rooijen N, Ran Rij G, Van der Gaag R: Prevention of corneal allograft rejection in rats treated with subconjunctival injections of liposomes containing dichloromethylene diphosphonate. Invest Ophthalmol Vis Sci 1994;35:3505–3561.

58   Billingham RE, Boswell T: Studies on the problem of corneal homografts. Proc R Soc Lond [B] 1953;141:392–406.

59   Treseler PA, Foulks GN, Sanfilippo F: The expression of HLA antigens by cells in the human cornea. Am J Ophthalmol 1984;98:763.

60   Whitsett CF, Stulting RD: The distribution of HLA antigens on human corneal tissue. Invest Ophthalmol Vis Sci 1984;25:519.

61   Wang HM, Kaplan HJ, Chan WC, Jonson M: The distribution and ontogeny of MHC antigens in murine ocular cells. Invest Ophthalmol Vis Sci 1987;28:1383–1389.

62   Steinmuller D: Immunization with skin isografts taken from tolerant mice. Science 1967;158:127–129.

63   Lafferty KJ, Prowse SJ, Simeonovic CJ, Warren HS: Immunobiology of tissue transplantation: A return to the passenger leukocyte concept. Annu Rev Immunol 1983;1:142–173.

64   Lechler RI, Batchelor JR: Restoration of immunogenicity to passenger cell-depleted kidney allografts by the addition of donor strain dendritic cells. J Exp Med 1982;155:31–41.

65   Khaw PT, Schultz GS, MacKay SL, Chegini N, Rotatori DS, Adams JL, Shimizu RW: Detection of transforming growth factor-alpha messenger RNA and protein in human corneal epithelial cells. Invest Ophthalmol Vis Sci 1992;33:3302–3306.

66   Donnelly JJ, Xi MS, Rockey JH: A soluble product of human corneal fibroblasts inhibits lymphocyte activation. Enhancement by interferon-gamma. Exp Eye Res 1993;56:157–165.

67   Kawashima H, Prasad SA, Gregerson DS: Corneal endothelial cells inhibit T cell proliferation by blocking IL-2 production. J Immunol 1994;153:1982–1989.

68   Streilein JW, Bradley D, Sano Y: Immunosuppressive properties of tissues of the ocular anterior segment. Ocul Immunol Inflamm 1996;4:57–68.

69   Jager MJ, Bradley D, Streilein JW: Immunosuppressive properties of cultured human cornea and ciliary body in normal and pathological conditions. Transplant Immunol 1995;2:135–142.

70   Kennedy MC, Rosenbaum JP, Brown J, Planck SR, Huang X, Armstrong CA, Ansel JC: Novel production of interleukin-1 receptor antagonist peptides in normal human cornea. J Clin Invest 1995;95:82–88.

71   Bora NS, Gobleman CL, Atkinson JP, Pepose JS, Kaplan HJ: Differential expression of the complement regulatory proteins in the human eye. Invest Ophthalmol Vis Sci 1993;34:3579–3584.

72   Streilein JW, Niederkorn JY, Shadduck JA: Systemic immune unresponsiveness induced in adult mice by anterior chamber presentation of minor histocompatibility antigens. J Exp Med 1980;152:1121–1125.

73   Streilein JW: Immune regulation and the eye: A dangerous compromise. FASEB J 1987;1:199–208.

74   Sonoda Y, Streilein JW: Impaired cell mediated immunity in mice bearing healthy orthotopic corneal allografts. J Immunol 1993;150:1727–1734.

75   Yamada J, Streilein JW: Induction of anterior chamber-associated immune deviation by corneal allografts placed in the anterior chamber. Invest Ophthalmol Vis Sci 1997;38:2833–2843.

76   Young D, Stark WJ, Prendergast RA: Immunology of corneal allograft rejection: HLA-DR antigens on human corneal cells. Invest Ophthalmol Vis Sci 1985;26:571–574.

77   Gebhardt BM: The role of class II antigen-expressing cells in corneal allograft immunity. Invest Ophthalmol Vis Sci 1990;31:2254–2260.

78   Donnelly JJ, Li W, Rockey JH, Prendergast RA: Induction of class II (Ia) alloantigen expression on corneal endothelium in vivo and in vitro. Invest Ophthalmol Vis Sci 1985;26:575–580.

79   Sano Y, Ksander BR, Streilein JW: Minor H, rather than MHC, alloantigens offer the greater barrier to successful orthotopic corneal transplantation in mice. Transplant Immunol 1996;4:53.

80   Liu L, Sun YK, Xi YP, Maffei A, Reed A, Harries P, Suciu-Foca N: Contribution of direct and indirect recognition pathways to T cell alloreactivity. J Exp Med 1993;177:1643–1650.

81   Lee RS, Grusby MJ, Glimcher LH, Winn HJ, Auchincloss H: Indirect recognition by helper cells can induce donor-specific cytotoxic T lymphocytes in vivo. J Exp Med 1994;179:865–872.

82   Shoskes DA, Wood KJ: Indirect presentation of MHC antigens in transplantation. Immunol Today 1994;15:32–38.

83   Hori J, Streilein JW: Cornea tissue inherently possesses immune privilege, due in part to constitutive expression of Fas ligand. Invest Ophthalmol Vis Sci 1998;39:S455.

84   Sonoda Y, Sano Y, Ksander BR, Streilein JW: Characterization of cell mediated immune response elicited by orthotopic corneal allografts in mice. Invest Ophthalmol Vis Sci 1995;36:427–434.

85   Yamada J, Yoshida M, Taylor AW, Streilein JW: Mice with Th2-biased immune systems accept orthotopic corneal allografts placed in 'high-risk' eyes. J Immunol 1999;162:5247–5255.

86   Ksander BR, Sano Y, Streilein JW: Role of donor-specific cytotoxic T cells in rejection of corneal allografts in normal and high risk eyes. Transplant Immunol 1996;4:61–64.

87   Callanan D, Peeler J, Niederkorn JY: Characteristics of rejection of orthotopic corneal allografts in the rat. Transplantation 1988;45:437–443.

88   Ross J, He Y, Pidherney M, Mellon J, Niederkorn JY: The differential effects of donor versus host Langerhans' cells in the rejection of MHC-matched corneal allografts. Transplantation 1991;52:857–861.

89   Dana MR, Yamada J, Streilein JW: Topical interleukin-1 receptor antagonist promotes corneal transplant survival. Transplantation 1997;63:1501.

90   Yamada J, Dana MR, Zhu SN, Alard P, Streilein JW: Interleukin-1 receptor antagonist suppresses allosensitization in corneal transplantation. Arch Ophthalmol 1998;116:1351.
91   Dana MR, Dai R, Zhu S, Yamada J, Streilein JW: Interleukin-1 receptor antagonist suppresses Langerhans' cell activity and promotes immune privilege. Invest Ophthalmol Vis Sci 1998;39:70–77.
92   Streilein JW, McCulley J, Niederkorn JY: Heterotopic corneal grafting in mice. A new approach to the study of corneal alloimmunity. Invest Ophthalmol Vis Sci 1982;23:489–500.
93   She SC, Steahly LP, Moticka EJ: Intracameral injection of allogeneic lymphocytes enhances corneal graft survival. Invest Ophthalmol Vis Sci 1990;31:1950–1956.
94   Okamoto S, Hara Y, Streilein JW: Induction of anterior chamber-associated immune deviation with lymphoreticular allogeneic cells. Transplantation 1995;59:377–381.
95   Niederkorn JY, Mellon J: Anterior chamber-associated immune deviation promotes corneal allograft survival. Invest Ophthalmol Vis Sci 1996;37:2700–2707.
96   Sano Y, Okamoto S, Streilein JW: Induction of donor-specific ACAID can prolong orthotopic corneal allograft survival in high risk eyes. Curr Eye Res 1997;16:1171–1174.
97   Streilein JW: ACAID: A treatment option for the immunological ocular disorders; in Ohno S, Oaki K, Usui M, Uchio E (eds): Uveitis Today. Proceedings of the Fourth International Symposium on Uveitis. Amsterdam, Elsevier, 1998, pp 297–302.
98   He YG, Mellon J, Niederkorn JY: The effect of oral immunization on corneal allograft survival. Transplantation 1996;61:920–926.
99   Holan V, Haskova Z, Filipec M: Transplantation immunity and tolerance in the eye: Rejection and acceptance of orthotopic corneal allografts in mice. Transplantation 1996;62:1050–1054.
100 Pleyer U, Milani JK, Dukes A, Chou J, Lutz S, Ruckert D, Thiel HJ, Mondino BJ: Effect of topically applied anti-CD4 monoclonal antibodies on orthotopic corneal allografts in a rat model. Invest Ophthalmol Vis Sci 1995;36:52–61.
101 Arancibia-Carcama CV, Oral HB, Haskard DO, Larkin DFP, George AJT: Lipoadenofection mediated gene delivery to the cornea endothelium. Transplantation 1998;65:62–67.

J. Wayne Streilein, Schepens Eye Research Institute, Harvard Medical School,
20 Staniford Street, Boston, MA 02114-2500 (USA)
Tel. +1 617 912 7422, Fax +1 617 912 0115, E-Mail waynes@vision.eri.harvard.edu

Streilein JW (ed): Immune Response and the Eye.
Chem Immunol. Basel, Karger, 1999, vol 73, pp 207–219

....

Retinal Transplantation

Henry J. Kaplan[a], *Tongalp H. Tezel*[a], *Adam S. Berger*[a],
Lucian V. Del Priore[b]

[a] Department of Ophthalmology and Visual Sciences Washington University
School of Medicine, St. Louis, Mo., and
[b] Center for Retinal Cell Transplantation, UMDNJ-NJMS, Newark, N.J., USA

Introduction

The historical success of allogeneic corneal transplantation established the eye as a unique site for tissue transplantation [see chapter 10 – M. Reza Dana for more details]. The distinctive immunologic characteristics of the eye, particularly the anterior chamber, were well documented several decades ago and led to the concept of immunologic privilege [see chapter 1 – Regional Immunity and Ocular Immunoprivilege, J. Wayne Streilein; chapter 3 – ACAID, Jerry Y. Neiderkorn, and chapter 4 – Ocular Immunosuppressive Environment, Andrew W. Taylor for more details]. Only recently have the techniques been developed to harvest and transplant either photoreceptor or retinal pigment epithelial (RPE) cells into the subretinal space. Thus, the survival, biologic function and immune protection afforded tissue transplanted to the subretinal space has only recently received attention.

The immune protection afforded allogeneic retinal cells transplanted into the subretinal space will be influenced by both the existence of immunologic privilege in that compartment, as well as the immunogenicity of the transplanted tissue. Recent information which addresses both of these issues will be presented. Additionally, the rationale for and clinical experience with retinal transplantation in the treatment of two diseases – age-related macular degeneration (AMD) and retinitis pigmentosa (RP) – will also be reviewed.

Immunologic Privilege in the Subretinal Space

Concept of Immune Privilege

Since immune privilege within the eye is presented in detail in other chapters, it will only be briefly summarized here. Immune privilege refers to the prolonged survival of tissue grafts or tumor cells when placed within a site, such as the anterior chamber of the eye, compared to the more abrupt homograft reaction observed when placed in more conventional sites, such as subcutaneous tissue [1]. The high success rate of allogeneic, orthotopic corneal grafts in the presence of major histocompatibility differences is another example of immunologic privilege in the eye [2].

The presence of immunologic privilege in the eye is thought to be the result of both unique anatomic features, as well as a special molecular milieu. Anatomic features that contribute to immune privilege within the anterior chamber include an absence of lymphatic drainage, the isolation created by the blood-ocular barrier, the presentation of antigen to the host via the circulation (i.e. the spleno-cameral axis), and the reduced expression of MHC class I and II molecules on resident cells [3]. It is well established that the subretinal space in a like manner, is protected by a blood-ocular barrier, via tight junctions between RPE cells, as well as the vascular endothelium of the retinal circulation. The subretinal space has no demonstrable lymphatic drainage and has reduced expression of MHC class I and II molecules on parenchymal cells of the neurosensory retina [4]. However, there is no evidence that antigen placed within the subretinal space gains direct access to the circulatory system. Thus, several anatomic features thought to be important for the development of immune privilege within the anterior chamber exist for the subretinal space.

Many of the molecular mechanisms of immune suppression identified as important for the development of immune privilege within the anterior chamber also exist in the subretinal space.

(1) *Complement inhibition:* Several complementary regulatory proteins, the putative role of which is to protect intraocular tissue from complement-mediated destruction, have been identified immunohistologically in the eye. In the neurosensory retina there is the selective expression of CD59, but not membrane cofactor protein (MCP) or decay-accelerating factor (DAF), which are expressed within the anterior chamber [5].

(2) *Fas ligand-mediated apoptosis:* Fas ligand is constitutively expressed in various ocular tissues, including the RPE and neurosensory retina. Evidence in vivo, as well as in vitro, suggests that constitutive expression of Fas ligand in a tissue leads to a deletion of Fas$^+$ T cells that enter the tissue [6, 7].

(3) *Immunosuppressive molecules:* It is well documented that aqueous humor contains severely immunomodulatory substances, including TGF-β_2,

free cortisol, IL-1 receptor antagonist, substance P and vasoactive intestinal peptide [8, 9]. Although the complete profile of immunosuppressive molecules secreted by the RPE has not been as well characterized, several such as TGF-β_2, have been demonstrated [7, 10–13].

Immune Privilege in the Subretinal Space

Several laboratories have demonstrated the existence of a limited immune privilege in the subretinal space. It is characterized by the antigen-specific inhibition of both the cellular and humoral immune response. Suppression of delayed-type hypersensitivity to histoincompatible tumor cells and soluble protein antigens [14, 15], as well as the delayed rejection of transplanted allogeneic RPE cells across either MHC class I or II disparities [16], demonstrates the inhibition of cell-mediated immunity after the introduction of antigen into the subretinal space. Antibody production to E1-deleted adenovirus [17], as well as the P-815 mastocytoma tumor [pers. observ.], is also markedly diminished after inoculation into the subretinal space. Thus, an important difference exists between immunologic privilege within the anterior chamber and the subretinal space. In the anterior chamber, delayed-type hypersensitivity is inhibited while the cytotoxic antibody response is enhanced. In the subretinal space, antibody production, as well as delayed-type hypersensitivity, is inhibited.

Although immunologic privilege exists within the normal subretinal space, an important question with respect to the transplantation of allogeneic tissue is the effect of disruption of the blood-ocular barrier on immune protection. Several diseases, e.g. AMD and RP, are associated with disruption of the RPE layer which may compromise the integrity of this barrier. If the blood-ocular barrier is artificially disrupted by the injection of sodium iodate [14] or naturally disrupted as in the RD mouse [18], abrogation of immune privilege within the subretinal space appears to occur. It still remains to be demonstrated whether allogeneic tissue transplanted into a compromised subretinal space will undergo a more abrupt homograft reaction.

The true nature of immune privilege within the subretinal space, is unknown because experimental studies have only been performed in either the rodent or outbred species. The subretinal space of the rodent is very difficult to study since access is only possible via a trans-scleral route because of the large rodent lens. The injection of an antigenic inoculum via this approach invariably results in both a breach of the RPE barrier, as well as placement of part of the inoculum in the suprachoroidal space. This complicates study of the true extent of immunologic privilege in the subretinal space. These problems can be avoided using a transvitreal approach in a larger species. Unfortunately, a transvitreal approach in larger species, such as the rabbit, has not employed inbred strains. Consequently, the immunogenetic disparity between donor and host is unknown and an analysis of the true extent of immunologic privilege in the subretinal space is again hindered. This is an important issue since meaningful clinical studies can only be conducted if the necessity for immunosuppression at the time of allogeneic RPE or photoreceptor transplantation in the subretinal space is precisely defined.

Immunogenicity of Retinal Tissue

The immunologic survival of an allogeneic transplant in the subretinal space is dependent upon both the presence of immune privilege in that space, as well as the immunogenicity of the transplanted tissue. There is ample evidence to suggest that RPE cells constitutively express MHC class I but not class II molecules; however, they can express the latter when stimulated with interferon-γ in culture [19, 20]. The RPE also constitutively express ICAM-1 [21], an important accessory molecule for T-cell activation. The expression of MHC class II and ICAM-1 predominately on the apical plasma membrane of cultured RPE [16] suggests these molecules may play an important role in the presentation of antigen to the host [22, 23].

The immunogenicity of adult murine RPE cells was studied to determine their ability to stimulate primed splenocytes both in vitro and in vivo. Freshly isolated adult murine RPE were immunogenic across both MHC class I and minor HC loci when tested by the CTL ^{51}Cr-release assay and T-cell clones. However, no expression of MHC class II molecules could be detected using a standard MLC [24]. In contrast, isolated adult murine photoreceptor cells were not immunogenic in similar studies, suggesting that they are less immunogenic than RPE cells. Since immune privilege within the subretinal space appears limited and allogeneic RPE cells are immunogenic, transplantation of RPE cells into the subretinal space will likely require the use of concomitant immunosuppression or autologous RPE cells. The need for immunosuppression following transplantation of allogeneic photoreceptor cells is less well defined.

RPE Transplantation – AMD

Rationale

The leading cause of severe visual loss in patients over age 55 is AMD. When choroidal neovascularization develops in AMD and extends beneath the center of the foveal avascular zone, the outcome is dismal. Seventy percent of eyes with subfoveal membranes secondary to AMD will develop a visual acuity of 20/200 or worse within 2 years [25]. Laser photocoagulation has been advocated for the treatment of subfoveal neovascularization, but laser treatment destroys the foveal photoreceptors and eliminates the recovery of central vision [26].

In 1989, Thomas and Kaplan [27] reported 2 patients with loss of central vision from subfoveal neovascular membranes and ocular histoplasmosis who improved dramatically to 20/20 and 20/40 following surgical excision. However, submacular surgery in patients with choroidal neovascularization and AMD has not met with similar success [28–31]. Clinical and laboratory studies suggest that a limiting factor in visual recovery following surgical excision of subfoveal choroidal neovascularization in AMD is atrophy of the subfoveal choriocapillaris. It has been demonstrated that removal of RPE with the choroidal neovascular complex will lead to secondary atrophy of the choriocapillaris [32–39]. Unfortunately, the adjacent RPE in AMD will not repopulate the area of Bruch's membrane that has been denuded (fig. 1). Consequently, RPE transplantation at the time of submacular surgery is being considered in an attempt to prevent postoperative atrophy of the subfoveal choriocapillaris, while simultaneously providing the appropriate support for the overlying foveal photoreceptors [33, 40, 41]. The ultimate objective is the recovery of lost central vision.

RPE Transplantation in Exudative AMD

Two clinical centers have performed RPE transplantation in AMD. The first clinical results came from surgery performed by a Swedish group using a patch of fetal RPE cells cultured in vitro for 1 week prior to transplantation [42]. Five patients had RPE placed beneath the neurosensory retina at the time of removal of subfoveal choroidal neovascularization. The preoperative visual acuity of the patients was severely compromised. The RPE transplant was successfully placed beneath the fovea in 3 patients, but was extrafoveal in the other 2. Several surgical complications were encountered including cystoid macular edema and macular pucker.

Scanning laser ophthalmoscopy demonstrated that all 5 patients were able to fixate over the area of the RPE graft immediately after surgery, but an absolute scotoma developed in this region within several months. The patients were not immunosuppressed at the time of surgery, and the changes observed following transplantation raise the suspicion that the allogeneic RPE cells were immunologically rejected.

Additionally, the transplants may not have survived because of the status of the underlying Bruch's membrane. Reattachment of transplanted RPE to this structure is important because RPE cells will undergo apoptosis if they do not attach to a suitable substrate [43].

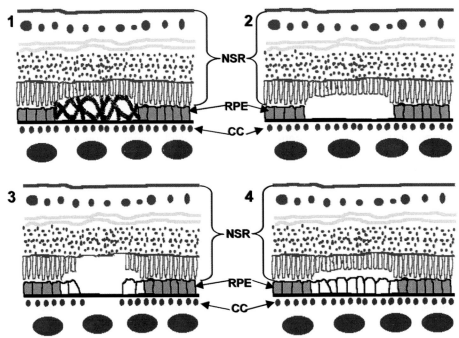

Fig. 1. Schematic representation of the neurosensory retina (NSR), retinal pigment epithelium (RPE) and choriocapillaris (CC). *1* A new vessel complex is depicted beneath the NSR in place of the RPE lying on Bruch's membrane (the solid line). *2* Immediately after removal of the new vessel complex by submacular surgical techniques there is mild disruption of the photoreceptors in the NSR, with frequent integrity of the CC. *3* If the RPE is removed at the time of surgery, and the residual RPE (nonpigmented) does not repopulate the denuded area of Bruch's membrane, the CC and overlying photoreceptors in the NSR rapidly atrophy. *4* If transplanted RPE cells (nonpigmented) attach to the denuded area of Bruch's membrane, the CC will remain intact and the overlying photoreceptors will be preserved.

We have also studied the effects of RPE transplantation at the time of submacular surgery for subfoveal choroidal neovascularization in exudative AMD. Twelve patients with subfoveal neovascularization underwent membranectomy with transplantation of a sheet of adult human cadaveric RPE [44]. Eligibility criteria included: drusen, age > 60, ETDRS visual acuity of ≤ 20/63, and subfoveal neovascularization ≤ 9 disc areas. All patients were immunosuppressed with oral prednisone, cyclosporine, and azathioprine immediately postoperative. Ten of 12 transplants were placed beneath the fovea and remained there postoperatively. Surgical complications observed postoperatively included rhegmatogenous retinal detachment (two eyes; repaired with scleral buckling surgery) and macular pucker (two eyes; with subsequent surgical removal).

The RPE transplants showed no signs of rejection within the first 6 months following surgery when the patients were maintained on immunosuppression. Two patients developed complications postoperatively which were possibly attributed to the immunosuppression; in 1 of the patients the medication was discontinued. Additionally, 2 other patients required an adjustment in their postoperative immunosuppressive regimen. The most appropriate immuno-suppressive regimen in this elderly population, which is more vulnerable to the side effects of these drugs, is still to be determined. These patients constitute a fragile study population. Two of the patients died within 7 months of surgery (ages 85 and 86) from heart disease.

There was a transient worsening of visual acuity, contrast sensitivity and reading time at the 1-month visit, with recovery to baseline levels by 3 months postoperatively.

These studies demonstrate that human RPE can be harvested from cada-veric eyes and transplanted into the subretinal space of patients with AMD at the time of submacular surgery. Further observation and investigation is needed to determined whether these transplants will improve the visual progno-sis in exudative AMD.

Clinical Implications

The development of submacular surgery to remove subfoveal choroidal neovascularization introduced the possibility of anatomically reconstructing the subretinal space. Simple excision of a choroidal neovascular membrane can be accompanied by the recovery of central vision if the subfoveal RPE is not removed at the time of surgery, or if the RPE is removed and adjacent RPE repopulates the denuded area, shortly thereafter (fig. 1). The presence of native or regenerated RPE is essential to prevent postoperative atrophy of the subfoveal choriocapillaris. Persistent bare areas of Bruch's membrane are observed in AMD after submacular surgery, presumably the result of the reduced ability of senescent RPE to divide and migrate, as well as the presence of residual abnormalities in the inner layers of Bruch's membrane. Thus, transplanted RPE cells will probably have to reattach to an abnormal substrate. Successful RPE transplantation will require understanding the ultrastructural and molecular composition of Bruch's membrane following submacular sur-gery in AMD, as well as the precautions necessary to prevent immunologic rejection of the allogeneic RPE cells.

Photoreceptor Transplantation – RP

Rationale

RP is a common hereditary disease that frequently results in legal blindness [45]. Rod photoreceptors degenerate early in the course of the disease, with the subsequent degeneration of cone photoreceptors as a late complication. Genetic studies demonstrate multiple gene mutations associated with both the photoreceptors, as well as the RPE [46–55]. Most of these genes encode proteins in the rod phototransduction cascade and in the photoreceptor outer segment disc structure. Although somantic gene therapy has been accomplished in the RD mouse, an animal model of the phosphodiesterase enzyme abnormality, it will probably be several years before gene transfer is a therapeutic option in RP [56].

Within the past few years, techniques have been developed to harvest and transplant organized sheets of photoreceptors into the subretinal space [57–59]. The therapeutic benefit of such transplants in RP has not been established. However, there are two potential mechanisms by which photoreceptor transplantation may have a therapeutic role. The first is reconstitution of the retinal neural network by the replacement of destroyed rod photoreceptor cells with transplanted normal rod photoreceptor cells. Stone et al. [60] demonstrated in postmortem eyes from patients with advanced RP and severe visual loss that only 4% of photoreceptors were retained, but 66% of the bipolar cells and 28% of the retinal ganglion cells remained. More recently, it has been demonstrated that focal light perception still persists in patients with blindness from advanced RP following electrical stimulation of the inner retina. These observations suggest the functional integrity of the inner retinal neural network in RP [61]. Thus, the neural network might be reconstituted after photoreceptor transplantation if synapses develop between transplanted photoreceptor cells and residual host bipolar cells.

Neonatal rodent photoreceptor cells have been observed to survive for up to 12 months when transplanted into the rodent subretinal space [57, 62]. We recently observed the survival of transplanted human adult xenogeneic photoreceptors within the subretinal space of the non-human primate for 6 months [pers. observ.]. The biological function of the rodent transplant has been inferred from the presence of synaptic ribbons with synaptic vesicles at the bipolar cell–outer nuclear layer interface, as well as from a physiological response to light [57, 62–64]. However, the definitive proof of functional new synapses following photoreceptor transplantation remains to be demonstrated.

A second mechanism by which photoreceptor transplantation may be beneficial in RP is through the rescue of cone photoreceptors by a soluble factor(s) elaborated by rod photoreceptors. Cone degeneration in the RD

mouse may be inhibited by the transplantation of normal rod-rich photoreceptor cells [65]. This observation suggests that cone survival may require a soluble
factor, which may be released from transplanted photoreceptor cells.

Clinical Studies in Man

We have previously demonstrated the technical feasibility of harvesting
and transplanting a sheet of adult human allogeneic photoreceptor cells
into the subretinal space of 2 patients with advanced RP and no light
perception [57]. It is noteworthy that the retinal transplant did not elicit
inflammation in either patient, even though they were not given systemic
immunosuppression postoperatively. This observation is consistent with the
concepts that adult human photoreceptor cells are minimally immunogenic,
since they do not possess detectable MHC class I molecules [24], and that
the subretinal space, like the anterior chamber of the eye, is immunologically
privileged. Thus, immunosuppression of the host may not be required to
prevent the rejection of transplanted allogeneic photoreceptor cells into the
subretinal space.

More recently, we operated on 8 patients with RP and functional vision.
They underwent retinal transplantation with adult human cadaveric photoreceptor sheets harvested with the excimer laser. No immunosuppression was
used postoperatively and the patients were followed for 12 months.

Patients with RP met the following inclusion criteria: age between 18 and
65 years; a central visual field $\leq$ a radius of $20°$ by Goldmann perimetry
using a V_4e target, an ETDRS visual acuity $\geq 20/400$, and an extinguished
rod response and cone B-wave >1 μV on full-field ERG or >0.10 μV on
maculoscope examination.

Best corrected ETDR visual acuity, median reading speed and contrast
sensitivity for the operated eye was unchanged at 12 months. The log threshold
for dark adaptation did not change appreciably for either the study eye or the
control eye. Both the amplitude and latency of the maculoscope ERG was
significantly decreased in the operated eye at 1 month but returned to preoperative levels by the 6-month evaluation. There was no apparent rejection of
the graft and no surgical complications. However, 1 patient did complain of
monocular torsional diplopia postoperatively, following a subsequent cataract
extraction.

Our clinical experience suggests that allogeneic photoreceptor transplantation within the subretinal space is feasible in man and is not associated with
apparent immediate immune rejection or other significant adverse events. The
ability of isolated sheets of adult human allogeneic photoreceptor cells to
reestablish the retinal neural network or rescue residual cones prior to degeneration remains to be demonstrated.

Conclusion

Important information has been learned establishing the existence of immune privilege in the subretinal space, as well as the variable immunogenicity of the neurosensory retina and RPE. There appears to be a need for immunosuppression following allogeneic RPE transplantation into the subretinal space and it may also be necessary for photoreceptor cells. This is an important issue which must still be clarified. A major problem in the determination of the need for immunosuppression following retinal transplantation is the difficulty in performing surgery in the rodent. The large lens of the rodent mandates a transcleral approach, with the inevitable breach of the RPE, as well as difficulty in placing the inoculum solely in the subretinal space. These obstacles compromise our ability to define the true extent of immunologic privilege in the subretinal space. It is imperative that these studies be repeated using a transvitreal approach in larger inbred species.

There are several retinal diseases for which we presently have no effective treatment. The potential usefulness of retinal transplantation as a treatment modality is now being explored in AMD and RP. A better understanding of the parameters determining the immunologic rejection of allogeneic retinal tissue, as well as the biologic function of transplanted cells within the subretinal space, will be necessary to successfully achieve this goal.

References

1   Medawar PB: Immunity to homologous grafted skin. III. The fate of skin homografts transplanted to the brain, to subcutaneous tissue, and to the anterior chamber of the eye. Br J Exp Pathol 1948; 29:58–69.
2   Sonoda Y, Streilein JW: Orthotopic corneal transplantation in mice – Evidence that the immuno-genetic rules of rejection do not apply. Transplantation 1992;54:694–704.
3   Streilein JW, Takeuchi M, Taylor AW: Immune privilege, T-cell tolerance, and tissue-restricted autoimmunity. Hum Immunol 1997;52:138–143.
4   Wang HM, Kaplan HJ, Chan WC, Johnson M: The distribution and ontogeny of MHC antigens in murine ocular tissue. Invest Ophthalmol Vis Sci 1987;28:1383–1389.
5   Bora NS, Gobleman CL, Atkinson JP, Pepose JS, Kaplan HJ: Differential expression of the complement regulatory proteins in the human eye. Invest Ophthalmol Vis Sci 1993;34:3579–3584.
6   Griffith TS, Brunner T, Fletcher SM, Gren DR, Ferguson TA: Fas ligand-induced apoptosis as a mechanism of immune privilege. Science 1997;270:1189–1192.
7   Jorgensen A, Wiencke AK, la Cour M, Koestel CG, Madsen HO, Hamann S, Lui GM, Scherfig E, Prause JU, Svejgaard A, Odum N, Nissen MH, Röpke C: Human RPE cell-induced apoptosis in activated T cells. Invest Ophthalmol Vis Sci 1998;39:1590–1599.
8   Streilein JW: Regulation of ocular immune responses. Eye 1997;11:171–175.
9   Ferguson TA, Griffith TS: A vision of cell death: Insights into immune privilege. Immunol Rev 1997;156:167–184.
10 Elner VM, Elner SG, Standiford TJ, Lukacs NW, Strieter RM, Kunkel SL: Interleukin-7 induces retinal pigment epithelial cell MCP-1 and IL-8. Exp Eye Res 1996;63:297–303.

11   Elner SG, Elner VM, Bian ZM, Lukacs NW, Kurtz RM, Strieter RM, Kunkel SL: Human retinal pigment epithelial cell interleukin-8 and monocyte chemotactic protein-1 modulation by T-lymphocyte products. Invest Ophthalmol Vis Sci 1997;38:446–455.

12   Elner VM, Burnstine MA, Strieter RM, Kunkel SL, Elner SG: Cell-associated human retinal pigment epithelium interleukin-8 and monocyte chemotactic protein-1: Immunochemical and in-situ hybridization analyses. Exp Eye Res 1997;65:781–789.

13   Bian ZM, Elner SG, Strieter RM, Kunkel SL, Elner VM: Synergy between glycated human serum albumin and tumor necrosis factor-α for interleukin-8 gene expression and protein secretion in human retinal pigment epithelial cells. Lab Invest 1998;78:335–344.

14   Wenkel H, Streilein JW: Analysis of immune deviation elicited by antigens injected into the subretinal space. Invest Ophthalmol Vis Sci 1998;39:1823–1834.

15   Sohn JH, Kaplan HJ, Bora NS: A 55 kD complement inhibitory protein is present in normal human intraocular fluid. Invest Ophthalmol Vis Sci 1998;39:S911.

16   Zhang X, Bok D: Transplantation of retinal pigment epithelial cells and immune response in the subretinal space. Invest Ophthalmol Vis Sci 1998;39:1021–1027.

17   Bennett J, Pakola S, Zeng Y, Maguire A: Humoral response after administration of E1-deleted adenoviruses; immune privilege of the subretinal space. Hum Gene Ther 1996;7:1763–1769.

18   Suber ML, Hurwitz MY, Aguilar-Cordova E, Hurwitz RL: The generation of delayed type hypersensitivity in rd mice signals a breakdown of ocular immune deviance. Invest Ophthalmol Vis Sci 1998; 39:S910.

19   Liversidge JM, Sewell HF, Thomson AW, Forrester JV: Lymphokine-induced MHC class II antigen expression on cultured RPE cells and the influence of cyclosporine A. Immunology 1988;63:313–317.

20   Liversidge JM, Sewell HF, Forrester JV: Human RPE cells differentially express MHC class II (HLA DP, DR and DQ) antigen in response to in vitro stimulation with lymphokine or purified IFN-γ. Clin Exp Immunol 1988;73:489–494.

21   Liversidge JM, Sewell HF, Forrester JV: Interaction between lymphocytes and cells of the blood-retina barrier: Mechanisms of T lymphocyte adhesion to human retinal capillary endothelial cells and RPE cells in vitro. Immunology 1990;71:390–396.

22   Percupo CM, Hooks JJ, Shinohara T, Caspi R, Detrick B: Cytokine-mediated activation of a neuronal retinal resident cell provokes antigen presentation. J Immunol 1990;145:4101–4107.

23   Osusky R, Dorio RJ, Arora Y, Ryan SJ, Walker SM: MHC class II positive RPE cells can function as antigen-presenting cells for microbial superantigen. Ocul Immunol Inflamm 1997;5:43–50.

24   Silbert JE, Gao EK, Yu XH, Kaplan HJ: Adult murine pigment epithelium is immunogenic. Invest Ophthalmol Vis Sci 1994;35:S1525.

25   Bressler SB, Bressler NM, Fine SL, Hillis A, Murphy RP, Olk RJ, Patz A: Natural course of choroidal neovascular membranes within the foveal avascular zone in senile macular degeneration. Am J Ophthalmol 1982;93:157–163.

26   Macular Photocoagulation Study Group: Laser photocoagulation of subfoveal neovascular lesions in age-related macular degeneration. Results of a randomized clinical trial. Arch Ophthalmol 1991; 109:1220–1231.

27   Thomas MA, Kaplan HJ: Surgical removal of subfoveal neovascularization in the presumed ocular histoplasmosis syndrome. Am J Ophthalmol 1991;111:1–7.

28   Berger AS, Kaplan HJ: Clinical experience with the surgical removal of subfoveal neovascular membranes. Ophthalmology 1992;99: 969–976.

29   Thomas MA, Grand MG, Williams DF, Lee CM, Pesin SR, Lowe MA: Surgical management of subfoveal choroidal neovascularization. Ophthalmology 1992;99:952–968.

30   Lopez PF, Grossniklaus HE, Lambert HM, Aaberg TM, Capone A Jr, Sternberg P Jr, L'Hernault N: Pathologic features of surgically excised subretinal neovascular membranes in age-related macular degeneration. Am J Ophthalmol 1991;112:647–656.

31   Lambert HM, Capone A Jr, Aaberg TM, Sternberg P Jr, Mandell BA, Lopez PF: Surgical excision of subfoveal neovascular membranes in age-related macular degeneration. Am J Ophthalmol 1991; 113:257–262.

32   Adelberg DA, Del Priore LV, Kaplan HJ: Surgery for subfoveal membranes in myopia, angioid streaks, and other disorders. Retina 1995;15:198–205.

33 Del Priore LV, Kaplan HJ, Silverman MS, Valentino TL, Mason G, Hornbeck R: Experimental and surgical aspects of RPE cell transplantation. Eur J Implant Ref Surg 1993;5:128–132.

34 Pollack JS, Kaplan HJ, Del Priore LV, Smith MS: Choriocapillaris atrophy following subfoveal membrane excision in exudative age-related macular degeneration. Ophthalmology 1993;100(9A).

35 Pollack JS, Del Priore LV, Smith ME, Feiner MA, Kaplan HJ: Postoperative abnormalities of the choriocapillaris in exudative, age-related macular degeneration. Br J Ophthalmol 1996;80:314–318.

36 Nasiir M, Sugino I, Zarbin MA: Decreased choriocapillaris perfusion following surgical excision of choroidal neovascular membranes in age-related macular degeneration. Br J Ophthalmol 1997; 81:481–489.

37 Akduman L, Desai V, Del Priore LV, Olk RJ, Kaplan HJ: Visual improvement after subfoveal surgery in POHS depends on perfusion of subfoveal choriocapillaris. Am J Ophthalmol 1997;123: 90–96.

38 Desai VN, Del Priore LV, Pollack JS, Kaplan HJ: Choriocapillaris atrophy after submacular surgery in the presumed ocular histoplasmosis syndrome. Arch Ophthalmol 1995;113:409–410.

39 Del Priore LV, Tezel TH, Berger AS, Kaplan HJ: Retinal pigment epithelial transplantation for subfoveal choroidal neovascularization. Vitreo-retinal and uveitis update. 47th Annual Symposium of the New Orleans Academy of Ophthalmology, 1999, pp 65–81.

40 Del Priore LV, Hornbeck R, Kaplan HJ, Jones Z, Swinn M: RPE debridement as a model for the pathogenesis and treatment of macular degeneration. Am J Ophthalmol 1996;122:629–643.

41 Del Priore LV, Kaplan HJ, Berger AS: RPE transplantation in the management of subfoveal choroidal neovascularization. Semin Ophthalmol 1997;12:45–55.

42 Algvere PV, Berglin L, Gouras P, Sheng Y: Transplantation of fetal retinal pigment epithelium in age-related macular degeneration with subfoveal neovascularization. Graefes Arch Clin Exp Ophthalmol 1994;232:707–716.

43 Tezel TH, Del Priore LV, Kaplan HJ: Reattachment to a substrate prevents apoptosis of human retinal pigment epithelium. Graefes Arch Clin Exp Ophthalmol 1997;235:41–47.

44 Tezel TH, Del Priore LV, Kaplan HJ: Harvest and storage of adult human RPE sheets. Curr Eye Res 1997;16:802–809.

45 Berson EL: Retinitis pigmentosa: Unfolding its mystery. Proc Natl Acad Sci USA 1996;93:4526–4528.

46 Kajiwara K, Berson EL, Cryja TP: Digenic retinitis pigmentosa due to mutations at the unlinked peripherin/RDS and ROM-1 loci. Science 1994;264:1604–1608.

47 Dryja TP, McGee TL, Reichel E, Hahn LB, Cowley GS, Yandell DW, Sandberg MA, Berson EL: A point mutation of the rhodopsin gene in one form of retinitis pigmentosa. Nature 1990;343: 364–366.

48 Farrar GJ, Kenna P, Jordan SA, Kumar-Singh R, Humphries MM, Sharp EM, Sheils DM, Humphries P: A three-base-pair deletion in the peripherin RDS gene in one form of retinitis pigmentosa. Nature 1991;354:478–480.

49 Kajiwara K, Hahn LB, Mukais S, Travis GH, Berson EL, Dryja TP: Mutations in the human retinal degeneration slow gene in autosomal dominant retinitis pigmentosa. Nature 1991;354:480–483.

50 McLaughlin ME, Sandberg MA, Berson EL, Dryja TP: Recessive mutations in the gene encoding the beta-subunit of rod phosphodiesterase in patients with retinitis pigmentosa. Nat Genet 1993; 4:130–134.

51 Dryja TP, Finn JT, Peng YW, McGee TL, Berson EL, Yau KW: Mutations in the gene encoding the alpha subunit of the rod cGMP-gated channel in autosomal recessive retinitis pigmentosa. Proc Natl Acad Sci USA 1995;92:10177–10181.

52 Huang SH, Pittler SJ, Huang X, Oliveira L, Berson EL, Dryja TP: Autosomal recessive retinitis pigmentosa caused by mutations in the alpha subunit of rod cGMP phosphodiesterase. Nat Genet 1995;11:468–471.

53 Bascom RA, Liu L, Heckenlively JR, Stone EM, McInnes RR: Mutation analysis of the ROM-1 gene in retinitis pigmentosa. Hum Mol Genet 1995;4:1895–1902.

54 Weil D, Blanchard S, Kaplan J, Guilford P, Gibson F, Walsh J, Mburu P, Varela A, Levilliers J, Weston MD, Kelley PM, Kimberling WJ, Wagenaar M, Levi-Acobas F, Larget-Plet D, Munnich A, Steel KP, Brown SDM, Petit C: Defective myosin VIIA gene responsible for Usher syndrome type 1B. Nature 1995;374:60–61.

55   Maw MA, Kennedy B, Knight A, Bridges R, Roth KE, Mani EJ, Mukkadan JK, Nancarrow D, Crabb JW, Denton MJ: Mutation of the gene encoding cellular retinaldehyde-binding protein in autosomal recessive retinitis pigmentosa. Nat Genet 1997;17:198–200.

56   Bennett J, Tanabe T, Sun D, Zeng Y, Kjeldbye H, Gouras P, Maguire AM: Photoreceptor cell rescue in retinal degeneration mice by in vivo gene therapy. Nat Med 1996;2:649–654.

57   Silverman MS, Hughes SE, Valentino TL, Liu Y: Photoreceptor transplantation: Anatomic electro-physiologic, and behavioral evidence for the functional reconstruction of retinas lacking photoreceptors. Exp Neurol 1992;115:87–94.

58   Silverman MS, Hughes SE: Transplantation of photoreceptors to light-damaged retina. Invest Ophthalmol Vis Sci 1989;30:1684–1690.

59   Kaplan HJ, Tezel TH, Berger AS, Wolf ML, Del Priore LV: Human photoreceptor transplantation in retinitis pigmentosa. A safety study. Arch Ophthalmol 1997;115:1168–1172.

60   Stone JL, Barlow WE, Humayun MS, de Juan E Jr, Milam AH: Morphometric analysis of macular photoreceptors and ganglion cells in retinas with retinitis pigmentosa. Arch Ophthalmol 1992;110: 1634–1639.

61   Humayun MS, de Juan E Jr, Dagnelie G, Greenberg RJ, Propst RH, Phillips DH: Visual perception elicited by electrical stimulation of retina in blind humans. Arch Ophthalmol 1996;114:40–46.

62   Gouras P, Du J, Gelanze M, Lopez R, Kwun R, Kjeldbye H, Krebs W: Survival and synapse formation of transplanted rat rods. J Neurol Transplant Plast 1991;2:91–100.

63   Del Cerro M, Ison JR, Brown GP, Lazar E, del Cerro C: Intraretinal grafting restores visual function in light-blinded rats. Neuroreport 1991;2:529–532.

64   Adolph AR, Zucker CL, Ehinger B, Bergström A: Function and structure in retinal transplants. J Neurol Transplant Plast 1994;5:147–161.

65   Mohand-Said S, Deudon-Combe A, Hicks D, Simonutti M, Forster V, Fintz AC, Leveillard T, Dreyfus H, Sahel JA: Normal retinal releases a diffusible factor stimulating cone survival in the retinal degeneration mouse. Proc Natl Acad Sci USA 1998;95:8357.

Henry J. Kaplan, MD, Washington University Eye Center, Washington University Medical Center, Campus Box 8096, 660 S. Euclid Avenue, St. Louis, MO 63110-1093 (USA)
Tel. +1 314 362 3144, Fax +1 314 362 2315, E-Mail kaplan@am.SEER.WUSTL.EDU

Author Index

Subject Index

Lacrimal gland
  anatomy 4
  infection 4, 5
Lymphocyte function-associated antigen-1,
  uveitis role 96
Lymphocytic choriomeningitis virus,
  immunopathology 120

Mast cell, allergic conjunctivitis
  response 51, 52
Melanin protein-induced uveitis, see Uveitis
α-Melanocyte-stimulating hormone,
  immune suppression in aqueous
  humor 79, 80
Molecular mimicry
  Mooren's ulcer autoimmunity 7
  uveitis role 171
Mooren's ulcer, molecular mimicry and
  autoimmunity 7
Mucosal-associated lymphoid tissue,
  features 25, 26
Murine ocular toxoplasmosis
  cytokine expression 108
  induction 108, 110
  posterior uveitis pathology
    comparison 168

Nerve growth factor, expression in vernal
  keratoconjunctivitis 50, 51

Ocular histoplasmosis syndrome, causes
  169

Pathogen-associated molecular patterns
  expression on apoptotic cells 12
  receptors 12, 13
  types 12
Photoreceptor transplantation, see
  Retinal transplantation
Posner-Schlossman syndrome, etiology 4
Pseudotumor orbitae, histology 3

Regional immunity, see also
  Immune privilege
  components 25
  examples 25–27
  overview 24, 25

Retina
  blood-ocular barrier 3, 92, 94
  damage from inflammation 91
  subretinal space immune privilege
    28, 29, 209, 210
Retinal transplantation
  immunogenicity of retinal tissue 210
  immunosuppression therapy 216
  overview 207
  photoreceptor transplantation in retinitis
    pigmentosa
    clinical studies 215
    rationale 214, 215
  retinal pigment epithelial transplantation
    in age-related macular degeneration
    clinical implications 213
    exudative disease 211–213
    rationale 210, 211
Retinitis pigmentosa
  course 214
  gene mutations 214
  photoreceptor transplantation
    clinical studies 215
    rationale 214, 215
River blindness, corneal scarring 34, 35

Skin-associated lymphoid tissue,
  features 26, 27

T cell
  allergic conjunctivitis response
    activation 48, 49
    chemokine expression 51
    cytokines 48, 50
    subtypes 49
  apoptosis 23, 24
  clonal deletion 22
  corneal transplantation rejection role
    190, 192–196
  cytokines
    anterior chamber-associated immune
      deviation 61, 62
    immunosuppression 73, 74, 77–79, 83
    production and functions 19, 20, 49
    synergism and regulation 98, 99
    T helper cell subsets 72, 82, 83
  damage in autoimmune disease 170

T cell (continued)
  immune privilege 32
  killer inhibitory receptor expression in
    tumor escape 148–150
  uveitis response 170–172, 174, 176–178
Tear fluid, viruses 4, 5
Tolerance
  antigen-presenting cell mechanisms 23
  autoimmune disease development
    102, 103, 170
  definition 16
Toxoplasmosis, see Murine ocular
  toxoplasmosis
Transforming growth factor-β
  experimental endotoxin-induced uveitis
    role 101
  immune suppression in aqueous
    humor 77–79
  tumor secretion and
    immunosuppression 144
Transplantation, see Corneal
  transplantation, Retinal transplantation
Tumor antigens, see also Immune privilege,
  tumors
  differentiation antigens 140
  identification 139, 140
  immunogenicity 137
  intron transcription abnormalities 142
  melanoma antigen gene 141, 142
  mutant antigens 141
  overexpression of normal antigens 141
  tumor escape following cancer
    immunization
    cytotoxic T lymphocyte response 148
    killer inhibitory receptor expression on
      T cells 148–150
    tumor antigen downregulation 148
Tumor necrosis factor-α, experimental
  endotoxin-induced uveitis role 99

Uveitis, see also Experimental autoimmune
  uveitis, Experimental endotoxin-induced
  uveitis, Murine ocular toxoplasmosis
  anterior uveitis
    features 163
    pathology
      infectious disease 163

      noninfectious disease 165
    autoimmunity 161, 163, 169–171
    blood-ocular barrier permeability
      93, 94
    causes 90, 160, 161, 163
    cell adhesion molecules
      fractalkine role 97
      functions 94–96
      intercellular adhesion molecule-1
        role 96
      lymphocyte function-associated
        antigen-1 role 96
    chemokine roles 97, 98
    classification 90
    clinico-pathological features 159, 160, 175
    complement activation 97
    damage mechanisms
      antigen-presenting cells 172, 173
      bystander damage 173
      clinical spectrum 175
      cytokines 174, 175
      effector cells 174
    definition 159
    genetic susceptibility 177, 178
    immune response regulation and
      dysfunction 175–178
    infectious disease 160, 161
    intraocular inflammation
      nomenclature 159
    lens-induced uveitis 103, 105
    melanin protein-induced uveitis
      103, 167
    posterior uveitis
      features 165
      pathology
        infectious disease 165, 166
        noninfectious disease 166
    T cell response 170–172, 174, 176–178

Vascular endothelial growth factor 144, 145
Vasoactive intestinal peptide, immune
  suppression in aqueous humor 80
Vernal keratoconjunctivitis, see also
  Allergic conjunctivitis
  clinical presentation 38, 39
  course 5
  nerve growth factor expression 50, 51